Practical Imaging Inform

Barton F. Branstetter IV
Editor

Katherine P. Andriole • Sylvia Devlin
Erik R. Ranschaert
Associate Editors

Practical Imaging Informatics

Foundations and Applications for Medical
Imaging

Second Edition

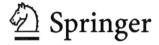 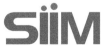

Editor
Barton F. Branstetter IV
Department of Radiology
University of Pittsburgh
Pittsburgh, PA
USA

ISBN 978-1-0716-1755-7   ISBN 978-1-0716-1756-4   (eBook)
https://doi.org/10.1007/978-1-0716-1756-4

Cover image by Leah Lynne Branstetter

This Springer imprint is published by the registered company Springer Science+Business Media, LLC part of Springer Nature.
The registered company address is: 1 New York Plaza, New York, NY 10004, U.S.A.

First Edition Dedication (2009)

For the four who laid the flagstones
And the three who walk behind,
*   Eyes wide with wonder*
And for Cara
Always for Cara

BFB

To my wife Terry, a font of affection and
inspiration.

DLR

This book is dedicated to my family, your
love and support strengthens me.
Philippians 4:13.

DSG

To my wife Janet, for her transcendent love,
encouragement, and support.

DLW

The Editors are indebted to Ms. Caroline
Wilson; without her tireless efforts, this book
never would have come to fruition.

Second Edition Dedication

For my parents,
*   who set me on this path;*
For my mentors,
*   who lit the way;*
And for Cara,
*   who walks along beside me*
*   hand in hand*

BFB

To my mom Patricia Corrigan Andriole
for her constant and unconditional love
and support

KPA

To my husband Vincent,
whose love and support made this possible

SD

My deep appreciation and thanks for all
those within and outside EuSoMII who
supported me in successfully further
expanding international cooperation in the
field of imaging informatics

ERR

The editors are indebted to Ms. Nikki Medina
for her guidance and support in the creation
of this book.

Introduction

The Evolution of the Imaging Informatics Professional

When the first edition of this book was published, medicine had just undergone a revolution. The digital age had swept through healthcare, transforming virtually every aspect of medical practice. This transformation brought with it new frustrations and new opportunities. One of those opportunities was a career path for people who wanted to manage the new digital environment. In radiology, in particular, there was a sudden need for a team of individuals who would ensure that the PACS functioned continuously and reliably.

But where to find these individuals? A strong computer background would be essential, but a computer programmer or IT professional might not understand the clinical needs that underlie the PACS. After all, most IT systems do not require support that is timely and urgent, with patient care decisions hanging in the balance. Changing from the IT culture to the medical culture can be difficult. So, a clinical background (e.g., technologists, nurses) is also critical. But relatively few people in clinical careers had the computer skills to maintain a system as complex as a PACS. Even fewer had an interest in switching to an untested and uncertain career path.

Thus was born the PACS administrator – that rare breed with knowledge of both clinical workflow and information technology. Unfortunately, there weren't enough people with the requisite skills to fill these roles. A few motivated, self-taught individuals from a variety of backgrounds found ways to fill the gaps in their own knowledge and become a bridge between the clinical and IT communities.

As PACS evolved, so did the training and background required of a PACS administrator. Keeping the PACS working was no longer sufficient -- the ability to improve the PACS, work with the vendors, and even make the PACS communicate with other IT infrastructure in the hospital became critical to the job. Other specialties outside of radiology began to need similar services, and the obvious person to play that role was the PACS administrator.

But this transition was not easy. Not only was the traditional training inadequate, the terminology describing the job was also inadequate. Seeing that the knowledge base developed in radiology was becoming needed throughout the medical enterprise, the Society for Computer Applications in Radiology transformed itself into the Society for Imaging Informatics in Medicine, and the PACS administrator was transformed into the Imaging Informatics Professional (IIP), who has responsibilities far beyond the boundaries of the PACS itself.

With the new terminology, the core knowledge needed for the job had widened. The clinical knowledge base now included medical specialties outside of radiology, and the IT knowledge base required an understanding of software interactions, networking, and security across the entire enterprise. Who can fill this role? Who has the skills and knowledge to do the job? How can employers be sure that applicants for an IIP position will be able to serve the physicians and patients who are the ultimate clients of the digital infrastructure?

That's where certifying organizations such as the American Board of Imaging Informatics (ABII) come in. This organization, and others like it, were created to certify individuals from varying backgrounds in IT and clinical care, and to ensure that everyone who calls themselves an IIP has the knowledge and skills needed not just to keep the PACS afloat, but to keep the entire medical imaging infrastructure running smoothly and improve efficiency for the whole medical enterprise.

Who Should Read This Book

The primary audience for this book is Imaging Informatics Professionals (and those who want to become one). Certification tests such as the Certified Imaging Informatics Professional (CIIP) test offered by the ABII is certainly a good reason to master the wealth of information in this book! But it is worth noting that this book, like all educational programs offered by the Society for Imaging Informatics in Medicine (SIIM), is independent of the ABII and the CIIP certification program. The authors of this book were trying to provide practical, useful information for everyday IIP practice, not to just teach to the test.

Hopefully, this book will also be useful to IIPs long after the test is completed and passed, as a reference and troubleshooting guide for everyday imaging informatics. The layout and format of the book is designed with one major purpose in mind: quick reference. Our goal was to make sure that anyone who had read the book could look up a critical piece of information in the minimum amount of time. If you flip to the correct chapter, the key words and key concepts should jump out at you, and hopefully, the information you need should be right there, easy to find. Important definitions, checklists, and concepts are set off in color-coded boxes that draw the reader's eye. Sources of additional information are clearly highlighted. IIPs are masters of workflow efficiency, so the textbook that supports them had better be efficient to use!

Although IIPs are the primary audience for this book, other professionals will hopefully find it useful. IT staff working in medicine, even if not in the formal role of PACS administrator, will benefit from understanding the clinical milieu that pervades their work. Physicians and trainees interested in informatics will find the information pertinent to their practice, and the knowledge base formed by reading this book can serve as a basis for more in-depth study. Administrators supervising or hiring IIPs may also find the book useful, to better communicate with those who are maintaining the digital infrastructure.

The Organization of This Book

The second edition of the textbook has some familiar elements and also some new material. (Back then, artificial intelligence was for chess matches, not medical imaging. And no one's medical data had been ransomed!) But the organization has been entirely re-designed to follow IIPs through their workday.

The book is divided into seven parts. The first two parts are Foundations, in which the basics of medical imaging and information technology are introduced. Depending on your background, some of these chapters may seem overly simplistic. The goal of these parts is to bring everyone up to speed on areas of knowledge that they might not bring with them from their previous fields of study.

The third part of the book builds on the IT foundation to bring us into the world of imaging informatics. We then switch back to the clinical realm to talk about how medical images are interpreted and used. The fifth part is devoted to the people in the reading room (mostly, how to make their workday better). In the sixth part, we discuss daily operations, including events that happen every day and events that hopefully never happen. The last part takes us to the proverbial 30,000 foot view, in which we plan for the long-term success of the entire healthcare enterprise.

As it has been for the past 20 years, the field of imaging informatics is rapidly changing. As with all technological fields, newer and better software and solutions are continually developed. No printed textbook can be completely current or exhaustive on topics such as these. The purpose of this book is to answer commonly asked questions and provide a basis for continued learning. To this end, many of the suggested readings in the chapters are links to web sites that are likely to be updated as technology improves.

It is important to remember that every hospital or imaging site is unique. Solutions that work in one location may be totally inappropriate for other enterprises, or even elsewhere within the same enterprise. But some shared themes run through all of medical imaging; hopefully, we have focused on those in this book.

The bottom line – our main goal – was to provide pertinent information to IIPs at the point when it matters most (in medical terminology, "support at the point of care"). With this book at your desk, you should be able to rapidly find the information you need to troubleshoot urgent situations – the sorts of situations faced every day by Imaging Informatics Professionals.

Barton F. Branstetter IV
University of Pittsburgh
Pittsburgh, PA, USA
BFB1@pitt.edu

Contents

Contributors

Katherine P. Andriole, PhD, FSIIM Brigham and Women's Hospital, Harvard Medical School, MGH & BWH Center for Clinical Data Science, Boston, MA, USA

William F. Auffermann, MD, PhD University of Utah, Salt Lake City, UT, USA

Kimberly A. Barnett, RT (R) (M) (MR) (CT), CIIP ExecuPharm, Voorhees, NJ, USA

Fred M. Behlen, Ph.D Medical Physics and Informatics, Laitek Inc., Homewood, IL, USA

Barton F. Branstetter IV, MD, FACR, FSIIM Department of Radiology, University of Pittsburgh, Pittsburgh, PA, USA

David E. Brown, CIIP, FSIIM Los Angeles, CA, USA

Guillaume Chassagnon, MD Université de Paris, AP-HP, Hopital Cochin, Paris, France

Robert M. Coleman, BS Maine Medical Center, Portland, ME, USA

Jeremy Collins, MD Mayo Clinic, Rochester, MN, USA

Tessa S. Cook, MD, PhD, CIIP, FSIIM University of Pennsylvania School of Medicine, Philadelphia, PA, USA

Dawn Cram, RT (R)(M), CIIP Healthcare Development Advisory Services, The Gordian Knot Group, LLC, Fort Lauderdale, FL, USA

Thomas Jay Crawford, DHA, CIIP University of North Carolina School of Medicine, Department of Radiology, Chapel Hill, NC, USA

Sylvia Devlin, MS, RT (R)(M)(QM), CIIP Medical Imaging Information Technology, Johns Hopkins Medicine, Baltimore, MD, USA

Keith J. Dreyer, DO, PhD, FACR, FSIIM Informatics Massachusetts General Hospital and Brigham and Women's Hospital, Boston, MA, USA

Harvard Medical School, Boston, MA, USA

ACR Data Science Institute, Boston, MA, USA

Bradley Erickson, MD, PhD Mayo Clinic, Rochester, MN, USA

Nikki Fennell, CIIP Radiology Partners, El Segundo, CA, USA

Adam E. Flanders, MD, FSIIM Thomas Jefferson University, Philadelphia, PA, USA

Laure Fournier Université de Paris, AP-HP, Hopital européen Georges Pompidou, PARCC UMRS 970, INSERM, Paris, France

Brad Genereaux, NVIDIA Corporation, Santa Clara, CA, USA

Douglas S. Griffin, BSRT, (R)(CIIP), MBA Oncology Services, Southeast Health, Dothan, AL, USA

Safwan S. Halabi, MD Ann & Robert H. Lurie Children's Hospital of Chicago, Chicago, IL, USA

Matthew Hayes, CIIP PACS, Radiology Partners, Orland Park, IL, USA

Janice Honeyman-Buck, PhD, FSIIM Society for Imaging Informatics in Medicine, Leesburg, VA, USA

Steven C. Horii, MD, FACR Department of Radiology, University of Pennsylvania Medical Center, Philadelphia, PA, USA

Department of Radiology, Hospital of the University of Pennsylvania, Philadelphia, PA, USA

Center for Fetal Diagnosis and Treatment, Children's Hospital of Philadelphia, Philadelphia, PA, USA

R. L. "Skip" Kennedy, MSc, CIIP Imaging Informatics, The Permanente Medical Group, Kaiser Permanente, Sacramento, CA, USA

Woojin Kim, MD VA Palo Alto, Palo Alto, CA, USA

Elizabeth A. Krupinski, PhD Department of Radiology & Imaging Sciences, Emory University, Atlanta, GA, USA

Kevin W. McEnery, MD UT M.D. Anderson Cancer Center, Houston, TX, USA

Matthew B. Morgan, MD Department of Radiology, University of Utah, Salt Lake City, UT, USA

Jason Nagels, CIIP, PMP Department of Clinical Informatics, HDIRS, Markham, ON, Canada

Gary S. Norton, RT(R) (ARRT), BS Defense Health Agency, Integrated Clinical Systems, Program Management Office, Fort Detrick, MD, USA

Matthew D. Ralston, MD Maine Medical Center, Portland, ME, USA

Erik R. Ranschaert, MD Ghent University, Ghent, Belgium

J. Robert Huber Jr, MBA, PMP Medical Imaging Information Technology, Johns Hopkins Medicine, Baltimore, MD, USA

Karen J. Roberts Enterprise Medical Imaging, MGB Mass General Brigham, Boston, MA, USA

Andrea G. Rockall, MRCP, FRCR Department of Cancer and Surgery, Imperial College London, London, UK

Bill Rostenberg, FAIA Emeritus Architecture for Advanced Medicine, Greenbrae, CA, USA

Christopher J. Roth, MD, MMCI, CPHIMS, CIIP Department of Radiology, Duke University, Durham, NC, USA

Duke Health, Durham, NC, USA

Ann Scherzinger, PhD Radiology-Radiological Sciences, University of Colorado School of Medicine, Aurora, CO, USA

Tom Schultz Enterprise Medical Imaging and Clinical Data Science Office, Mass General Brigham, Boston, MA, USA

Rasu B. Shrestha, MD MBA Strategy and Transformation Office, Atrium Health, Charlotte, NC, USA

Eliot L. Siegel, MD, FACR, FSIIM Diagnostic Radiology and Nuclear Medicine, University of Maryland, School of Medicine, Baltimore, MD, USA

Edward M. Smith, ScD (Deceased)

Erik S. Storm, DO, MBI, CIIP Departments of Radiology and Medical Education, Salem VA Medical Center, Salem, VA, USA

James Whitfill, MD Internal Medicine and Biomedical Informatics, University of Arizona College of Medicine Phoenix, Phoenix, AZ, USA

Charles E. Willis, PhD, DABR, FAAPM, FACR Department of Imaging Physics, University of Texas MD Anderson Cancer Center, Houston, TX, USA

Part I
Medical Imaging

Chapter 1
Introduction to Medical Images

William F. Auffermann

Contents

1.1 Healthcare and Medical Imaging

- Healthcare is defined as "efforts made to maintain or restore physical, mental, or emotional well-being, especially by a trained and licensed professional" [1].
- The endpoint for healthcare is health and well-being.
- Healthcare workers include professionals with a wide range of skills, most of whom are licensed by the government to provide care. Patient-facing roles include:
  - Physicians
  - Physician assistants
  - Registered nurses
  - Nurse practitioners
  - Technologists
  - Support personnel and assistants

> **DEFINITION: Medical Imaging**
>
> Several different technologies that are used to visualize the human body in order to diagnose, monitor, or treat medical conditions [2].

W. F. Auffermann (✉)
University of Utah, Salt Lake City, UT, USA
e-mail: WILLIAM.AUFFERMANN@hsc.utah.edu

© The Author(s), under exclusive license to Springer Science+Business Media, LLC, part of Springer Nature 2021
B. F. Branstetter IV (ed.), *Practical Imaging Informatics*,
https://doi.org/10.1007/978-1-0716-1756-4_1

DEFINITION: Patient-Facing

Healthcare providers who directly interact face-to-face with patients are called "patient-facing." In medical imaging, the technologists who create the images are usually patient-facing, but the radiologists who interpret the images may or may not be.

- Medical imaging is a branch of healthcare where associated personnel may or may not have significant patient-facing roles.
- Healthcare support workers, including information technology professionals, often have very specialized roles.
  - They may become focused on specific tasks entailed in one's job such that the big picture of achieving positive health goals for patients is lost.
  - Remember that having an imaging study acquired and presented for interpretation is only one part of the patient care pathway.

    FURTHER READING: FDA Web Site on Medical Imaging

    https://www.fda.gov/radiation-emitting-products/radiation-emitting-products-and-procedures/medical-imaging.

  - The sequence of events that are related to healthcare and medical imaging may be well considered as a chain, where breaking any one link causes failure of the entire system.
  - This chapter is intended to provide the imaging informatics professional (IIP) with a big picture overview of the role of medical images and health data in healthcare.

1.2 Why Medical Images Are Helpful in Healthcare

Medical images have two primary uses in healthcare: to establish a diagnosis in a patient with symptoms or signs of illness and to screen asymptomatic patients (those without symptoms). Failure to accurately identify and report the presence of disease may lead to misdiagnosis and delayed diagnosis, which may contribute to patient injury and/or death. Secondary uses include guiding patient management (e.g., evaluating a patient's response to chemotherapy), guiding surgeons through complex operations, and direct treatment (image-guided procedures).

1.2.1 Establishing a Diagnosis and Misdiagnosis

- Prior to medical imaging, a physician relied on the history elicited from the patient and their physical examination.
- Unfortunately, many medical conditions share similar signs and symptoms.
  - For example, a cough can be the presenting symptom for ailments ranging from seasonal allergies to cancer.

- Physical examination may add some useful information to establish a diagnosis, but often it is inconclusive.
- It is difficult to estimate the degree to which medical imaging has improved the timely diagnosis of diseases.
- Patients' lives are directly saved with medical imaging, often by establishing a correct diagnosis and avoiding misdiagnosis.

> **HYPOTHETICAL SCENARIO: Saving Lives with Imaging**
>
> Aortic dissection is a life-threatening disease of the main artery carrying blood out of the heart to the body. Based on history and physical examination alone, physicians may correctly suspect this diagnosis in as low as 15%–43% of patients. If left untreated, the death rate is near 50% at 48 hours. The accuracy of a CT scan for detection of aortic dissection is 98–100%. Consequently, CT (and medical imaging in general) plays a crucial role in the timely identification and treatment of aortic dissection.

1.2.2 Screening and Delayed Diagnosis

- Medical imaging is also used for screening of asymptomatic patients.
- One common screening test is mammography for breast cancer.
  - Breast cancer is the most common form of malignancy in females, accounting for 30% of all new cancer.
  - However, breast cancer accounts for 15% of cancer-related deaths in females.
- While the reason for this difference in incidence and mortality is likely multifactorial, it is believed that breast cancer screening is contributory.
- For women 40–74 years of age who participate in screening, there is an estimated 40% reduction in breast cancer mortality.

DEFINITION: Screening

Using medical imaging to detect hidden (occult) disease in patients who do not feel sick. The goal of screening is to detect diseases in an early stage when they can be treated more successfully.

The Questions We Try to Answer with Medical Images

Medical imaging is used to extend the diagnostic capabilities of the physician beyond that which can be ascertained through a history and physical examination. Diagnostic imaging modalities generate images of processes occurring within the patient's body.

DEFINITION: Modality

A modality is a particular technology used to create medical images. Examples include CT scans and MRIs.

- The diagnosis of disease involves a combination of history, physical examination, laboratory testing, and imaging, but confirming the diagnosis of many diseases relies entirely on imaging.

CHECKLIST: Imaging Modalities and Abbreviations

Conventional radiography (X-rays)	XR
Ultrasound	US
Computed tomography (CT scans)	CT
Magnetic resonance	MR
Nuclear medicine	NM
Fluoroscopy (X-ray movies)	FL

HYPOTHETICAL SCENARIO: Relying on Imaging

A medical condition that is often difficult to diagnose is pulmonary embolism (PE). The symptoms of PE are often nonspecific (meaning that they can be seen with many different diseases). They include chest pain and shortness of breath. This disease is due to clot lodging in the pulmonary arteries (the arteries carrying blood to the lungs). PE is a potentially lethal disease if not diagnosed and treated expeditiously. Laboratory tests are of limited use in confirming the diagnosis. CT, however, can show the clots lodged inside the arteries and make a precise diagnosis (Fig. 1.1).

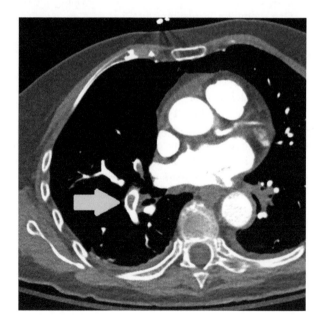

Fig. 1.1 Image from a CT of the chest showing a pulmonary embolism (PE) in right pulmonary arteries. A representative embolism is marked with a green arrow

1.3 The Chain of Events for Medical Imaging

The events that occur during the healthcare of any patient will differ by patient and visit.
- Each step may be divided into multiple smaller steps for completion of each task.
- The steps involved in a patient's passage through a healthcare encounter involve many nonimaging steps.
- While nonimaging aspects of a healthcare encounter are not typically the purview of the IIP, it is nonetheless important to recognize how they contribute to the overall patient experience.

STEP-BY-STEP: An Imaging Encounter

Step-by-step: Health system pathway of a patient with chest pain, potential aortic dissection:

1. Patient experiences chest pain.
2. Contact between the patient and healthcare provider is established.
3. Patient is scheduled for an appointment.
4. Patient arrives at their appointment and checks in.
5. Patient is shown to an examination room.
6. Preliminary information is collected by an assistant.
7. Patient is seen by a healthcare provider.
8. A full history is taken, and a physical examination is performed.
9. Imaging studies are ordered.
10. Patient is discharged with follow-up instructions for imaging and treatment.
11. Patient goes to radiology for the requested imaging study and checks in.
12. The patient's medical information is reviewed, and the appropriate imaging protocol is selected.
13. The patient is evaluated for contraindications to the requested study.
14. The imaging study is performed.
15. Images are collected and processed by the technologist.
16. Images are transmitted to PACS.
17. Imaging study is routed to the appropriate PACS worklist.
18. Radiologist reviews the images.
19. Radiologist generates a report of the imaging findings and sends the report to PACS and the electronic medical record (EMR). If there are urgent findings, the radiologist may also contact a provider caring for the patient by telephone.
20. The EMR provides the healthcare provider a notice that imaging study results are available for review.
21. Healthcare provider reviews report for the imaging study, possibly at a later time.
22. Healthcare provider revises their diagnosis and treatment plan as needed.
23. Healthcare provider instructs their office to contact the patient as needed for further follow-up and/or treatment.

1.4 Urgency in Radiology (Why Physicians Need the Results Now!)

People who work in healthcare but are not immediately involved in patient care often do not understand a physician's insistence that they need something "right now!" A few hypothetical scenarios are provided to illustrate why expeditious evaluation and reporting of medical studies is important.

HYPOTHETICAL SCENARIO: "The Images Are on the Way"

Ms. A is having chest pain and sees her physician, Dr. X. Dr. X orders a chest radiograph to evaluate. After the examination is performed, Dr. X has the patient wait in the office for the results. However, the PACS is having problems, and after waiting 2 hours for results, the patient leaves for home with a prescription for ibuprofen and instructions to follow-up next week or go to the emergency department if symptoms worsen. Two hours after the patient leaves, the images become available on PACS and the radiologist identifies a pneumothorax on the radiograph. A pneumothorax is a potentially lethal disorder in which air between the lung and chest wall can increase in size, compressing the lungs and heart. The radiologist calls Dr. X regarding these critical findings. Dr. X thanks the radiologist for the result and promptly hangs up to contact the patient for further emergent treatment. Then next day Dr. X calls back and expresses anger that it took 4 hours to receive these results. Dr. X says "Ms. A says she is considering suing the hospital! It's a good thing the she didn't die!".

If you speak with radiologists, they most will likely be able to relate similar stories to you. The patient care chain needs to function in a timely fashion. A break at any link of the patient care chain can delay care downstream and potentially result in patient harm and death. So when a physician says that they need the images "now," there could be a very good, life or death, reason for the urgency. In medicine, minutes can matter.

HYPOTHETICAL SCENARIO: "Have You Tried Rebooting?"

The radiologist, Dr. Y, is having a rough day. The day is busy, and there have been several urgent emergency department cases, two involving motor vehicle accidents. Each patient has multiple injuries making evaluation of the images complex. The last case, Mr. B, may have traumatic aortic injury (a potentially life-threatening injury). The problem is that the image series is very large, and every time Dr. Y tries to open the relevant series, the PACS application freezes. Mr. B's family members are beside themselves with worry and want to know if their husband/father is going to need emergent thoracic surgery to live. But Dr. Y still cannot look at the images. There is the other lower acuity trauma, but the radiologist is not able to look at those images either, with the PACS workstation down. The doctor has also heard that there may be a motor vehicle accident patient flown by helicopter to the hospital in the next hour. Just then the phone rings, it is the reading room assistant saying: "Surgery is on the phone about a STAT postoperative study. They are waiting for your report on Line 1." Frantic, Dr. Y calls the PACS team to let them know about the PACS problems and the urgency of this issue for patient care. The PACS professional responds by saying "Have you tried rebooting?"

The radiology reading room can be a very hectic environment. Decisions often need to be made quickly. For a patient in critical condition, minutes matter. The radiologist is very aware of this and can sometimes feel at a loss to help the patient when there are IT issues preventing timely image evaluation and reporting. Consequently, having one or more steps of the imaging chain break can be very stressful. It is important for the IIP to recognize this urgency and try to fix things with a priority proportional to their urgency. It is understood that one cannot do the impossible, but it is helpful to recognize why the radiologist and other healthcare providers may become stressed when things do not work as planned.

HYPOTHETICAL SCENARIO: "It's Only Been 15 Minutes"

Mr. C is having a sub-ideal experience at the medical center. He is experiencing abdominal pain and arrived on time for his appointment with Dr. Z. However, there were several urgent patients added to Dr. Z's schedule, and Mr. C is seen an hour late. After he is seen, his healthcare provider recommends a CT of the abdomen. The EMR was recently upgraded and the healthcare provider's office is having difficulty placing the order. After 30 minutes, the order for an add-on urgent CT is placed and the patient goes to radiology, where they are running behind. The patient waits an hour to be scanned. The scan takes 15 minutes. Mr. C was told to go back to Dr. Z's clinic to wait for results, and he does as instructed. Mr. C is getting anxious. He wants to wait for the results, but his child will be finishing school in 30 minutes and needs to be picked up. He thinks "If I can get here on time, why can't the hospital get its act together?". Mr. C is still in pain and gets increasingly irritated. There is some trouble sending the images from the CT to PACS. After a scanner-to-PACS image transmission delay of 15 minutes, the IT team gets a call that "the images need to get loaded right away, now!". The HIT professional is rather perplexed, after all, "It's only been 15 minutes."

It important to note that delays at any point in the patient management chain will cascade downstream. Multiple points of delay may aggregate to cause significant delays in patient care before a patient even reaches the radiology department. Consequently, even small delays in radiology may be the straw that breaks the camel's back for patient or provider patience.

These issues are sometimes referred to as "the primacy of patient care." In a hospital setting, the care of the patient takes precedence over the convenience and predictability that providers and support staff might otherwise prefer. This is unlike other work environments and is one of the most difficult cultural changes for IIPs who have not previously worked in a healthcare setting.

> **FURTHER READING: Introductory Texts on Medical Imaging**
>
> Herring W, Learning radiology: recognizing the basics. 4th ed., Elsevier; 2019, ISBN-13: 978-0323567299.
>
> Smith, Farrell T. Radiology 101: the basics and fundamentals of imaging. 4th ed. Lippincott Williams & Wilkins; 2013, ISBN-13: 978-1451144574.

> **KEY CONCEPT: The Primacy of Patient Care**
>
> It may seem to a new IIP that everything in the hospital is an emergency. Even tiny delays cause huge frustrations, and the IIP is expected to fix problems with a level of urgency that would be unnecessary in other work environments. If you are new to healthcare, be ready for this change in expectations.

1.5 Additional Healthcare Data Needed for Medical Imaging

The PACS, report-generation system, and radiology workstations are at the core of what an IIP working in medical imaging will be concerned with. However, there are several additional computer systems that radiology depends upon.

1.5.1 Relevant Clinical Information

In addition to high-quality image data, it is important for the radiologist to have accurate clinical information related to the indication for an examination. This information serves two main functions:

1. It helps the radiologist select the best imaging examination for the patient.
2. It helps the radiologist interpret the study and arrive at the correct diagnosis.

HYPOTHETICAL SCENARIO: History Matters

An imaging study is requested of the chest; the only indication provided is "cough." Now consider if the provider offered a more comprehensive history; two examples are shown below:

1. Seventeen-year-old with acute onset of fever and cough
2. Seventy-one-year-old with chronic cough, unintended weight loss, and history of heavy tobacco use

In the first case, the diagnosis is most likely to be pneumonia, and a chest radiograph is the most appropriate study to order. In the second instance, one should have a higher suspicion of cancer given the patient's age, chronicity of the condition, and smoking risk factor. Regardless of the findings on the X-ray, that patient may need a CT of the chest.

Clinical information related to the reason for the order should be automatically imported from the EMR to the PACS.
- While this is helpful, the ordering provider often does not provide complete information.
- The radiologist often will consult the EMR for further patient information.
- PACS integration with the EMR is very helpful.
- A radiologist may become impatient if the integration is not working or if the EMR is down entirely.

Availability of pertinent clinical information is an underappreciated aspect of medical imaging.
- IIPs are not responsible for the accuracy of the indication provided for an examination.
- However, IIPs may facilitate many aspects of the availability of clinical information.
- The PACS viewer may be integrated with the EMR, facilitating ready access.
  - If the integration is not working, the radiologist may need to manually search for a patient, which is inefficient.
- If the PACS-EMR integration is not working:
  - A radiologist can look up the information on the EMR manually. This would take a minute or two per case.
  - A few minutes here and a few minutes there may result in an outpatient CT not being read until after the patient has left the clinic.

1.5.2 Results Reporting

- The typical means of communicating routine nonurgent results is the EMR.

- The radiologist needs to notify relevant healthcare providers in an expeditious manner for unexpected and emergent findings on medical images.
  - Having a secretary or reading room assistant can make the radiologist much more efficient.
  - Some results need to be communicated over the course of minutes, in which case routine communications using the EMR are not adequate.
  - Urgent and emergent results historically have been communicated by the radiologist or support staff tracking down a healthcare provider to report the results in person or verbally over the telephone.
- Increasingly, there are computerized services supported by IIPs capable of automatically communicating unexpected or urgent findings.
  - Such services can markedly improve the radiologist's workflow, especially if they are integrated with the radiology workstation, the EMR, and the healthcare system's paging and telephone system.
  - These integrated critical results reporting systems represent another potential point of system failure and yet another piece of interconnected software that the HIT professional may need to manage.

PEARLS

- Medical imaging plays a central role in the delivery of healthcare and is critical to health system function.
- There are many complex interrelated steps involved in the passage of a patient through the healthcare system that may be considered analogous to a chain. A delay of any one step may cause delays in the whole system.
- Imaging studies can rapidly establish many diagnoses in a manner that may not be feasible without imaging.
- There is an expectation that medical images are acquired, available on PACS, and reported in a consistent and timely fashion.
- Clinical medicine can be very busy and stressful. When information technology systems do not work as planned or there are delays not related to imaging, it causes stress on the remainder of the system and a sense of urgency that may not be immediately apparent to an IIP.

References

1. Health Care, in Merriam-Webster. 2020, Merriam-Webster.com.
2. FDA Medical Imaging. 2018. Available from: https://www.fda.gov/radiation-emitting-products/radiation-emitting-products-and-procedures/medical-imaging.

Self-Assessment Questions

Please select the best answer to each question.

1. Health system workers who impact patient care include:

    (a) Physicians
    (b) Physician assistants
    (c) Nurses
    (d) Imaging informatics professionals
    (e) All of the above

2. Medical imaging can help with patient care because:

    (a) Health professionals really do not need them, but imaging can help if they are busy.
    (b) The symptoms and signs of many diseases are nonspecific by other diagnostic criteria.
    (c) They improve the revenue of a health system.
    (d) Medical imaging studies are amenable for data-mining.
    (e) All of the above.

3. It is important to recognize that there are many steps involved in providing healthcare to a patient because it helps one understand:

    (a) The more steps, the more you can bill.
    (b) The IIPs do not need to worry about the clinical aspects of patient management.
    (c) A delay at any point can have effects downstream.
    (d) IT systems are built to scale with increased complexity of patient throughput.
    (e) All of the above.

4. Delays in the availability of medical images on the institutional PACS can cause:

    (a) Delayed diagnosis of critical medical conditions
    (b) Stress for the patient, family members, and medical personnel
    (c) Delays in patient care downstream
    (d) Medicolegal issues if a patient is injured
    (e) All the above

5. The clinical information provided to a radiologist interpreting a study is important because:

    (a) It is required by the EMR for report creation.
    (b) Structured templates typically have a field for clinical information.
    (c) It is primarily useful for teaching institutions as an aid for trainee education.
    (d) It helps the radiologist formulate an accurate impression.
    (e) All the above.

6. Which is true regarding communicating urgent and emergent findings on medical imaging studies:

   (a) They are common and follow typical reporting mechanisms.
   (b) They are usually communicated verbally, but there are new IT-enabled solutions.
   (c) The EMR is the standard mechanism for communication of all medical results. Additional steps are not needed.
   (d) Face-to-face communication is typical.
   (e) All the above

Chapter 2
Medical Terminology

Kimberly A. Barnett

Contents

2.1 Introduction

Medical terminology creates a standard way for healthcare professionals to communicate effectively and efficiently. A common language allows medical professionals to accurately describe procedures and results regarding a patient's condition. Well-defined terms result in higher-quality patient care with fewer errors. This chapter will describe the medical terminology that directly impacts medical imaging.

2.2 Subspecialty Sections in the Radiology Department

There are divisions within the Radiology Department that facilitate specialization in specific areas of the body. Specializing permits the radiologist to provide the highest quality of care to patients.

K. A. Barnett (✉)
ExecuPharm, Voorhees, NJ, USA

B. F. Branstetter IV (ed.), *Practical Imaging Informatics*,
https://doi.org/10.1007/978-1-0716-1756-4_2

- Body imaging includes thoracic, abdominal, and pelvic imaging. Sometimes body imaging is subdivided into chest (thoracic) imaging and abdominopelvic imaging.
- Breast imaging is performed for either screening or diagnostic purposes. Breast imaging is sometimes its own division and sometimes part of a larger Women's Imaging Division that also includes obstetrics and gynecology.
- Cardiovascular imaging is imaging of the heart and the blood vessels of the heart.
- Emergency radiology is imaging that is performed for patients being seen in the Emergency Department (ED). Trauma and acute illnesses predominate. Interpretation is usually time sensitive. Some departments have a distinct Emergency Division, while other departments spread this responsibility among the other subspecialty divisions.
- Interventional radiology (IR) is a procedural division in which a radiologist uses images to guide treatment of medical conditions. These procedures are considered "minimally invasive" (compared to traditional surgery).
  - In some departments, IR includes procedures in the chest and abdomen, while in other departments, this division is exclusively devoted to vascular procedures.
  - Interventional neuroradiology is devoted to the vessels leading to the brain. It may be part of IR or part of neuroradiology (or may be run by a different department such as neurosurgery).
  - Spinal procedures may be performed by IR, neuroradiology, or MSK.
- Musculoskeletal (MSK) radiology focuses on imaging for disorders of the bones, joints, and associated musculature.
- Neuroradiology focuses on abnormalities of the central and peripheral nervous systems, head, neck, and spine. In some departments, imaging of the neck and skull base is in a separate Ear, Nose, and Throat Division.
- Nuclear medicine and PET imaging specialists use radioactive tracers (radio-pharmaceuticals) for diagnosis of disease and for therapy.
- Pediatric radiology focuses on children and adolescents. This division may practice in a separate children's hospital. Alternatively, smaller departments may divide this responsibility among the other divisions.

2.3 Positions, Planes, and Projections

Because body parts can move relative to one another, a standard body position is needed for anatomical reference. Directional terms, imaging planes, and imaging projections are all based on the patient in this **anatomical position** (Fig. 2.1). In the

> **KEY CONCEPT: Anatomical Position**
>
> All directional terms, imaging planes, and imaging projections are based on a patient in the anatomical position.

anatomical position, the body is upright facing the observer, with feet placed flat on the ground directed forward, with arms positioned at the body's sides, and with palms of hands facing forward.

Fig. 2.1 Anatomical position

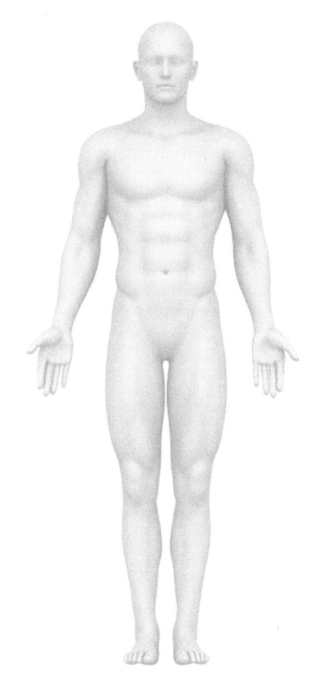

2.3.1 Directional Terms

Directional terms help explain the relative locations of structures in the body.
- **Anterior** or **ventral** is located to the front of the body. The nose is an anterior structure of the body. The pectoralis muscles are anterior to the heart.
- **Posterior** or **dorsal** is located near the back of the body. The shoulder blades are located on the posterior aspect of the body.
- **Superior** or **cranial** is toward the head. The neck is superior to the heart.
- **Inferior** or **caudal** is away from the head. The toes are inferior to the knees.
- **Medial** is toward the midline of the body. The big toe is medial to the little toe.
- **Lateral** is away from the midline of the body. The thumb is lateral to the pinky finger. (Reminder: These directional terms are based on the anatomical position – look back at Fig. 2.1.)
- **Proximal** is nearer to the center of the body. The elbow is proximal to the fingers; the neck is proximal to the head.
- **Distal** is further from the center of the body. The foot is distal to the knee.

2.3.2 Imaging Planes

Imaging planes (Fig. 2.2) are used extensively in cross-sectional imaging (Fig. 2.3).
- **Axial plane** (transverse plane) is a horizontal plane that divides the body into upper and lower parts.
- **Coronal plane** (frontal plane) is a vertical plane that divides the body into anterior and posterior parts.
- **Sagittal plane** (lateral plane) is a vertical plane that divides the body into right and left parts.
    - **Median** (midsagittal plane) is a sagittal plane through the midline of the body dividing it into equal right and left halves.

2.3.3 Body Positions

Body positions help us understand how the patient is positioned when the images are acquired.
- **Erect** – standing or sitting
- **Supine** – lying on back
- **Prone** – lying face down
- **Decubitus** – lying down
- **Lateral decubitus** – lying on side
    - **Right lateral decubitus** – right side is down on table
    - **Left lateral decubitus** – left side is down on the table

Fig. 2.2 Imaging planes

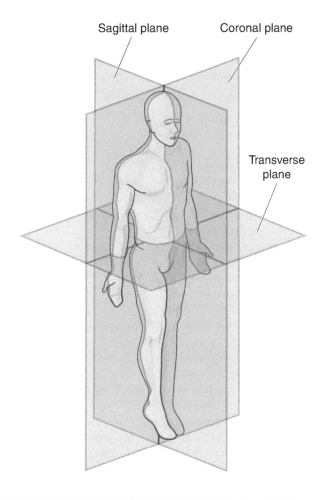

Fig. 2.3 Imaging planes – MRI example

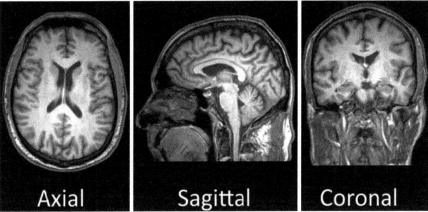

- **Trendelenburg position** – lying supine on an inclined table with head lower than feet
- **Reverse Trendelenburg position** – lying supine on an inclined table with feet lower than the head

2.3.4 Imaging Projections

Projections refer to the way the patient is positioned when the X-ray beam passes through the body. It is the direction of the beam as it passes through the patient.

FURTHER READING

Bruce Long, Jeannean Rollins, Barbara Smith. Merrill's Atlas of radiographic positioning and procedures. 3 volume Set, 14th ed. Mosby; 2018.

- **Frontal projections**
    - **AP** (anterior posterior) projection is when the X-ray beam passes from the front of the body to the back of the body (e.g., portable or bedside chest X-rays are taken AP).
    - **PA** (posterior anterior) projection is when the X-ray beam passes from the back of the body to the front of the body (e.g., upright ambulatory chest X-rays are taken PA).
- **Lateral** projection is when the X-ray beam passes from the left to right or right to left through the body.
- **Oblique** projection is when the X-ray beam is at an angle other than frontal or lateral.
- **Mammographic views**
    - **RCC** (right cranial caudal) is a view of the right breast from top to bottom.
    - **LCC** (left cranial caudal) is a view of the left breast from top to bottom.
    - **RMLO** (right mediolateral oblique) is a mammography view where the X-ray beam is at an angle to the right breast.
    - **LMLO** (left mediolateral oblique) is a mammography view where the X-ray beam is at an angle to the left breast.

2.4 Anatomical Terms in a DICOM Header

There are numerous anatomic terms that can be found in a DICOM header. Below are definitions for the most commonly used DICOM fields that contain anatomic terms.

FURTHER READING

DICOM Standard Browser. Innolitics. https://dicom.innolitics.com/ciods

Referencing the DICOM standard is highly recommended (see **Chap. 12**).

2.4.1 Image Laterality (0020,0062)

The image laterality field refers to one side of the body versus the other. The available values are:
- **Left side (L).**
- **Right side (R).**
- **Unpaired (U)** – structures that exist on only one side of the body.
- **Bilateral (B)** – both sides of the body are included.

2.4.2 Patient Orientation (0020,0020)

The patient orientation field defines the imaging plane by using two values that designate the anatomical directions of the rows and columns of pixels in the image.
- **Anterior (A)**
- **Posterior (P)**
- **Right (R)**
- **Left (L)**
- **Head (H)**
- **Foot (F)**

2.4.3 Body Part Examined (0018,0015)

This is a text description of the part of the body being examined, for example, "abdomen." For each body part being examined, there are corresponding SNOMED and RADLEX clinical terms (see **Chap. 18**).

> **FURTHER READING**
>
> DICOM Part 16, Chapter L: Correspondence of anatomic region codes and body part examined defined terms.

2.4.4 Study Description (0008,1030)

This DICOM tag is a description or classification of the study performed that is generated by the institution. This list of descriptions is variable and needs to be coordinated with the RIS (radiology information system) or EMR (electronic medical record).

2.4.5 Patient Position (0018,5100)

The position of the patient relative to the imaging equipment (i.e., how the patient goes into the scanner). This DICOM tag is used for annotation purposes. These are only some of the possible designations.

- **Head first – prone (HFP)**
- **Head first – supine (HFS)**
- **Feet first – prone (FFP)**
- **Feet first – supine (FFS)**

PEARLS

- Divisions in radiology allow radiologists to specialize in specific areas of the body so they can provide the highest quality of care to patients.
- Directional terms help explain the location of a structure in the body and where it is in relation to another structure in the body.
- Imaging planes figuratively divide the body in two.
- Body positions define how the patient is positioned as the images are acquired.
- Imaging projections refer to the way the patient is positioned when the X-ray beam passes through the body.

Self-Assessment Questions

1. What division in radiology specializes in imaging of the heart?

    (a) Breast
    (b) Cardiovascular
    (c) Musculoskeletal
    (d) Neuroradiology

2. Directional terms, imaging planes, and imaging projections are all based on what position?

    (a) Prone
    (b) Supine
    (c) Anatomical
    (d) Trendelenburg

3. What directional term is used to describe the position of the big toe to the body?

    (a) Superior
    (b) Lateral
    (c) Distal
    (d) Lateral

4. What imaging plane divides the body into anterior and posterior parts?

   (a) Coronal
   (b) Sagittal
   (c) Axial
   (d) Median

5. Lying face down is considered what position?

   (a) Supine
   (b) Lateral decubitus
   (c) Prone
   (d) Erect

6. List three imaging planes.

7. Describe the anatomical position.

8. What are the terms that can be displayed in the patient orientation field?

Chapter 3
Medical Imaging Modalities and Digital Images

Katherine P. Andriole

Contents

3.1 Introduction

3.1.1 Special Aspects of Medical Images

Medical imaging technologies enable views of the internal structure and function of the human body. Information obtained from the various modalities can be used to diagnose abnormalities, guide therapeutic procedures, and monitor disease

K. P. Andriole (✉)
Brigham and Women's Hospital, Harvard Medical School, Boston, MA, USA

MGH & BWH Center for Clinical Data Science, Boston, MA, USA
e-mail: kandriole@bwh.harvard.edu

B. F. Branstetter IV (ed.), *Practical Imaging Informatics*,
https://doi.org/10.1007/978-1-0716-1756-4_3

treatment. Medical images have unique performance requirements, safety restrictions, characteristic attributes, and technical limitations that often make them more difficult to create, acquire, manipulate, manage, and interpret. Some of these contributing factors include:

- Complexity of imaging situations:
  - Equipment size and available space,
  - Inaccessibility of the internal structures of the body to measurement,
  - Patient positioning,
  - Patient illness,
  - Procedure practicality.
- Variability of the data between patients; for example, between normal and abnormal anatomy and physiology, within normal ranges, and within the same patient at different times or body positions.
- Effect of imaging transducer on the image, including artifacts created by the imaging method or by something in the patient's body. A major source of artifact in images of living systems is **motion**.
- Safety considerations, patient discomfort, procedure time, and cost–benefit trade-offs.

DEFINITION: Artifact

Any component of the image that is extraneous to the representation of tissue structures; can be caused by a technique, technology, hardware, or software error.

3.1.2 Medical Imaging Terminology

- **Medical Imaging Hierarchy:** Patient – Examination (Study) – Series (Sequence) – Image. For example, a patient may undergo an imaging examination, also called a study, such as computed tomography (CT) of the abdomen. This study may include several sequences (a.k.a. series), such as a set of images with contrast and a set without contrast. A sequence or series may consist of a single image or multiple images.

CHECKLIST: Medical Imaging Hierarchy

1. Patient
2. Study or Examination
3. Series, Sequence or View
4. Image
5. Pixel

- Modalities can be characterized by whether their energy source uses **ionizing radiation** such as for radiography, fluoroscopy, mammography, CT, and nuclear medicine or nonionizing radiation such as for ultrasound and magnetic resonance imaging (MRI).
- **Projection** (planar) imaging, such as projection radiography in which X-rays from a source pass through the patient and are detected on the opposite side of the body,

produces a simple two-dimensional (2-D) shadow representation of the tissues lying between the source and the detector. Each point in the image has contributions from all objects in the body along a straight line trajectory through the patient. Overlapping layers of tissues can make planar imaging difficult to interpret.

- **Tomographic** (cross-sectional) imaging modalities include CT, MRI, and ultrasound. In CT, for example, the X-ray source is tightly collimated to interrogate a thin transverse section through the body. The source and detectors rotate together around the patient producing a series of one-dimensional projections at a number of different angles. The projection data are mathematically reconstructed to create a 2-D image of a slice through the body. Digital geometric processing can be used to generate a three-dimensional (3-D) image of the inside of objects from a series of 2-D image slices taken around a single axis of rotation. Historically, images have been generated in the axial (transverse) plane that is orthogonal to the long axis of the body. Today's modern scanners can reformat the data in any orientation (orthogonal or oblique to the body axis) or as volumetric representations due to the ability of modern scanners to acquire isotropic (equal dimensions in the x-, y- and z-planes) voxels.

- Medical modalities produce representations of anatomical (**structural**) or molecular/physiological (**functional**) information of the imaged body parts. For example, X-ray images are representations of the distribution of the linear attenuation coefficients of tissues and are largely images of anatomy or the structural nature of the tissues in the body. Radioisotope imaging of nuclear medicine produces images of the distribution of chemical, molecular, or physiological function of the tissue. Some modalities, such as ultrasound, can provide other types of functional measures, such as speed of blood flow through vessels.

DEFINITION: Ionizing Radiation

Radiation capable of producing energetically charged particles that move through space from one object to another where the energy is absorbed. Radiation is potentially hazardous if used improperly.

KEY CONCEPT: Imaging Modalities

Modalities can be characterized by their energy source as invasive (using ionizing radiation) or noninvasive. They are acquired in 2-D planar projection mode or tomographic cross section; and produce images representative of anatomical structure and/or physiological or molecular function.

KEY CONCEPT: X-Ray Attenuation

Attenuation of an X-ray beam is largely a function of tissue radiodensity. Bone, for example, has a higher attenuation coefficient than soft tissue. In a radiograph of the chest, bony structures highly attenuate (or absorb) X-rays, passing less signal through the body to the detector; whereas soft tissues are less attenuating, passing more signal through to the detector. Air is least attenuating, and thus high signal hits the detector and is represented as black in most images; no signal hitting the detector is usually represented as white. In a chest radiograph, the air spaces in the lungs appear black, soft tissues are lighter gray, and the bony ribs and spine are white.

3.2 Diagnostic Imaging Modalities

For each diagnostic modality given below, the energy source and detector used in image formation are listed along with the tissue characteristic or attribute represented by the modality. Advantages and disadvantages for each are included.

3.2.1 Projection Radiography

- Source: X-rays; ionizing radiation; part of the electromagnetic spectrum emitted as a result of bombardment of a tungsten anode by free electrons from a cathode. The source passes through the patient and X-rays are detected on the opposite side of the body.
- Analog detector: fluorescent screen and radiographic film; historical and rarely used today in developed countries with access to digital technology.
- Digital detector: **computed radiography (CR)** uses a photostimulable or storage phosphor imaging plate; direct **digital radiography (DR)** devices convert X-ray energy to electron–hole pairs in an amorphous selenium photoconductor, which are read out by a thin-film transistor (TFT) array of amorphous silicon (Am-Si). For indirect DR devices, light is generated using an X-ray sensitive phosphor and converted to a proportional charge in a photodiode (e.g., cesium iodide scintillator) and read out by a charge-coupled device (CCD) or flat panel Am-Si TFT array.
- Image attributes: variations in the **grayscale** of the image represent the X-ray attenuation or density of tissues; bone absorbs large amounts of radiation allowing less signal to reach the detector, resulting in white or bright areas on the image; air has the least attenuation causing maximum signal to reach the detector, resulting in black or dark areas of the image.

- Advantages: fast and easy to perform; equipment is relatively inexpensive and widely available; low amounts of radiation; high spatial resolution capability. Particularly useful for assessing the parts of the body that have inherently high contrast resolution but require fine detail such as for imaging the chest or skeletal system.
- Disadvantages: poor differentiation of low contrast objects; superposition of structures through projection of a 3D object (the patient) onto a 2D image makes image interpretation difficult; uses ionizing radiation.

3.2.2 Mammography and Tomosynthesis

- Source: X-rays; ionizing radiation as in other projection radiography examinations.
- Detector: analog film may still be used in some countries. However, specialty Digital Detectors made as dedicated systems for imaging the breast are available and in widespread use. CR can be used as a direct replacement for screen-film systems as it can be used with existing acquisition system infrastructure. Direct DR devices include CCD multi-detectors, slot-scanning CCD detectors, and Am-Si flat panel detectors. All acquire images at higher spatial resolution than for other digital projection radiographs. **Digital Breast Tomosynthesis (DBT)**

FURTHER READING: Physics of Medical Imaging

Bushberg JT, Seibert JA, Leidholdt EM, Boone JM. The essential physics of medical imaging. Philadelphia: Lippincott Williams & Wilkins; 2002.

Huda W, Slone R. Review of radiologic physics. Philadelphia: Lippincott Williams & Wilkins; 2003.

Sprawls P. Physical principles of medical imaging. New York: Aspen Publishers, Inc.; 1993.

HYPOTHETICAL SCENARIO: Radiation Dose

Exposure to radiation at excessive doses can damage living tissue. Note however that the radiation exposure for a chest X-ray is equivalent to the amount of radiation exposure one experiences over a 10-day period from natural surroundings alone.

devices generate 2D and pseudo-3D images of the breast by acquiring multiple 2D slice images at different angles as the X-ray source moves in an arc around the breast.

- Image attributes: variations in the grayscale of the image represent the X-ray attenuation or density of tissues; with calcifications appearing as white or bright areas in the image.
- Advantages: fast and easy to perform; equipment is relatively inexpensive and widely available; low amounts of radiation; high spatial resolution capability. Tomosynthesis has the advantage of improved visibility of superimposed structures as a pseudo-3D image and has been shown to assist in the detection of early breast cancers and decrease the call-back rate for additional tests.
- Disadvantages: traditional 2D mammography suffers from superposition of overlapping structures; uses ionizing radiation; image file sizes are large for mammograms and for breast digital tomosynthesis, and both require specialty display workstations.

KEY CONCEPT: Special Requirements for Mammography

Mammography has been among the last modalities to transition to digital acquisition, storage, and display. This may be due to a number of its special requirements including high spatial resolution (to enable visibility of fine spiculations and microcalcifications), high contrast resolution (to increase conspicuity among subtle differences in soft tissue, and the ability to visualize dense and overlapping tissues). Radiation dose must be kept low to be effective as a screening examination. Traditional mammography also has special display requirements that must accommodate very high spatial resolution (5 MegaPixel), ease of simultaneous display of the basic four-view examination (bilateral craniocaudal (CC) and mediolateral oblique (MLO) views) in addition to the ability to view prior historical examinations alongside the current study. The ability to apply masking and traditional markups is also required. Mammography detectors whether CR or DR have higher spatial resolution capabilities (50 to 100 micron pixel sizes) than for other projection radiography studies (200 micron pixel size), are sampled at roughly twice the frequency, and therefore generate much larger digital files (approximately 40 MB or more per image). Typical breast tomosynthesis examinations can range from approximately 450 MB to 3 GB, and require specialty acquisition and display devices. Computer-aided detection (CAD) algorithms are typically used with digital mammography and require either an additional stand-alone or integrated CAD system. Mammography is highly regulated and specific laws of the Mammography Quality Standards Act (MQSA) must be met with regard to acquisition and display workstation implementations [1].

3.2.3 Fluorography

- Source: continuous low-power X-ray beam; ionizing radiation.
- Detector: X-ray image intensifier amplifies the output image.
- Image attributes: continuous acquisition of a sequence of X-ray images over time results in a real-time **X-ray video**; may use inverted grayscale (white for air; black for bones).

SYNONYMS: Fluoroscopy
• Fluorography • Fluoro • Cine • Radiofluoroscopy • RF

- Advantages: can image anatomic motion and provide real-time image feedback during procedures. Useful for monitoring and carrying out studies of the gastro-intestinal tract, arteriography, and interventional procedures such as positioning catheters.
- Disadvantages: lower image quality than static projection radiographs; typically only a subset of key images are archived.

3.2.4 Computed Tomography (CT)

- Source: collimated high-power X-ray beam; X-ray tube and detector array rotate around the patient.
- Detector: early sensors were scintillation detectors with photomultiplier tubes excited by sodium iodide (NaI) crystals; modern detectors are solid-state scintillators coupled to photodiodes or are filled with low-pressure xenon gas. Data is collected and stored in a "sinogram" matrix from which tomographic slices are reconstructed using a "filtered back-projection" or "adaptive statistical iterative reconstruction" (ASIR) algorithm [1].
- Image attributes: thin transverse cross-sectional sections of the body are acquired representing the absorption pattern or X-ray attenuation of each tissue. Absorption values are expressed as **Hounsfield Units**, also called CT numbers, with water as the zero frame-of-reference. To highlight certain tissues, CT images are dynamically viewed with different Window (window width) and Level (window level) presets. Window width reflects the range of grayscales displayed with all pixels below the range appearing black and those pixels above the range appearing white in the image. Window reflects image contrast. Window level defines the center value of the width and reflects the perceived brightness in the image. Increasing the window width results in an image with perceived decrease in contrast (e.g., bone window/level ~2000/300, lung window/level ~1500/−700). Decreasing the window width results in an image with perceived increased contrast (e.g., abdominal window/level ~400/40, brain window/level ~80/35, liver window/level 200/50) [1].

KEY CONCEPT: Window and Level

Cross-sectional imaging modalities produce 12-bit data (4096 potential values) or more for each pixel. The human eye can only distinguish between 700–900 different shades of gray, and most display monitors are capable of producing only 8-bit grayscale (256 grays). Thus, when viewing images, the radiologist will focus on a portion of the data that falls within a defined range (the window). Any pixel with a value below the window will be displayed as black, and any pixel with a value higher than the window will be displayed as white. Pixels with values within the window will have different shades of gray. You could define the window by its upper and lower values, but it is more commonly defined by its center point (level) and extent (width). Adjusting the window on the fly is a routine part of image interpretation.

- Advantages: good contrast resolution allowing differentiation of tissues with similar physical densities; tomographic acquisition eliminates the superposition of images of overlapping structures; advanced scanners can produce images that can be viewed in multiple planes (multiplanar reformats) or as volumes due to the ability to acquire isotropic voxels using current multidetector row technology scanners. Any region of the body can be scanned; has become diagnostic modality of choice for a large number of disease entities; useful for tumor staging.
- Disadvantages: high cost of equipment and procedure; high dose of ionizing radiation per examination; artifacts from high contrast objects in the body such as bone or metallic devices; can generate large study file sizes for examinations such as CT angiography, cardiac CT, and perfusion studies (e.g., for stroke) [1].

DEFINITION: Hounsfield Unit

CT number representing absorption values of tissues; expressed on a scale of −1000 units for the least absorbent (air) to the maximum X-ray beam absorption of bone (+3000 for dense bone). Water is used as a reference material for determining CT numbers and is, by definition, equal to 0. Set ranges of CT numbers can designate tissue type, and differences in tissue Hounsfield units can indicate abnormal findings and/or pathology.

3.2.5 Magnetic Resonance Imaging (MRI) [1]

- Source: **high-intensity magnetic field** (1.5–3 Tesla and some 7T); typically, helium-cooled superconducting magnets are used today; nonionizing; gradient coils turn radiofrequency (RF) pulses on/off at different time sequences based on the desired image contrast and anatomical presentation; example **pulse sequences** include spin echo, fast spin echo, inversion recovery, STIR, FLAIR, gradient echo, etc. Manipulable acquisition parameters include TR (repetition time), TE (echo time), TI (inversion time), flip angle, and slice thickness.
- Detector: phased array receiver coils capable of acquiring multiple channels of data in parallel.

- Image attributes: produces images of the body by utilizing the magnetic properties of protons in tissues, predominately hydrogen (H^+) in water and fat molecules; the response of magnetized tissue when perturbed by an RF pulse varies between tissues and is different for pathological tissue as compared to normal. T1, T2, proton density, blood flow, perfusion, and diffusion are some of the tissue characteristics exploited by MRI to manipulate tissue contrast.
- Advantages: **nonionizing radiation**, originally called nuclear magnetic resonance (NMR) but because the word "nuclear" was associated with ionizing radiation, the name was changed to emphasize the modality's safety; can image in any plane; has excellent soft tissue contrast detail; visualizes blood vessels without contrast; no bony artifact since no signal from bone; particularly useful in neurological, cardiovascular, musculoskeletal, and oncological imaging.
- Disadvantages: high purchase and operating costs; lengthy scan time; more difficult for some patients to tolerate; susceptible to motion artifact; poor images of lung fields and bone; inability to show calcification; contraindicated in some patients with **pacemakers, hearing aids or metallic foreign bodies**; safety issues must be adhered to for hospital personnel working in the vicinity of MRI scanners.

KEY CONCEPT: MRI Procedure

The patient is subjected to a magnetic field, which forces the H^+ nuclei in tissues to align with the magnetic field. An excitation pulse of radiofrequency is applied to the nuclei, which perturbs them from their position (through energy absorption). When the pulse is removed, the nuclei return to their original state releasing energy (re-emission), which can be measured and converted to a grayscale image. Multiple pulse sequences are typically used in combinations specific to the diagnostic requirements.

3.2.6 Nuclear Medicine and Positron Emission Tomography (PET)

- Source: X-ray or γ-ray emitting radioisotopes are injected, inhaled, or ingested; most common isotopes are technetium-99, thallium-201, and iodine-131.
- Detector: gamma camera with NaI scintillation crystal measures the radioactive decay of the active agent; emitted light is read by photomultiplier tubes; pulse arithmetic circuitry measures number and height of pulses. Further, these pulses are converted to an electrical signal that is subsequently processed into a grayscale image.
- Image attributes: metabolic, chemical, or physiological interactions of the radioisotope are measured. The radioisotope chemical is distributed according to physiological function so the image primarily represents **functional information**; however, since function is distributed in the physical structures, recognizable anatomical images are produced, though at a lower quality.

- Advantages: measures targeted specific chemical-physiologic tissue function; valuable diagnostic tool particularly for imaging infarcts in the cardiovascular system, imaging uptake at sites of increased bone turnover as in arthritis and tumors, assessing the aggressiveness of small tissue nodules, and in oncologic assessment.
- Disadvantages: high cost of some radioisotopes; ionizing radiation; long scan times; patients must wait for the radiotracer to distribute before being imaged.

DEFINITION: SPECT

Single-Photon Emission Computed Tomography; a tomographic slice is reconstructed from photons emitted by the radioisotope in a nuclear medicine study.

DEFINITION: PET

Positron Emission Tomography uses cyclotron-produced positron-emitting isotopes including oxygen, carbon, nitrogen, and fluorine, enabling accurate studies of blood flow and metabolism (as with fluorine-19 fluoro-deoxyglucose (FDG)). Positron isotopes are short-lived positively charged antimatter electrons. The main clinical applications are in the brain, heart, and tumors.

3.2.7 Ultrasound

- Source: high-frequency sound waves produced by a transducer made of a piezo-electric crystal.
- Detector: the source **transducer** also functions as a receiver of reflected sound and converts the signal into an electric current, which is subsequently processed into a grayscale image.
- Image attributes: sound waves travel through the body, are affected by the different types of tissues encountered and reflected back; a real-time moving image is obtained as the transducer is passed across the body.
- Advantages: very low cost; safe nonionizing energy source; can scan in any plane; equipment is portable and can be used for bedside imaging; particularly useful for monitoring pregnancy, imaging the neonatal brain, visualizing the uterus, ovaries, liver, gallbladder, pancreas, and kidneys, confirming pleural effusions and masses, and assessing the thyroid, testes, and soft-tissue lesions; increasing use as the first imaging modality for triage at the point-of-care.
- Disadvantages: **operator-dependent**; poor visualization of structures underlying bone or air; scattering of sound through fat yields poor images in obese patients. Not all PACS (picture archiving and communication system) display stations are capable of displaying ultrasound video clips thus requiring specialty ultrasound "mini-PACS."

> **KEY CONCEPT: Doppler Ultrasound**
>
> A technique to examine moving objects in the body. Blood flow velocities can be measured using the principle of a shift in reflected sound frequency produced by the moving objects. Can be used to image the cardiac chambers and valves of the heart, arterial flow, particularly to assess the carotids and peripheral vascular disease, and venous flow studies for the detection of deep-vein thrombosis.

3.2.8 Visible Light

- Source: visible light spectrum; electromagnetic radiation wavelengths between approximately 380 (violet) to approximately 750 (red) nanometers.
- Detector: charge-coupled devices (CCD) and video cameras. Mobile phones may have adequate image quality but have security issues.
- Image Attributes: wavelength dictates the "color" while intensity, propagation direction, contrast, and polarization contribute to the perceived appearance.
- Advantages: uses a noninvasive energy source; visible light imaging is used in light microscopy for pathological diagnosis, hematology, dermatology to photograph skin lesions, gastroenterology (colonoscopy/endoscopy), ophthalmology to image the retina, and during surgical procedures.
- Disadvantages: has limited ability to penetrate tissues deeply like the energies used in radiological imaging.

3.3 Digital Images

3.3.1 Definition

- A continuous image $f(x,y)$ is a 2-D light intensity function f at spatial coordinates x,y; the value f at location x,y is proportional to the brightness or grayscale of the image at that point.
- A digital image is an image $d(x,y)$ that has been **discretized** (digitized) both in space (physical location) and in amplitude (gray level); it can be considered as a matrix whose row and column indices identify a point x_1, y_1 in the image, and the corresponding matrix element value $d(x_1, y_1)$

> **KEY CONCEPT: Pixels and Voxels**
>
> A pixel is the smallest discrete element in a digital image and it has a single color value. A voxel is a three-dimensional picture element in a 3-D image and represents a volumetric sample of the body.

identifies the gray level at that point. Elements in the digital array are called **pixels** (short for "picture elements") and each is represented by a numerical value. Three-dimensional images consist of **voxels** ("volume elements").
- The **matrix size** is the product of the number of pixels in each dimension.

3.3.2 Digital Image Formation

- To be suitable for computer processing, an image function must be digitized both spatially and in amplitude. Image sampling is the digitization of the spatial coordinates and is related to pixel size, reflective of matrix size and affects spatial resolution.
- Image gray level quantization is digitization of the amplitude or brightness, is determined by computer bit depth, and is reflected in the image contrast resolution.
- The process of digital image production includes scanning of the analog image line-by-line to obtain a continuous analog signal representing the variations in image brightness, followed by dividing the analog signal into individual pixels in a process known as spatial sampling, which is typically performed in equal intervals; this is followed by converting the amplitude into a digitized numerical pixel value in the process of contrast quantization; lastly, an analog-to-digital (ADC) converter turns the quantized level into binary code (Fig. 3.1).

3.3.3 Image Quality Factors

- **Spatial resolution** limits sharpness (edges separating objects in the image) or visibility of fine detail and is a function of sampling that affects matrix and pixel size. Since each pixel can have only one numerical value, it is not possible to observe any anatomical detail within a pixel. More frequent sampling that results in smaller pixels (larger matrix sizes) provides better visibility of fine detail and a better quality higher spatial resolution image. If images are insufficiently sampled, the poorer resolution images may have a characteristic blockiness or checkerboard artifact.
- **Contrast resolution** limits differentiation of detail within and between objects and is a function of the bit depth used to represent the grayscale quantization. Insufficient quantization can result in false contouring or ridges in which smoothly varying regions of an object within the image become undifferentiable.
- **The total resolution of a digital image is the combination of the spatial resolution and the contrast resolution.** An image file size is equal to the product of the matrix size (number of rows times number of columns) times the number of

> **KEY CONCEPT: Spatial Resolution vs. Contrast Resolution**
>
> Spatial resolution of an image limits visibility of fine detail and is reflected in matrix and pixel size. High spatial resolution enables visibility of small objects. Conventional X-rays and mammography have excellent spatial resolution. Contrast resolution limits the ability to distinguish between differences in object intensities in an image and is represented by the number of different colors or grays in the image. High contrast resolution enables differentiation of tissues with similar imaging characteristics. CT and MRI exhibit high contrast resolution.

8-bit bytes required to represent the image bit depth. For example, a CT slice is typically 512 rows by 512 columns and the grayscale is represented by 16 bits. It requires 2 bytes to account for 16 bits of grayscale, and therefore, a CT slice file size is $512 \times 512 \times 2 = 524{,}288$ bytes or approximately half a megabyte (MB). A single-view chest radiograph is approximately 10 MB.

- **Noise** is a characteristic of all medical images; increased noise can lower image quality; noise is sometimes referred to as image mottle and gives the image a textured, snowy, or grainy appearance that can degrade visibility of small or low contrast objects. The source and amount of image noise depend on the imaging method; nuclear medicine images generally have the most noise, followed by MRI, CT, and ultrasound; radiography produces images with the least amount of noise.

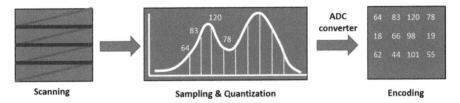

Fig. 3.1 The digital image formation process including scanning, sampling and quantization, and analog-to-digital conversion

KEY CONCEPT: Intrinsic Image Quality

A trade-off between spatial resolution and contrast or density resolution; an image with intrinsically poor spatial resolution can be made visually sharper by enhancing the contrast.

PEARLS

- Medical images have special features that make them difficult to create, acquire, manipulate, manage, and interpret. Complexities include human variability, performance requirements, safety considerations, motion artifacts, technical limitations, and cost.
- Diagnostic imaging modalities are categorized by their sources (ionizing or nonionizing radiation), acquisition mode (projection or cross-section), and tissue property measured (anatomic structure or molecular function).
- Medical imaging hierarchy includes patient, examination (study), series (sequence), image, and pixel.
- Digital images are discretized (digitized) by sampling in space (location) and quantizing in contrast (grayscale).
- Spatial resolution limits sharpness or visibility of fine detail and edges in the image; it is a function of sampling that affects matrix and pixel size.
- Contrast resolution limits the number of different colors or grayscales represented in the image and is a function of quantization bit depth.

Reference

1. Seibert JA. Modalities and Data Acquisition. Ch 4 in Practical Imaging Informatics First Edition, BF Branstetter, IV Editor, Springer, 2009.

Suggested Reading

ACR-AAPM-SIIM-SPR Practice Parameter for Digital Radiography (2017 Revision). Available at: https://www.acr.org/-/media/ACR/Files/Practice-Parameters/Rad-Digital.pdf. Accessed January 4, 2021.
ACR-AAPM-SIIM Practice Parameter for Determinants of Image Quality in Digital Mammography (2017 Revision). Available at: https://www.acr.org/-/media/ACR/Files/Practice-Parameters/Dig-Mamo.pdf. Accessed January 4, 2021.
Brown BH, Smallwood RH, Barber DC, Lawford PV, Hose DR. Medical physics and biomedical engineering. London: Institute of Physics Publishing; 1999.
Gonzalez RC, Woods RE. Digital image processing. Reading: Addison-Wesley Publishing Co.; 1993.
Rosenfeld A, Kak AC. Digital picture processing. San Diego: Academic Press, Inc.; 1982.
Webb A. Introduction to biomedical imaging. Hoboken: John Wiley & Sons, Inc.; 2003.

Self-Assessment Questions

1. Which of the following is the most significant source of artifact in medical images?

   (a) Human variability
   (b) Patient positioning
   (c) X-ray dose
   (d) Subject motion
   (e) Safety considerations

2. Which of the following imaging modalities use ionizing radiation as its source?

   (a) Magnetic resonance imaging
   (b) Computed tomography
   (c) Ultrasound imaging
   (d) All of the above
   (e) None of the above

3. Which of the following modality is most affected by the skill of the operator?

   (a) Projection radiography
   (b) Ultrasound
   (c) Computed tomography
   (d) Magnetic resonance imaging
   (e) Positron emission tomography

4. In the formation of a digital image, sampling affects which of the following?

   (a) Visible fine detail
   (b) Image matrix size
   (c) Spatial resolution
   (d) All of the above
   (e) None of the above

5. Which imaging modality provides higher spatial resolution?

   (a) Chest projection radiograph
   (b) Chest CT

Chapter 4
Image Post-Processing

Jeremy Collins and Bradley Erickson

Contents

4.1 Introduction

Nearly all images produced in a medical imaging department are processed to some extent. The ultimate goal of image post processing is to produce visually pleasing images and to increase conspicuity of findings. Processing is often performed to make digital images look more like their hard copy film predecessors, to accentuate

J. Collins · B. Erickson (✉)
Mayo Clinic, Rochester, MN, USA
e-mail: Collins.jeremy@mayo.edu; bje@mayo.com

© The Author(s), under exclusive license to Springer Science+Business Media, LLC, part of Springer Nature 2021
B. F. Branstetter IV (ed.), *Practical Imaging Informatics*,
https://doi.org/10.1007/978-1-0716-1756-4_4

certain features in the imaging data (e.g., bone and soft tissue kernels in CT), or to provide higher resolution (e.g., interpolation for MRA). However, post-processing can also be used to improve the performance of computer-assisted detection (CAD) algorithms and to produce visual representations of specific anatomic features of the imaging data that are more useful. This chapter will begin with very basic image processing functions and proceed to more advanced techniques that are increasingly being applied as a part of routine CT and MR post-processing pipelines.

4.2 Image Filtering

4.2.1 Histogram Manipulation

- Standard **window/level manipulation** may be considered manipulation of the histogram of an image. Reducing the window width stretches contrast, while wider windows compress contrast. These values are typically described as follows: (window width/window level). The level is positioned in the center of the histogram window with values extending beyond the window assigned to the maximum or minimum brightness. Standard window/level settings for CT include head (100/40), lung (1500,−750), soft tissue (400/40), and bone (2500/300). Figure 4.1 shows examples of window level applied

DEFINITION: Histogram

A graph that reflects how many pixels of each brightness are on the image. The horizontal axis is brightness, and the vertical axis is number of pixels.

DEFINITION: Hanging Protocol

By default, a PACS will display images in the order that they were produced on the scanner, using default windows from the scanner. But this may not be the most convenient way to interpret the images. A hanging protocol is a reproducible way of organizing images when they are displayed on the PACS. Hanging protocols are based on DICOM tags.

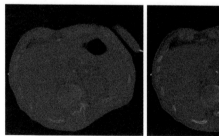 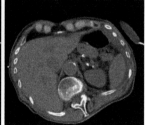

Full Window   Bone Window   Soft Tissue Window

Fig. 4.1 Window/level operations

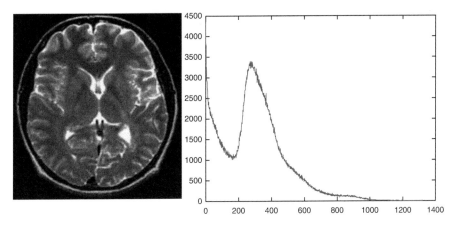

Fig. 4.2 An MRI image and its histogram. Note that the intensities for air have been excluded because they would have dominated the histogram, hiding the data of the brain itself

to the CT images of the abdomen. Although the histogram image filter can be manipulated in real-time on PACS workstations, such standard image filters are first applied in hanging protocols.

- Histograms may also be **matched** between images to produce similar contrast between images from different studies. This technique is useful for visual comparison across patients in MR exams (Fig. 4.2).

4.2.2 Enhancement

Many enhancement methods exist. Two commonly used in medical imaging are:

- **Unsharp mask filters** may be applied to images to bring out **features of details**. Unsharp masking is a standard enhancement filter that selectively subtracts a blurred image from the original. Pixels in the blurred image that differ from the original by an amount more than a user specified

> **KEY CONCEPT: Enhancement**
>
> When radiologists say "enhancement," they are usually talking about an intravenous injection of material that makes vascular tissues more visible. But it the context of image post-processing, enhancement refers to any method that makes particular elements in the image more conspicuous.

threshold are *considered* to be "masked." Any pixel under the mask is subtracted from the original, otherwise the pixel is unmodified.

- **Edge sharpening filters** selectively enhance edges in the image. These filters are demonstrated in Fig. 4.3.

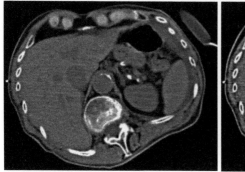
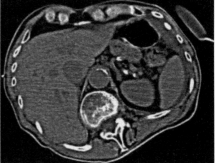

Unsharp masking   Edge sharpening

Fig. 4.3 Image enhancement filters

4.2.3 Frequency Filtering

Images may be decomposed into a collection of frequencies by the **Fourier transform**. Multiplication in the Fourier domain is equivalent to convolution in the image domain. Thus, all Fourier domain filters have equivalent convolution-based filters in the image domains. When convolution-based filters become too big, they are more efficiently implemented in the Fourier domain. Although difficult to understand and interpret, the Fourier transform is very useful for image processing and analysis. Examples are shown in Fig. 4.4.

4.2.4 Noise Reduction

Noise is present in all medical images. We can reduce the amount of noise by increasing radiation dose for imaging dependent on X-ray energy. On MRI, noise is reduced by increasing the MR field strength, number of imaging coils, or imaging time. Reducing spatial resolution improves noise in CT

DEFINITION: Convolution

The multiplication of a neighborhood of pixels by a "kernel." Each value in the kernel is the number by which the corresponding neighborhood pixel is multiplied. If all the values in the kernel are "1," the result is the mean.

DEFINITION: Fourier Transform

A Fourier transform converts an image from a familiar Cartesian matrix (the usual X-Y-Z coordinate space) to the frequency domain, where the image is represented by the summation of numerous sinusoidal patterns. Fourier space is hard to conceptualize.

DEFINITION: Noise

Random fluctuations in the image information that can obscure the true elements in the image. Noise reduction is synonymous with improving the signal-to-noise ratio (SNR) or contrast-to-noise ratio (CNR).

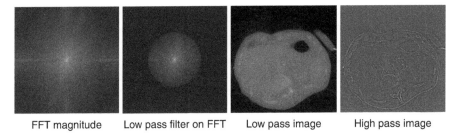

FFT magnitude   Low pass filter on FFT   Low pass image   High pass image

Fig. 4.4 Frequency domain spectra and filtering. FFT = Fast Fournier Transform

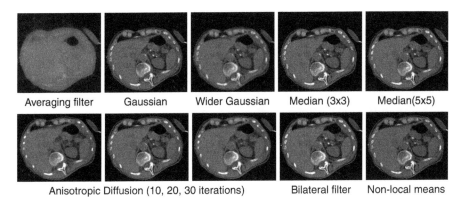

Averaging filter   Gaussian   Wider Gaussian   Median (3x3)   Median(5x5)

Anisotropic Diffusion (10, 20, 30 iterations)   Bilateral filter   Non-local means

Fig. 4.5 Filtering and de-noising algorithms

and MRI but reduces image sharpness. Image processing also offers ways to reduce noise, but these methods may introduce artifacts. Several common filters for noise reduction are described below and demonstrated in Fig. 4.5.

- The simplest filter for noise reduction is **averaging**, sometimes called **block filtering**. Each pixel is replaced by the average of its neighbors. The filter considers neighboring pixels with a user-specified radius. A radius of 1 is a 3×3 block of pixels, centered at the output pixel. Averaging may unfortunately smooth out edges or fine detail as it removes high-frequency noise elements.

> **DEFINITION: Filter**
>
> A processing method that enhances or removes a specific component in a signal or image. The name could reflect what is removed, what is enhanced, or the calculation that is used.

- Slightly more complex is the **Gaussian filter**. The Gaussian filter averages the pixels, but the contribution of neighborhood pixels is weighted by their distance from the output pixel (pixels further away are weighted less, and the weight is the Gaussian function value). Hence, Gaussian filtering blurs the image. An equivalent result is achieved with low pass filtering using a Gaussian filter in the Fourier domain. Gaussian filters are classified by their sigma, or width.

- **Median filtering** considers a patch of neighborhood pixels. The intensities in the patch are sorted, and the median value is chosen in the output. Median filters are simple and efficient noise reduction filters with good performance. They exhibit less blurring than averaging and Gaussian filters.
- **Anisotropic diffusion filtering** smooths the image while preserving strong edges. This filter iteratively solves the solution to a partial differential equation modeling heat flow. The smoothing caused by the "heat" does not flow across regions of large image changes or gradients. This filter has several parameters controlling the rate of heat flow and the amount of smoothing to apply.
- **Bilateral filtering** is similar to the Gaussian filter. Both spatial distance and intensity distance are specified when setting weights for a pixel in the neighborhood. Near an edge, neighborhood pixels will have a large difference ("intensity distance") from the output pixel and have a smaller weight. Bilateral filtering produces results similar to anisotropic diffusion without the need for iteration. Hence, bilateral filtering is more efficient than anisotropic diffusion filtering and is a better choice.
- The recently proposed **non-local means filter** examines a "patch" centered about each pixel. The output pixel is a weighted average of center pixels from patches in a user-specified search region. Patches of similar contrast and intensity are more heavily weighted. Through this approach, regions of the image with similar patches will wash out noise when averaged. Both the patch size and search region influence the output quality and processing time.

4.2.5 Practical Considerations

- Though sometimes used for display, filtering is often used as a preprocessing step for segmentation, classification, and computer-aided diagnosis. Many algorithms do not consider effects of noise and therefore produce better results on preprocessed images.
- Filters may be applied to each image independently, or may be applied in a 3D mode, incorporating pixel information from neighboring images. 3D filtering may cause unwanted artifacts when applied to thicker images. In general, 3D filters are much slower to apply than single slice filtering.
- Simple filters such as averaging, Gaussian, and median are generally implemented as kernel operations sliding over each pixel in the image. On modern workstations, these filters operate in near real-time. Better noise reduction can be obtained with more complex filters such as the anisotropic, bilateral, and nonlocal means filters, but at the expense of computation time. Consequently, complex filters are often performed through batch processing and stored in PACS as secondary capture series.

4.3 Segmentation

Segmentation is an essential step if one wishes to perform automated measurements on organs or diseases (Fig. 4.6).

DEFINITION: Segmentation

The separation of an image into meaningful components. In most medical applications, this refers to an anatomic structure (e.g., blood vessels, bone, lung) or a disease process (e.g., a tumor).

4.3.1 Basics

- A basic segmentation algorithm is **global thresholding**. A pixel is considered foreground if its intensity is equal to or higher than the threshold value and background if lower than the threshold value. Bones in CT images are easily segmented with thresholding, though contrast material and calcifications may sometimes be erroneously included in the foreground.
- The Otsu algorithm automatically determines a threshold such that the foreground and background have low variation in intensity and are as widely separated as possible. The Otsu algorithm can reliably segment tissue from air on CT images, and can also be useful for MRI images where the intensity scale is not consistent.
- To segment individual objects, a set of "seed pixels" are selected. Each neighboring pixel is classified as foreground or background based on some criteria, usually intensity value. The neighbors of the neighbors are checked, and the process of **"region growing"** continues until no new neighbors meet the inclusion criteria. Region growing is used to interactively segment organs.

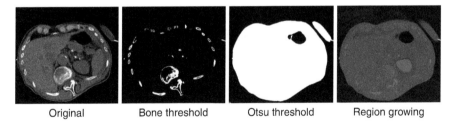

Original   Bone threshold   Otsu threshold   Region growing

Fig. 4.6 Segmentation examples

4.3.2 Morphological Operators

- **Morphological image filtering** is a technique for processing of geometrical structures as applied to images. While morphological operators may be applied to grayscale images, they are most often applied to binary images (black and white).
- The **structuring element** probes the image with a shape, deciding how the shape fits or misses the shapes in the image. "Square" and "jack" are common shapes for structuring elements. Specialized structuring elements (such as tubular shapes for vessels) may be constructed for image post-processing. Examples of the square and Jack structuring elements are shown in Fig. 4.7.
- Two common morphologic operations are **erosion** and **dilation**. Erosion can be thought of as moving the structuring element around the inside of the segmented region. Border pixels are "eroded" away from the border to where the structuring element completely fits within the object. Dilation is best thought of as moving the structuring element around the outside of the segmented object, making the object bigger (dilating) by adding the center voxel of the structuring element anytime it touches a voxel in the segmented region. The effects of dilation and erosion on an object depend heavily on the structuring element chosen as is seen in Fig. 4.7.
- Frequently, segmentations generated using thresholding contain "**holes**," regions or voxels outside the intensity range that are not included in the object. Holes may be filled using a combination of erosion and dilation, a morphologic operation called **closing**. Dilation is applied first, followed by erosion. Closing has the effect of filling small holes in the segmentation while smoothing the border region. "**Opening**" applies erosion followed by dilation. Opening enlarges holes in the segmentation while smoothing the border region.

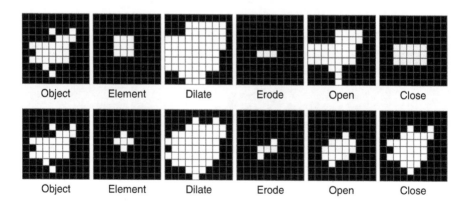

| Object | Element | Dilate | Erode | Open | Close |

| Object | Element | Dilate | Erode | Open | Close |

Fig. 4.7 Morphological operations with square (top row) and jack (bottom row) elements

4.3.3 Classification

- In contrast to segmentation, classification algorithms assign a
voxel to one or more "classes" of
tissue. Segmentation can be
thought of as classification of
image data into two classes:

> **DEFINITION: Classification**
>
> The assignment of a meaningful name like "lung" to a group of pixels or voxels.

object (foreground) and excluded imaging data (background). **Semantic
Segmentation** is a term used when one simultaneously performs segmentation
and then assigns a label or class to the segmented object.
- **Multispectral classification** utilizes data from two or more images of the same
anatomy to assign class labels to voxels. A common example is using T1- and
T2-weighted MRI scans to distinguish white matter and gray matter. Such
schemes can be augmented with **prior probabilities**. Prior information is often
spatial, indicating the frequency at which a voxel is white matter or gray matter.
This information is compiled from a population into an **atlas**. For example, a
well-known atlas of neuroanatomy is available in the Statistical Parametric
Mapping (SPM) package (http://www.fil.ion.ucl.ac.uk/spm/).

4.4 Registration

- Registration may be intra-subject
(within the same patient), inter-
subject (across different patients),
intra-modality (using images
from one imaging modality), or
inter-modality (using images from
multiple modalities). Algorithms
for registration are loosely classified by **transforms** allowed, **similarity metric**, and **minimization**.
To register two images, a minimization algorithm tries different

> **DEFINITION: Registration**
>
> The process of aligning images with one another. This means that the same anatomic tissue exists at a given X, Y, Z location on all registered images.
>
> **DEFINITION: Transform**
>
> A mapping from the space of one image to the space of another image.

transformations and evaluates each of these transformations using a similarity
metric. The minimization process tries to find the global minimum of the similarity metric; the transformation at that minimum should bring the two images into
alignment. This process is graphically shown in Fig. 4.8. The moving image is
transformed by rigid transformation onto a fixed image. The metric used is a
squared difference metric. Difference images are useful ways to evaluate the success of registration for images of the same modality and signal weighting.

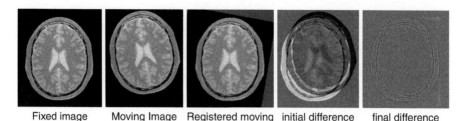

| Fixed image | Moving Image | Registered moving | initial difference | final difference |

Fig. 4.8 Registration example. (Images courtesy of Insight Software Guide)

4.4.1 Transforms

- Transforms have one or more parameters. The number of parameters for a transform is referred to as the dimension of the transform. For example, for a simple rigid 2D transform there is one rotation parameter and one or two translation parameters. Simple transformations generally have fewer parameters while more complex or deformable transformations have many parameters.

- **Rigid-body transforms** allow rotation and translation, but not scale or deformation. In 3D, there are three rotations and three translation parameters comprising a six-dimensional space. Rigid-body transformations are used in neuroimaging. Patients are often imaged in different positions and rigid-body transforms are used to align images acquired at different times to aid radiologic interpretation.

> **KEY CONCEPT: Rigid Transforms**
>
> Rigid image registration is useful for images of structures that do not deform substantially (e.g., the brain) or images of structures that move with predictable motion (e.g., the heart when electrocardiographic gating is applied). Rigid transforms do not work well for structures that move without a consistent shape, like the small bowel.

- **Affine transforms** add scaling and shearing to rigid-body transforms and are useful for inter-subject registration. Often, registration using an affine transform is used as input to high-dimensional deformable transformation registration. Affine transforms are 12-dimensional transforms.

- **Deformable transformations** are often called high-dimensional transforms and allow many possible deformations of one image into another. Deformable transforms are applied inter-subject (mapping subjects to one another), and intrasubject in regions of high motility, for example, abdomen, lungs, or after surgery that changes the shape of anatomic features. For each continuous point in one image, a deformation may be calculated and applied to move the point onto the corresponding point in the second image. Deformable transformations are commonly classified by the type of **kernel** or **basis** used (e.g., B-spline, thin-platespline, cosine).

4.4.2 Similarity Metrics

- Similarity metrics quantitatively score the "goodness-of-fit" of two images related by a transformation. The score produced by a similarity metric indicates how well the images are aligned with a lower score indicating a better

> **DEFINITION: Similarity Metrics**
>
> Quantitative measures of how well two images are matched. They are an essential element of image registration.

agreement between the two images. A similarity metric with an analytic gradient allows optimizers (discussed in the next section) to rapidly find a global minimum. Metrics without analytic gradients may also be used in optimizers but the gradients must be found numerically.
- One of the most basic similarity metrics is **mean squared differences**. The goodness of fit in the mean squared differences metric is measured by the summation of the squared differences between the two images. This metric requires the images to be from the same patient in the same modality. The mean squared difference similarity metric is computationally challenging because each voxel in the image is used in the calculation.
- The **normalized correlation** similarity metric is independent of contrast differences in the two images and may be used cross modality. Normalized correlation is also computationally demanding.
- Statistical based similarity metrics do not require each voxel in the image to be used in the computation but rather take a statistical sampling of the voxel set in the image. Most statistical metrics are based on image entropy. Entropy is the measure of information content in a signal, the joint entropy between two images is used as a similarity metric. This is known as **mutual information** and is the most common statistical similarity metric.

4.4.3 Optimization

- Optimization is a very active area of research in the medical imaging community. Optimization is also a very difficult problem, and solutions that work in one imaging domain may not work in others. An optimization algorithm tries to find a global solution to an energy function. The similarity metrics and the parameters to the transformation are what the optimization algorithm is modifying in an attempt to find a global solution.
- A simple optimization algorithm is **gradient descent**. The gradient descent algorithm begins with a certain set of transformation parameters and uses the analytic gradient of the similarity metric on the transformation parameters to follow the gradient down to the global minimum. Gradient descent is susceptible to local minima where a less than optimal solution is found.

- If analytic gradients cannot be computed for the similarity metric, a **line search algorithm** such as the Powell optimizer is useful. Each parameter of the transform is optimized in turn in a greedy fashion. In a greedy algorithm, one parameter is changed, until a local minimum is found, then the next parameter is changed until all have been optimized in turn.
- For high dimensional transformations, **statistical optimization algorithms** are effective at finding global minima. A statistical optimization algorithm attempts to find a local gradient at a given transformation by probing in random directions in the parameter search space. The Evolutionary Powell method is an example of a statistical optimization algorithm that can be applied to 2D or 3D data.

HYPOTHETICAL SCENARIO: Image Post-processing

Describe a sequence of steps for improving the quality of MIP renderings of MRA data for intracranial vessels.
Possible answer:

1. Apply a noise reduction filter like a non-local means filter
2. Compute the histogram, and find the peak representing brain. Do this by finding the biggest peak which is above air (air intensity is found by sampling image corners)
3. Segment the image into vessels by setting a threshold above brain intensity. Have this image be binary—'1' or '0'.
4. Multiply this "mask" with the original image so that non vessels have 0 intensity, while vessels have original MRA intensity.
5. Render the MRA.

4.5 3D Visualization

Modern medical modalities such as CT and MRI generate large amounts of 3D volumetric data in the form of 2D slices. Post-processing techniques, including volume rendering, allow this data to be displayed in a variety of useful ways.

DEFINITION: Volume Rendering

A visualization technique to display a 2D image of a 3D data set that retains access to the original voxel data. Commonly referred to as a "3D reconstruction."

- **Projection rendering** is the simplest and fastest volume rendering method, and maximum intensity projection (**MIP**) is a commonly used example. Though commonly used, MIPs do not provide depth information and may obscure important structures. MIPs of vascular anatomy created from CTA and MRA generate post-processed images that have a similar appearance to digital subtraction (x-ray) angiography. As such this projection rendering technique is easily understood by referring physicians.

- Another option is to extract the surface of interesting object(s) and then render accordingly. Shading methods are used with this technique, generating a shaded surface display (**SSD**) rendering. Different shading models may be used, changing the appearance of the rendered surface. By taking advantage of widely available rendering hardware (Graphical Processing Units) surface rendering can be performed very efficiently. One shortcoming of SSD rendering is that internal features of the objects are obscured. In addition, surface rendering requires **segmentation** (see previous section). Historically anatomic segmentation was a manual, labor-intensive process. Machine learning and deep learning-based methods facilitating anatomic segmentation are increasingly available, enabling automatic anatomic visualization using the SSD rendering method.
- **Direct volume rendering** produces images of 3D volume data sets directly from the 3D volume data without extracting any geometrical information about the objects captured. When rendering a data set, optical properties (color and opacity) are accumulated along each viewing ray. The optical properties are specified by using transfer functions that are applied to the volume data.
- **Cinematic rendering** is a novel post-processing technique for 3D visualization of complex anatomy from CT imaging data. This method generates life-like anatomic images with shading and texturing. This technique generates images which are photo-realistic and mimic dissections in the anatomy lab or the surgeon's view of anatomy in the operating room.

4.5.1 Volume Data and Its Grid Structure

In medical imaging, 3D volume data is usually in a rectangular format grid, consisting of multiple "slices," where each slice often has a dimension of 1024×1024, 512×512, or 256×256. While each 2D image slice is generally isotropic (in 2D coordinate system), the whole 3D volume data is generally anisotropic (in 3D coordinate system). Resampling the data to produce **isotropic voxels**

DEFINITION: Isotropic

Having the same size in each dimension.

DEFINITION: Voxel

A portmanteau of the words volumetric and pixel, used to represent the individual elements of a 3D volume data set.

before volume rendering is optional, but maybe useful. Conversely, 3D imaging data is often reconstructed into (thicker) overlapping 2D slices to improve volume rendered image quality by reducing noise; 40–50% slice overlap is commonly applied.

4.5.2 Projection Rendering

Multi-planar Reconstruction (MPR)

- MPR is the reconstruction of images in orientations other than how the images were acquired (typically axial). The new orientations are most commonly coronal or sagittal, but sometimes more arbitrary orientations such as oblique or even curved planar orientations. This method allows real-time review of imaging data in any plane and is commonly used when reviewing volumetric data of sufficiently high spatial resolution. Consequently, this method is commonly applied to CT or MR angiographic data.
- A common application is creating **coronal and sagittal** reformatted images from axial datasets. MPR can sometimes provide better demonstration and additional diagnostic information, particularly in the evaluation of complex anatomical structures or areas that are traditionally difficult to evaluate on axial images. The spatial resolution and noise metrics are important considerations when generating MPR images. To generate pleasing MPR data, the original 3D dataset should be isotropic or reconstructed with overlapping slices to eliminate gaps in the data.
- State-of-the-art PACS systems now have built-in MPR capability, enabling users to generate these other viewing planes without them being generated at the modality console and sent to PACS as secondary DICOM series.

Maximum Intensity Projection (MIP)

- MIP is the projection of voxels with **highest intensity** onto an arbitrarily oriented plane. MIP is commonly used in angiography to extract **vascular structures** from CT or MRI data sets.

Minimum Intensity Projection (MinIP)

- In contrast to MIP, MinIP is the projection of voxels with **lowest intensity** onto an arbitrary plane. At each voxel along a viewing ray the lowest data value encountered is recorded.
- MinIP is often used for rendering low density structures such as the **lungs and airways**.

> **KEY CONCEPT: MIP and MinIP**
>
> The lack of depth information is a limitation of the MIP and MinIP techniques. As a result, objects lying in the same projection plane of high or low intensity structures are partially or completely obscured. Both MIP and MinIP can be regarded as simplified volume ray casting algorithms, and thus a form of direct volume rendering.

4.5.3 Surface Rendering

- Surface-rendering, also known as shaded surface display (SSD), produces images that look like pictures of three-dimensional **solid objects**.
- Surface rendering refers to a class of techniques that use surface primitives (or patches) such as polygons (typically triangles) to fit the isosurface inside a vol-

ume data, and then use shading models to render the surface. Surface rendering treats the object inside a volume as having a uniform value.

- Before the isosurface is fitted, segmentation algorithms may be optionally used to extract the structure or mask of the interested object. By doing segmentation, unwanted overlying structures can be eliminated, and the fitting process can also be simplified.
- After the isosurface is fitted, we calculate the normal at each patch's vertex by interpolating the gradient at voxels. Normals are then used in the shading process. Three most commonly used shading models are: Constant, Gouraud, and Phong.
- **Marching Cubes** is a famous algorithm for building polygonal (triangular) patches of an isosurface from a 3D volume. The algorithm assumes that, with the specified value, there is a continuous isosurface inside the volume.
- Shading models are used to describe how light interacts with objects and reflects to our eyes. Shading models include models of illumination. The **Phong illumination model** is the most widely used illumination model. All shading models, such as Constant and Gouraud, are based on the Phong illumination model.

> **FURTHER READING: Marching Cubes**
>
> Marching Cubes on Wikipedia: http://en.wikipedia.org/wiki/Marching_cubes.
> Open source implementation using VTK: http://www.vtk.org

4.5.4 Direct Volume Rendering

- There are two classes of direct volume rendering techniques: image order (or image based) techniques and object order (or object based) techniques.
  - **Image order techniques** use rays casting from some point (e.g., human eye) through each pixel in the resulting image to the 3D volume data, resampling points along the ray from the volume data, and compositing the contribution of each resampling point in each ray as the resulting pixel.
  - **Object order techniques** compute the projection and contribution of each voxel in 3D volume data set to the pixels in the image plane.
- A typical **pipeline** of direct volume rendering includes the following operations: *segmentation, gradient computation, resampling, classification, shading, and compositing.* Different algorithms and implementations may have more or less operations, as well as differing sequences.

> **DEFINITION: Pipeline**
>
> A sequence of stages that performs a task in several steps, like an assembly line in a factory. Each stage takes inputs and produces outputs which are stored in its output buffer. One stage's output is the next stage's input.

- The **gradient** is the normal of the local surface near a resampling point used to calculate diffuse reflection and specular reflection of light.
- There are several ways to approximate the gradient in a discrete 3D volume. **Central difference** and **intermediate difference** are most commonly employed approaches.
- Central difference approach is commonly applied because it also smooths noise, generating visually pleasing images. However, intermediate differences are more accurate and therefore preserve more imaging detail.
- As imaginary rays pass through the block of voxels, samples will be taken along each ray for accumulation. Because these sample points are seldom located exactly in the voxel locations, estimation is needed to get the desired sample according to the voxels surrounding it. This process is called **resampling** or **interpolation**. Resampling is computationally intensive—if too much resampling is needed, it can greatly decrease the performance of the rendering algorithms.
- The **classification stage** in the volume rendering pipeline allows you to see inside of an object in a volume without explicitly defining the shape and boundary of that object. This is one of the main advantages of direct volume rendering over surface volume rendering. A special property, called **opacity** (or alpha), is assigned to each voxel in the volume.
- In the shading stage, a first step called **coloring** is executed. Coloring is the process of assigning colors to voxels. This is realized by a function called color transfer function. The

> **DEFINITION: Opacity**
>
> A measure for how transparent a voxel is, ranging from 0 (completely transparent) to 1 (completely opaque).

  second step in the shading stage is to apply a **shading model** to the colors. Since most medical modalities only generate gray-level image data sets, shading is very useful in enhancing the realism of the image.
- **Compositing** is the process of accumulating multiple RGBA (short for RGB and alpha) value pairs calculated along a specific ray to one single RGBA value pair representing a pixel in the resulting image. After a composition is done for all possible rays, the final image is formed.
- Two popular configurations of the volume rendering pipeline exist, pre-shaded and post-shaded configurations.
  - In the **pre-shaded configuration**, classification and shading are done for all voxels initially, and then interpolations are implemented for the resulting RGBA values down to the sample points on a ray
  - In the **post-shaded configuration**, interpolations are executed first for gradient and intensity values down to the sample points on the ray, and then classification and shading are performed on the sample points.
- Based on the two configurations, three important volume rendering methods exist: volume ray casting, splatting, and Shear-Warp. It is important to note that each of these methods has many variations when implemented.

– **Volume ray casting** is a class of image order volume rendering techniques that can provide results of very high quality at the price of long runtime. It computes 2D images from a 3D volumetric data set by casting an imaginary ray from some point (human's eye, for example) to the volume. Volume ray casting, which processes volume data, must not be confused with the traditional concept of ray casting found in computer graphics, which processes surface data only.

– **Splatting** is a class of algorithms that computes the contribution of a voxel to the image by convolving the voxel with a reconstruction kernel that distributes the voxel's value to a neighborhood of the

> **FURTHER READING: Splatting**
>
> Westover L. Interactive volume rendering, Chapel Hill Workshop on Volume Visualization, Chapel Hill, NC; 1989. p. 9–16.

pixel. The distribution area and data are called the footprint of the voxel. Because there is no resampling or interpolation process, the splatting algorithm is faster than the ray casting algorithm, but it generally suffers from lower rendering quality.

– The **Shear-Warp algorithm** absorbs the advantages of both image-order algorithms and object-order algorithms and is considered to be the fastest of the three methods. The core idea of the Shear-Warp algorithm is the introduction of an

> **FURTHER READING: Shear-Warp**
>
> Lacroute P, Levoy M. Fast volume rendering using a shear-warp factorization of the viewing transformation. Proc. SIGGRAPH '94, Orlando, FL, July, 1994; p. 451–8.

intermediate object space, called sheared object space. Volume data is first resampled and transformed to this space, where simple ray casting method is then applied.

4.5.5 Cinematic Rendering

Interest in cinematic rendering for imaging visualization came from the success of computer graphical animation methods in the entertainment industry. Cinematic rendering expands on direct volume rendering to generate photo-realistic images of 3D imaging CT data in real-time (Fig. 4.9).

- This recently introduced, novel vendor-specific method implemented currently for CT data extends other volumetric rendering methods by applying texture and realistic shadowing to patient anatomy.
- This technique is best applied to high density and high contrast structures (e.g., contrast-enhanced vessels or bones).

Fig. 4.9 Cinematic rendering of the abdomen. The lighting model produces images that look life-like. These depend on having some recognition of what structures likely are and applying color models commonly used ("learned") for that structure, such as bones being light beige, heart, arteries and kidneys being red, and veins being blue

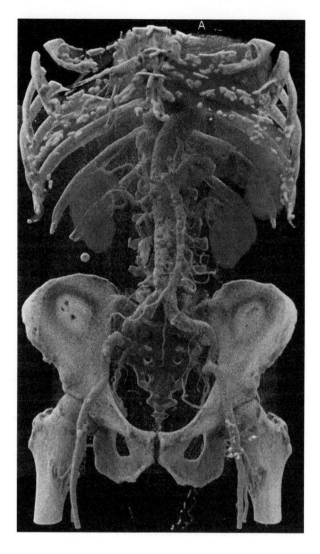

- Cinematic rendering is useful to show the relationship between multiple different anatomic structures at once, such as vascular anatomy, bony anatomy, and the solid abdominal organs or the relationships of mediastinal structures in congenital heart disease. Hollow lower density structures such as subcutaneous/mesenteric fat, bowel, or airways are not well depicted with this method.
- Cinematic rendering uses computational algorithms with random sampling and different light mapping techniques to create a more visually realistic volume rendered output from CT data and could be applied to MR data in the future.

- Cinematic rendering integrates the more complex high dynamic range rendered light paths (reflection, scattering, light extinction) to include all light scattered along possible directions of a ray. Monte Carlo simulations are used to generate a subset of randomized light paths with an acceptable distribution to reduce computation time to enable real-time rendering during image manipulation. Structure transparency in cinematic rendering is handled similarly to other volumetric rendered methods and is based on a transfer function. This transfer function assigns a unique color and opacity to each attenuation value.

FURTHER READING: Cinematic Rendering

Dappa E, Higashigaito K, Fornaro J, Leshka S, Wileermuth S, Alkadhi. Cinematic rendering – an alternative to volume rendering for 3D computed tomography imaging. Insights Imaging. 2016;7(6):849–56.

Elshafei M, Binder J, Baecker J, Brunner M, Uder M, Weber GF, Grutzmann R, Krautz C. Comparison of cinematic rendering and computed tomography for speed and comprehension of surgical anatomy. JAMA Surg. 2019;154(8):738–44.

4.6 Post-processing and Billing

Despite significant advancements in post-processing technology post-processing of imaging data commonly requires dedicated time and effort by technologists, radiologists, or other imaging specialists. The separate billing process for such efforts are intended to offset the hardware, software, and personnel costs of providing these services, beyond interpreting the imaging alone. The CPT codes specify software and hardware configurations for billing.

KEY CONCEPT: 3D Post-processing CPT Codes

There are two 3D current procedural terminology (CPT) codes: 76376 and 76377. The distinction is determined by the location where the post-processing occurs. 76376 includes post-processing performed on the imaging modality console. 76377 includes post-processing performed on a dedicated, independent workstation. Angiographic CT and MR CPT codes are inclusive of any post-processing as part of the "technical" charge. The dedicated 3D post-processing CPT codes cannot be billed with angiographic codes; such angiographic codes are often termed "bundled" codes.

PEARLS

- Image filtering reduces noise in images, while preserving edge information. Image filtering may be used as a preprocessing step or in real time during image review.
- Segmentation is the process of identifying regions of interest within an image and is often used for quantification of size and shape of structures.
- Registration algorithms are composed of transformations, similarity metrics, and optimization of algorithms. Registration is useful for comparing studies through time and is easily applied in rigid structures such as the brain, but is more difficult to apply to body imaging.
- Volume rendering is a visualization technique to display a 2D image of a full 3D dataset.
- MIP and MinIP are the simplest and fastest volume rendering methods.
- Direct volume rendering can give users details of the objects inside a volume, whereas surface rendering shows only the exterior of objects.
- Cinematic rendering is a new technique that generates life-like, photo realistic 3D anatomic images.

Suggested Readings

Bankmann I. Handbook of medical imaging. San Diego, Academic Press; 2000.
Barthold L, et al. Introduction to volume rendering. Hoboken, Prentice Hall; 1998.
Insight Software Guide, http://www.itk.org/ItkSoftwareGuide.pdf.
Vis5D homepage: http://www.ssec.wisc.edu/~billh/vis5d.html.

Self-Assessment Questions

1. Which of the following de-noising algorithm does not use a convolution kernel?

    (a) Averaging filter
    (b) **Non-local means**
    (c) Gaussian filter
    (d) Median filter

2. Morphological filtering is commonly used for?

    (a) Registration
    (b) De-noising
    (c) **"Cleaning up" segmentation**
    (d) Image display

3. Which of the following filters is the simplest to compute?

   (a) **Averaging**
   (b) Non-Local means
   (c) Gaussian
   (d) Anisotropic diffusion

4. In a registration algorithm, the metric is used to:

   (a) Filter the images
   (b) Find the global minimum
   (c) Segment the images
   (d) **Determine how well the images are aligned**

5. Which registration transform is most suitable for intra-examination brain registration?

   (a) Thin plate spline
   (b) Affine transformation
   (c) **Rigid body transformation**
   (d) Deformable registration

6. Which of the following is *not* a direct volume rendering technique?

   (a) MIP
   (b) **Marching Cubes**
   (c) Volume ray casting
   (d) Splatting
   (e) Shear-Warp

7. To render more than one object in a volume simultaneously, which of the following volume rendering techniques will lead to the best rendering quality?

   (a) MIP
   (b) **Cinematic rendering**
   (c) Volume ray casting
   (d) Splatting
   (e) Shear-Warp

8. Describe situations in which MIP is preferable to MinIP.

9. Describe situations in which MinIP is preferable to MIP.

Chapter 5
Incorporating Nonimage Data

Matthew Hayes

Contents

5.1 Introduction

There are several types of DICOM objects that can be inserted into an examination in addition to the diagnostic images themselves. These objects may contain information regarding the study or patient that may assist the interpreting physician by adding supporting information. Thus, we must have a method for capturing data that may not represent an image directly but is associated with and informs key details about a study.

5.2 Sources of Non-Image Objects

5.2.1 Scanned Documents

Scanned documents are paper sheets that are run through a scanner, digitized, converted to DICOM, then sent as an image to a PACS repository. From there, they can be retrieved and displayed within the PACS application. Historically, paper

M. Hayes (✉)
PACS, Radiology Partners, Orland Park, IL, USA

B. F. Branstetter IV (ed.), *Practical Imaging Informatics*,
https://doi.org/10.1007/978-1-0716-1756-4_5

documents were often scanned and saved as PDF (Portable Document Format) files, but these could not be displayed on PACS workstations.

- **Patient Documents** consist of process paperwork generated as a part of the visit workflow for an imaging procedure. Examples of patient documents include privacy disclosures and consent forms. For some examinations, patients may be asked to document where they are feeling pain or discomfort either on a diagram or in words. This information may be useful to the technologist and/or the interpreting radiologist.
- **Exam Documents** are directly related to the exam itself. Examples include protocoling forms, tech worksheets, and physician orders. These forms directly reflect characteristics of the performed procedure. Also, in terms of protocols and orders, they may direct what type of exam is performed.
  - A practice may deploy procedure-specific paper note templates to be filled out by the acquiring technologist. Technologist written notes about the procedure may contain qualitative observations as well as quantitative measurements of certain anatomy or pathologies. The results of these documents will inform and guide the interpreter's diagnostic findings.

5.2.2 External Sources

- External processing sources and applications are not a part of the main PACS, such as
  - Other software applications based within the home institution
  - Output from other institutions
  - External cloud-hosted programs that have linkages back to the home system
- Image post-processing (see **Chap. 4**) yields additional images for diagnostic purposes. Some of these functions are embedded in the PACS display software, while some require separate systems which may or may not be integrated (stand-alone) with the PACS. Examples include
  - 3D volume rendering
  - Multi-planar reformatted images
  - Variable intensity projections
  - Quantitative measurement methods

DEFINITION: RECIST

The Response Evaluation Criteria in Solid Tumors is an imaging-based system for determining whether a cancer treatment has been successful. Based on changes in size of tumor, the patient is classified as having stable disease, complete response, partial response, or progression.

There are automated post-processing systems that can assist with this analysis.

- Measurements may be exported and processed within structured reporting applications or speech recognition report generation systems that automatically embed them within the final report.

FURTHER READING: RECIST

https://www.ncbi.nlm.nih.gov/pmc/articles/PMC5737828/.

- Machine learning and artificial intelligence applications have generated another novel vector for the post-processing of imaging datasets (see **Chap. 14**).
- The output of external software may take the form of
  - Annotations highlighting findings on an existing image
  - Additional image sets derived from the original input data
  - A narrative textual report
  - Quantitative metrics
- Any of these data can be placed in the PACS, where they are most conveniently viewed during image interpretation.

HYPOTHETICAL SCENARIO: Examples of External Software

- Response Evaluation Criteria in Solid Tumors (RECIST)—The logging and tracking of cancerous lesions based on imaging sets for a unique patient. The AI software independently identifies lesions on an imaging set. Each lesion identified by the application is assigned a unique identifier. As the application is used over time and applied to additional studies, the unique identifier can be then collated with the lesion measurements projected over a chronological progression providing an interpreter an indication lesion response of treatment over time. This data helps to tell if a particular treatment is working.
- Vendor hosted patient screening tools—A vendor may host a processing engine either on or off premises, separate from the PACS. The PACS routes image data and measurement files to the system for processing. Within the vendor's application, the images are processed based on specific criteria. The analytic output can then be compared against clinical indications, trial criteria, or pathological thresholds by the software. If the criteria are met and accepted, feedback can be given back to a practice for additional follow-up with the patient. The feedback can be delivered through secure web portals, email alerts or further integration with the clinic's applications. Some use cases for this method include cardiac screenings and prosthetic device fittings. These screening tools can be used where there is no available in-house expertise for a given clinical application.
- Vendor hosted imaging analytic tools—Similar to the above use case, the system analyzes source data and produces a set of new secondary annotated images. The system then routes the new data back to the source PACS as an additional image series within the original exam. Electronic alerts are delivered back to an interpreter, alerting them to newly available diagnostic data. Additionally, the application may produce quantitative imaging measurement overlays, indices measurements, and send back data. Result formats include DICOM Measurement SR, textual report, or annotated image.

5.2.3 Modalities

The third common source of non-imaging data comes from the imaging modalities themselves. Commonly, these objects have the benefit of classification and structure according to DICOM.

- DICOM Structured Reporting (SR) objects come codified with the DICOM modality code SR.
- Instead of containing pixel data, the contents can be either textual or numerical data.
- DICOM SR structure and content are outlined by different templates types, depending on the specific medical subspecialty in which the images are acquired.
- Two common examples of DICOM SR use cases are modality dose reporting and ultrasound measurements.
- Dose reporting centers around the effort to estimate the amount of radiation a patient is exposed to. The long-term effort is to improve patient safety by determining methods and opportunities to lower the cumulative dose administered to patients. This keeps alignment with the ALARA principle: As Low As Reasonably Achievable. By deploying a collection of DICOM Dose SR reports, a system can perform statistics around specific patients and devices. Collective comparison can be performed, and individual modality dose performance can be compared to its peer devices. An

> **FURTHER READING: DICOM SR Templates**
>
> http://dicom.nema.org/medical/dicom/current/output/html/part16.html.

> **KEY CONCEPT: Dose Reporting**
>
> Total lifetime radiation dose is a well-recognized measure of potential harm done by medical imaging. Automated modality dose reporting ensures that the radiation dose for every exam is logged in the patient's medical record. There are PACS add-ons that can continuously tally a patient's total lifetime dose, drawing attention to patients who may be at risk.

> **FURTHER READING: DICOM Dose SR**
>
> https://www.dicomstandard.org/using/radiation.

> **FURTHER READING: ALARA**
>
> Centers for Disease Control and Prevention Radiation safety guidelines https://www.cdc.gov/nceh/radiation/alara.html.

identified modality may be delivering higher radiation for a certain procedure compared to other devices. That machine may be further investigated for deviations and fixed to lower the amount of radiation given to patients. Modality protocols in the case of CT can also be evaluated for dose optimization.

HYPOTHETICAL SCENARIO: Echocardiography

Ultrasound machines in cardiology contain libraries of specific named measurements. The libraries are crafted around the American Society of Echocardiography reporting guidelines. As a cardiac sonographer performs an exam, they choose from a picklist the specific label and tag their measurements. The ultrasound machine stores those values until the exam acquisition is complete. Then the measurements are compiled into a DICOM SR format and transmitted with the images at the end of the acquisition. Many cardiac-based PACS have SR parsing processes that read the SR objects and automatically insert the tagged numbers into the final diagnostic report.

- Since the objects are standardized, originating and receiving applications should have a DICOM Conformance statement that outlines how the SR objects are ingested and processed. Additional support documents of the consuming application should explain the sequence by which results are processed with respect to a workflow. Such documents are necessary due to the nature of textual data versus clinical specialty labeled measurements and may not be covered in a DICOM conformance statement.

5.3 Data and Workflow Considerations

As with any imaging information data set, an assessment of the end-user workflow should be performed before deploying any solution (see **Chap. 25**). The end goal of these nonimage objects should be to enhance the interpreter's knowledge about a particular set of images with the least impact on their productivity or disruption to workflow.

KEY CONCEPT: DICOM Wrapper

Many PACS can only consume and display data if it arrives in DICOM format, with all the appropriate DICOM headers. There are software applications that add DICOM headers to data that is not natively in DICOM format. The data can then be interpreted by the PACS and included in patients' imaging studies. This makes the data readily accessible to the physician interpreting the study.

A DICOM wrapper can often be applied by the scanner computer software.

5.3.1 Paper Scanned Documents

- Paper is typically white or light-colored with black text imprinted on it. When scanned directly and viewed on a diagnostic monitor with DICOM conformant luminance levels, the distinct contrast of the paper at high luminance can disrupt a viewer's ocular photosensitivity. Set the scanning application to invert scans to produce **black background with white text**.
- Be sure to thoroughly understand how every scanning device operates. There may be variability in paper orientation and which side of the physical paper the scanner first processes between different makes and models of scanners.
- Standardize scanner configurations by make and model and keep them digitally accessible. Having ready access to the configuration files will reduce the likelihood of a newly installed or repaired device deviating from expected behavior. Reduced deviations equal reduced workflow impact.

5.3.2 DICOM SR

- Application vendors should disclose which SR templates they can process. It is the job of the processing application to understand multiple vendor formats and implementation methods.
- Implementation of DICOM SR can vary from manufacturer to manufacturer. Verify documentation and test the modality's functionality before putting it into patient use.
- Design image routing carefully. Begin by understanding the capabilities and functions of both the source system and the receiving system. Certain implementations may require high volumes of traffic in and out of a PACS as the SR's get processed. These additional transactions may impact the overall processing burden of a PACS.

5.3.3 AI applications

- Artificial Intelligence applications often require images to work. A key consideration for feeding information into an AI system should be architecture. The combination of hardware and software that hosts the applications needs to be robust enough to handle the imaging requests while accommodating the resource needs of the production PACS.
- The use of AI applications will increase the processing burden of a PACS. The additional routing of images in and out of the system requires a proportional increase of processing threads to accommodate the traffic. During implementa-

tion, the maximum processing capacities of both the source image repository and the AI system need to be defined and tested. Violations of those limits may have negative impact on PACS functionality, negatively impacting usability and potentially causing an increase in result turnaround times.

- Common information interchange formats have not been formalized. Every vendor may have different system requirements as well as feedback mechanisms to the end user. If multiple applications are being used, consider options to consolidate communications paths as possible. The potential additive effect of each application notification mechanism may be overwhelming and distracting to an interpreting physician. These distractions affect efficient workflows. Notification should blend in and enhance workflow, not distract or detract.

5.3.4 Shared Considerations

1. Check conformance statements and test functionality before deploying any solution into a patient care setting. By utilizing DICOM conformance statements for all applications involved, specific handling exceptions can be identified early. Assess the impact of the exceptions against anticipated workflows to determine if adjustments are required.
2. Maintain continuity of DICOM study unique identifiers (SUID)
    - Turn off application-assigned SUIDs. Choose a single "source of truth" to assign unique study instance identifiers. This may come from a system such as a RIS. This eliminates the chance any post-processed or scanned data will register as an additional new study in a PACS or DICOM Archive.
    - If available, consider turning on PACS post-processing workflow so that the system can accept data in any study state before "Final."
3. High numerical series number
    - When incorporating nonimage data, apply series numbers that allow for a clear delineation from diagnostic images in the study.
    - Series numbers for raw data are usually enumerated directly (1,2,3…). Using numbers above 1000 will ensure that there is no overlap with the raw data.
    - If done properly, scanned paperwork and SR objects will appear in PACS lists in a consistent manner.
4. Use consistent, informative DICOM series descriptions. Note these are typically input at the scanner but can be unified across devices.
    - Clear descriptions enhance hanging protocols.
    - Clear labels can be used for filtering during database mining operations.
5. Monitor exception queues for objects that fail to merge back into the source exam.

PEARLS

- It is much more efficient for the interpreting physician if all the relevant non-imaging data is within the PACS. If the physician must go to another data system, that is wasted time.
- Paper tokens and physical objects can be digitized and added to the PACS, where they are less likely to be lost or mismanaged.
- DICOM Structured Reporting Objects often flow with a study's images; IIPs should understand the end points
- Identify the end consumer, then design workflows to their needs.
- With any DICOM implementation, two vendors may not perform the same execution. *Test* before you use!
- White text on a black background will coexist with radiologic images better than traditional black-on-white text.

Self-Assessment Questions

1. Which of these is considered a nonimage object?

   (a) CT Reconstruction
   (b) CT Reformat
   (c) Volumetric Rendering
   (d) AI interpretation

2. How can you make scanned paper document more readable in a PACS environment?

   (a) Use white-on-black text
   (b) Use very large font
   (c) Disallow all compressed file types
   (d) Apply optical character recognition to all documents

3. Where does a DICOM wrapper live?

   (a) In the PACS
   (b) On the modality
   (c) On the scanner computer
   (d) Outside the firewall

4. When applying a series number to digitized nonimage data, use

   (a) The smallest number that is not already in use in the study
   (b) A large number that will not conflict with series numbers from raw data
   (c) A random number generator
   (d) Your birthday

5. Identify paper objects in your own department that could be digitized and incorporated into a PACS.

6. Consider the security requirements needed for incorporation of output from a cloud-based third-party post-processing application.

Part II
Information Technology

Chapter 6
Computers and Networking

Adam E. Flanders

Contents

A. E. Flanders (✉)
Thomas Jefferson University, Philadelphia, PA, USA
e-mail: Adam.Flanders@jefferson.edu

© The Author(s), under exclusive license to Springer Science+Business Media,
LLC, part of Springer Nature 2021
B. F. Branstetter IV (ed.), *Practical Imaging Informatics*,
https://doi.org/10.1007/978-1-0716-1756-4_6

6.1 Introduction

The core infrastructure of any modern radiology department is made up of computers and the connectivity or *networking* capability between these devices. All transactions between modalities, PACS, scheduling, billing, dictation, and reporting systems are made possible through specialized computer programs or *applications* that are executed by computers. Computer systems are quite diverse and are often designed to augment a specific task, whether it is to support image reconstruction for a modality such as computed tomography (CT) or digital radiography (DR) or rapid image display as in PACS workstations. Fundamentally, all computers are built around a similar base design with enhancements in specific areas to address certain needs such as rapid storage access and data transfer for file servers or improved video characteristics for PACS client display stations. The purpose of this chapter is to familiarize the reader with the fundamentals of computer architecture, networking, and computer applications.

6.2 Computers 101: Hardware

6.2.1 Hardware Elements of Computers

- There are five **core hardware components** of the modern digital computer system: the central processing unit (CPU), memory, input devices, output devices, and a bus. These are all part of a **physical machine** or a single computer.
- While some components are given greater emphasis for a particular computer design (e.g., a faster CPU for computationally intensive tasks), virtually all types of computers have these five key components represented. Most of the hardware components in the modern digital computer are contained within small modular semiconductor packages (**integrated circuits [ICs] or chips**) that, in turn, contain millions of discrete components.

> **KEY CONCEPT: Software vs. Hardware**
>
> The fundamental distinction between software and hardware is that hardware exists as the tangible physical components and connections inside of a computer. Software is a set of instructions that are performed on the hardware.

> **KEY CONCEPT: Core Computer Hardware Components**
>
> - CPU (central processing unit)
> - Memory
> - Input devices
> - Output devices
> - Bus

- Numerous ICs are interconnected on a large circuit board, frequently referred to as the **motherboard**. The motherboard is interfaced with other outside components (e.g., disk drives, power supply, keyboard, network, etc.) using specialized couplers providing necessary power and connectivity to **peripheral devices** such as disk drives (storage), video displays, and keyboards.

- The **central processing unit (CPU)** or **microprocessor** is typically the largest integrated circuit on the motherboard, and its role is to execute specific commands or instructions/machine code dictated by a computer program and to orchestrate the movement of data and instructions through the entire computer system.
- Although the CPU is frequently personified as the "brain" of the computer, it has no innate "intelligence" or inherent ability to make decisions. The CPU's strength is in its ability to process instructions and manipulate data at amazing speeds. In this regard it is the perfect soldier; it follows all commands presented to it with blazing efficiency.
- The number of instructions that a CPU can perform per second is expressed as its **clock speed**. Typical personal computer CPUs can perform over three billion instructions per second or three gigahertz (3 GHz). Modern CPUs actually contain 2–12 CPUs or **cores** in 1 IC (**multicore CPU**). This provides unparalleled computational speed as each core shares the processing tasks formerly assigned to one CPU.
- While the strength of the CPU is in its ability to process instructions, it has limited capability to store data before or after execution. The CPU relies on **physical memory** to store this information and provide it to the CPU on demand.

6.2.2 GPUs/TPUs

- A graphics processing unit (GPU) is a specially designed microprocessor that handles graphics and display operations that are sent to the video display with the capability for high volume and low precision computing.
- Early computers did not require GPUs because the demand for graphics operations and calculation was small and could be shared by the CPU.
- Today's high-resolution 3D graphics require off-loading the computational burden for graphical display on these specialized microprocessors that are integrated into a separate graphics card specifically designed to manage all graphics operations.
- A side benefit of GPU architecture is that they are intrinsically very powerful; they may contain hundreds of internal computing cores that are capable of extremely efficient number crunching. This made them a very inexpensive means to achieve supercomputing power and handle the demands inherent to the growing field of **machine learning**.
- A tensor processing unit (TPU) is a specially designed integrated circuit for processing related to neural networks and machine learning. It is a proprietary technology developed by Google Inc for their TensorFlow AI software platform.

6.2.3 Memory Types

- **Memory** is a computer component that is principally used to
temporarily store data (and
results) and applications or programs. In contrast to the CPU, a
memory module has no capability
to process instructions; instead

  > **SYNONYMS:**
  > - Software
  > - Application
  > - Program
  > - Process

  memory is designed to reliably store large chunks of data and then release this
  data on command (often at the behest of the CPU).
- Physical memory can exist in **solid-state** form as an integrated circuit or as **physical media** (spinning magnetic disk or hard disk drive [HDD], compact disc
[CD], digital versatile disk [DVD], or solid-state drive [SSD]).
- **Nonvolatile memory** will retain data written to it until it is erased or overwritten.
Examples include USB memory sticks and disk drives [HDD and SSD]. Since
the inherent speed of nonvolatile memory is substantially slower than that of
volatile memory, volatile RAM is typically employed on the motherboard to augment data processing.
- A solid-state memory module that can be erased and rewritten an unlimited number of times is generically referred to as **random-access memory or RAM**.
- **Read-only memory (ROM)** is memory that has pre-stored instructions/data that
is nonvolatile (persists without power applied). EPROM or erasable programmable read-only memory is a type of ROM that can be erased and reused. This is
often how patches/updates are applied to hardware devices.
- Memory that can only retain data with power applied to it is referred to as **volatile memory** – most RAM motherboard memory modules are of this type. These
are rated by their **storage capacity** (given in mega- or gigabytes), **access speed**
(in nanoseconds), **data rate** (DDR2), and **configuration** (single in-line memory
module or dual in-line memory module SIMM or DIMM).
- Some forms of memory are designed for specific tasks. **Video memory (VRAM)**
is employed on video graphics cards to store graphical information to improve
video display performance. A specialized form of high-performance memory is
found on most CPUs to help efficiently buffer data that moves in and out of the
microprocessor core (**L2 cache memory**).

6.2.4 Storage

- There are additional forms of
computer memory that are classified simply as **storage**, principally
because they are characterized by
slower speed compared to solid-
state memory and nonvolatile

  > **CHECKLIST: Types of
  > Data Storage**
  > - Online
  > - Near-line
  > - Off-line

characteristics (data persists indefinitely until erased/overwritten). These are made up of spinning media (disk drives, CDs, and DVDs) and linear media (tape). Strategy for storage is a balance of cost versus demand for access; data that has a high probability for immediate future use (e.g., recent relevant prior imaging studies) should be kept in an online state.

- **Online storage** refers to high-performance, nonremovable media that requires no human or mechanical intervention to retrieve. Data on spinning hard disk arrays is an example of online storage. As storage costs have decreased, most data is kept in online storage.
- **Near-line storage** consists of removable media (e.g., tapes, CDs, or DVDs) that are made available through mechanical means such as a robotic tape or optical disk jukebox. The efficiency of data retrieval with a near-line system is dependent upon the mechanical speed of the robotic system and the queuing mechanism of the media.
- **Off-line storage** is removable media that requires human intervention to load and retrieve data. As a result, performance is lowest for off-line storage. While off-line storage is the least expensive storage strategy, it is otherwise quite inefficient and is therefore reserved for data that has a low probability for future use.

6.2.5 Input/Output

- **Input/output devices** are hardware extensions that allow humans (or other devices) to interact with a computer. Examples of input devices include the keyboard, touch screen, mouse, microphone, and camera. Typical output devices include the video display, printer, plotter, and speaker.

6.2.6 Data Bus

- The **data bus** is the physical data chain built into the motherboard that allows for efficient data transfer. This is supported by several integrated circuits, known as the **chipset**, which coordinates uninterrupted data transfers through the bus. The chipset performs an essential role as the typical microprocessor can execute several billions of commands per second; it is highly dependent upon an efficient mechanism for delivering instructions and data to it. This requires that there is a well-orchestrated method for moving data between motherboard components and the CPU. Multiple different designs have been developed; the most common in use today is PCI (peripheral component interconnect) and PCI Express. The data bus is defined by a **data width** (typically 32 or 64 bits), which specifies how much data is delivered across the bus per cycle and a **clock speed** (given in megahertz).

6.2.7 BIOS

- Another key component to the typical computer motherboard is the **BIOS (basic input/output system)**. The BIOS is comprised of a non-erasable ROM chip that contains the minimal amount of software necessary to instruct the computer how to access the keyboard, mouse, display, disk drives, and communications ports.

- When the power is first applied to the computer, the motherboard relies on the BIOS to tell it what additional components are available to the motherboard for input and output (e.g., disk drives, memory, keyboard, etc.) The motherboard "becomes aware" of what is available and how to access it, each and every time the computer is restarted.

> **KEY CONCEPT: Booting Up**
>
> The motherboard, CPU, and memory retain no previous information about how the computer is configured. Every time the computer turns on, it pulls itself up by its bootstraps ("booting up").

- The BIOS also provides information to the motherboard on where to find the first piece of software to load during the startup process. The startup process is also known as the **boot process**. The first piece of software to load is usually a portion of the **operating system** that will coordinate the other software programs.

6.2.8 Virtual Machine

- While all of the components are components of a single computer, the outdated notion of a one-for-one relationship between CPU, memory, and storage has evolved into an abstraction known as a **virtual machine**.

- A **virtual machine (VM)** is a software representation of hardware. It is an **image file** of a single computing environment that is all encapsulated in software yet performs exactly like a physical machine. Multiple virtual machines can co-exist and run on a single physical computing environment sharing resources. The user of these **guest** systems has the identical experience as that of using an independent physical device.

> **KEY CONCEPT: Virtual Machine vs. Physical Machine**
>
> Multiple virtual machines can be supported on a single piece of hardware allowing for economies of scale with decreased maintenance, backup, and recovery costs. Each virtual machine acts like a distinct computer, but several virtual machines can exist on a single piece of hardware.

- A VM environment offers tremendous economies of scale, allowing multiple operating systems to run simultaneously on a single physical device. VMs are easier to maintain, manage, back up, and restore and can be cloned at will. Most modern data centers use VMs to support vendor software solutions rather than installing physical devices for each company.

6.3 Computers 101: Software

- Hardware can be seen and handled. **Software**, on the other hand, is a virtual concept. While we can handle the media that software is written on, we cannot actually "see" the software.
- The term "software" applies both to **application programs** and **data**.
- Software at its lowest level (the level at which it interacts with the CPU) consists of a long series of **bits** or binary digit (ones and zeros). All data written to physical media, whether it is magnetic disk, USB stick, CD, DVD, or RAM, is stored as an orderly series of bits. A **byte** of data is eight sequential bits.
- Software is divided into operating **system software**; **application software**, programs which help users perform specific tasks; and **programming or development software**, programs that aid in the writing (i.e., coding) of other software.
- All software consists of individual procedures that command the computer to follow a precisely orchestrated series of instructions. The number of individual instructions specified in any one program varies depending upon the type

> **FURTHER READING: Core Computer Components**
>
> How Computers Work (10th Edition). White R, Downs TE. Que Publishing, Indianapolis, 2014.

  and complexity of the software – from ten to one hundred million lines of code. (The Windows X operating system, for example, contains approximately 50 million lines of code.) By comparison all of the code hosted by Google approximates two billion lines of code!
- All computer software must be moved into storage (i.e., disk drive) or physical memory (RAM) before it can be **executed** by the microprocessor. The instructions are passed through a series of software layers where they ultimately reach the microprocessor. Executing an instruction causes the computer to perform one or more operations.

6.3.1 Computer Operating System

- The **operating system (OS)** is the underlying software that integrates the hardware with software applications. It is distinguished from the essential hardware components in that it consists entirely of *software* – millions of lines of machine commands that are understood and obeyed by the microprocessor. The OS actually consists of hundreds or thousands of individual programs **(executables and libraries)** that are bundled together. Many of these individual programs are designed to work cooperatively with each other (libraries), whereas single executable files may be run on demand by the user of another **process** on the system.
- The OS is automatically executed each time the computer is started, and it is the *most* important software component running on any computer. A modern computer cannot operate without an operating system.

- Although the CPU is frequently personified as the "brain" of the computer, it is really the OS software and the CPU acting together that provides the underlying "intelligence" of system. The OS and the CPU are inexorably linked; therefore, the distinction between software and hardware is sometimes blurred.
- The OS is designed to automatically manage nearly every task (or **process**) including maintenance of the files on the disk, tracking input from peripheral devices like keyboards or network cards, displaying output on printers and video displays, and controlling **memory allocation**. Memory allocation is crucial to maintaining stability of the system because if two programs try to use the same area of memory, both programs will usually fail.
- Two of the most critical jobs of the OS are ensuring that programs do not unintentionally interfere with each other, adjudicating limited resources (e.g., memory), and maintaining security.
- A function paramount to the modern OS is the support of the **graphical user interface (GUI pronounced "gooey")**. A GUI replaces typed computer commands with a graphical representation of the task (e.g., moving a file). This is accomplished by creating a visual representation of the computer file system (the desktop), icons, and windows and linking them to the movements of a pointing device such as a mouse or trackball.
- The OS also provides a foundation or **software platform** for all other software (application programs). Therefore, the choice of operating system to a large extent determines which application software can be used on a particular system.
- There are several operating systems in use today. The most popular is the Windows OS (Microsoft, Redmond, Washington) which runs on the majority of computers worldwide, especially business computers. Other choices include UNIX, Linux, DOS, and the macOS (Macintosh).
- A **multiprocessing OS** supports use of more than one CPU. A **multitasking OS** allows more than one program to run simultaneously. A **multithreading OS** allows different parts of a program to run concurrently, and a **multiuser OS** allows two or more individuals to run programs concurrently on the same computer system.
- An OS includes hundreds of small programs called **drivers**. Drivers enable software to interact with the ubiquitous hardware devices attached to the motherboard and between components on the motherboard itself. In other instances, drivers allow one software component to safely interact and exchange data with another piece of software.

> **KEY CONCEPT: Drivers**
>
> Drivers are small programs that enable the operating system and application programs to interact with each other and with peripheral hardware devices. They require periodic upgrades, especially when the OS changes.

- From the user perspective, the OS provides the framework in which the application software runs. All application software runs **on top of** the OS; the OS, in turn, exchanges data/instructions directly with the hardware. In general, application software cannot interact directly with the hardware; it must be brokered through the OS. The OS essentially adjudicates allocation of resources to meet the demands of the user and applications. The modern OS is intentionally designed to sustain itself automatically with minimal user interaction. The software that is designed to perform real work for users is the application software.

6.3.2 Application Software

- OS software is designed to run autonomously with little interaction from the individual user. The OS monitors all internal functions of the computer, maintains stability of the hardware components, and regulates the processing of data in the microprocessor.
- **Application software** is a program designed to do *real work* for a user. Application software does not supplant the base OS software. Instead, application software runs *on top of* the OS such that an application is written (or coded) to work with a specific OS. The application is coded with OS-specific instructions to request specific actions such as opening a window, writing text, drawing objects, etc.
- Examples of application software include word processors, Internet browsers, PACS viewers, dictation systems, and spreadsheets.

6.3.3 Software Containers

- **Containers** are often compared to VMs as both allow multiple kinds/types of software to be run in a contained or isolated environment.
- While VMs are an abstraction of the hardware layer of a computer, a **container** is an abstraction of an application. One or more containers can share a single OS.

> **KEY CONCEPT: Virtual Machines vs. Containers**
>
> A virtual machine (VM) is an abstraction of the hardware layer of a computer, whereas a container is an abstraction of an application.

- **Containerizing** an application involves bundling the application, its configuration files, all needed libraries, and dependencies into an isolated self-sustaining file running inside of an OS.
- The application container allows specific inputs to go in and specific outputs to come out. This provides for a very secure and stable environment.
- Unlike a VM, a container does not include an entire OS to function, only the essential components (i.e., dependencies).
- Two of the most popular container systems are **Docker** and **Kubernetes**.

6.3.4 Programming Languages

6.3.4.1   Low-Level Programming Language

- **Low-level programming language** is the software language that is **directly** understood by a microprocessor and is termed **machine code or machine language**. Every CPU model has its own native machine code or **instruction set**. The instruction set consists of a limited number of relatively primitive tasks, like adding or subtracting data in specialized memory placeholders called registers or moving data from one register to the next.
- Despite their enormous processing speed, the intrinsic mathematical capabilities of a microprocessor are quite limited; a CPU cannot perform simple multiplication or division on its own – it has to be *taught how to do it.* By stringing a series of machine codes together, more complex processing (e.g., multiplication) is possible.
- Both machine code and its symbolic representation (**assembly language**) are considered low-level languages because they are the closest command analog to the actual functional details of the microprocessor. Low level does not imply diminished quality or efficiency; in fact, programs written directly in machine code or assembly language are very efficient.
- Although low-level programming instructions produce efficient programs, programming in machine code or assembler is difficult, tedious, and very time-consuming.

6.3.4.2   High-Level Programming Language

- **High-level programming language** is an abstraction of machine code programming because it uses natural language elements instead of arcane numbers and abbreviations. This makes the process of programming simpler, intuitive, and more understandable to the human programmer.
- High-level programming is the foundation of most software development projects. There are many high-level languages in common use today. Some of the popular languages currently include C, BASIC, Python, JavaScript, Java, Go, R, PHP, and Swift.
- Using high-level programming languages, programmers (or "coders") type out individual lines of the **source code** for an application, using a development software program.

6.3.4.3   Integrated Development Environment

- An **integrated development environment (IDE)** is a toolset that facilitates programming by providing a workspace that makes coding more efficient.

- The lines of the source code need to be translated into **machine code** before the program can be understood and tested on the microprocessor.
- This conversion process is known as **compiling** a program, and the software that converts the source code to machine code is known as a **compiler.**
- Most software development platforms include one or more compilers. The compiler turns the source code into an **executable** program which is customized for the specific OS/microprocessor combination for which the program was developed.
- The compiler saves the programmer a substantial amount of time and effort by constructing the sequence of machine codes that accurately represents each source code command.
- Programmers must follow a tedious sequence of compiling, testing, identifying errors, correcting errors, re-coding, and re-compiling a program in a process known as **debugging** the program. Most of the time devoted to programming is spent debugging the code.
- **Scripting languages** differ from compiled languages in that the source code is **interpreted** and converted into machine code at the time of execution – obviating the compiling process. The development process with scripted languages is typically more rapid than with compiled code since it can be tested while written; however, because scripting languages are interpreted at the time of execution, they are typically slower to execute. Therefore, scripted language is often reserved for smaller programs that are not computationally intensive. Scripting languages include JavaScript, VBScript, Python, and ASPX.

6.4 Computer Networking

- A **computer network** is a group of two or more interconnected computers that are capable of sharing data and resources. Networking allows multiple independent users to share the same resources (i.e., applications and data) and work with this data simultaneously.
- Fast, reliable networks form the backbone of a digital radiology department and allow large quantities of imaging data to be efficiently transported between modalities, archives, and viewing stations.
- Computer networks can be classified on the basis of scale (i.e., size, complexity), scope, topology, architecture, and connection method.
- The most common network is the **local area network (LAN)**. A LAN is characterized by serving computers in a small geographic area such as a home or office.
- A network which is comprised of two or more LANs is termed a **wide area network (WAN)**. Although the term is somewhat ambiguous, it is more commonly used to describe networks with a broad geographic coverage – metropolitan, regional, or national. The largest WAN is the public **Internet**, which is a global system of interconnected computer networks.

- A typical radiology department network would consist of at least one LAN which may be interconnected to a larger WAN (e.g., a hospital or enterprise network).
- Connection of two or more networks (i.e., **internetworking**) changes the scope of network resources available to any computer on the network. An **intranet** is one or more networks that are under control of a single administrative authority. Access to any external or unregulated networks is either not provided or is limited to authorized users.
- An **extranet** is an internally managed network (intranet) that maintains limited connectivity to networks that are neither managed, owned, nor controlled by the same entity. An extranet is typically isolated from the public Internet with security measures such as **firewalls** which regulate connectivity to outside or unmanaged networks. Most hospitals and business organizations configure their internal network in this way.
- Many home networks (wireless or wired) are extranets that consist of a LAN with access provided to the public Internet (WAN) via an **Internet service provider (ISP)**.

> **FURTHER READING: Networking**
>
> Computer Networking: A Top-Down Approach (7th Edition). Kurose JF, Ross KW. Addison Wesley, 2017.

- A **virtual private network (VPN)** is a method for including a distant device into an intranet with nearly the same level of security as if it were on the premises.

6.4.1 Physical (Hardware) Networking Components

- Basic components of a computer network include the network card, cabling, and a point of connection (e.g., hub, repeater, bridge, router, or network switch).
- The **network interface card (NIC)** is the piece of computer hardware that provides the capability for a computer to communicate over a network. Every NIC possesses a unique number, its **medium access control (MAC) address**. This number can be used to help route data to and from other computers.
- The physical connection of the computer to the network is usually accomplished through specialized cabling that contains four pairs of simple copper wires (twisted pair) in a configuration

> **DEFINITION: Bandwidth**
>
> The maximum amount of data that can be transmitted over a medium, usually measured in bits per second.

known as category 5 or **Cat5**, or its enhanced version Cat5e. Cat5 cabling frequently terminates in special rectangle plastic connectors that resemble oversized telephone connectors.

- Other forms of physical connection used less often include **fiber-optic cables (optical fiber)** and **wireless** (802.11x). Fiber optic provides greater transmission capacity (**bandwidth**) than Cat5, and wireless affords greater access where physical connections are not readily available.

- The term **Ethernet** describes the wiring and signaling schema for the NIC and the cabling between devices on the network.

6.4.2 Network Switches, Hubs, Bridges, and Routers

- The cornerstones of the computer network are **switches**, the devices that connect other devices together on the network. Switches vary in the degree of functionality by which they manage the data traffic that passes through them. The term *switch* is an imprecise term that refers to many types of network devices.
- The simplest and most inexpensive of network switches is the network **hub**. The hub provides a simple and passive method for all computers connected to it to transmit and receive data to each other. Each computer network

CHECKLIST: Types of Network Switches

- Hub
- Bridge
- Router

cable has an individual connection to the hub. The hub creates a shared medium where only one computer can successfully transmit at a time and each computer (**host**) is responsible for the entire communication process.
- The hub is a passive device. The hub merely replicates all messages to all hosts connected to it and does not have any capability to route messages to a specific destination. A network hub is the most basic and inefficient means of connectivity. For this reason, simple hubs are rarely used today.
- The network **bridge** improves upon the design of the basic network hub by providing a level of active management of the communication between attached hosts. The bridge is capable of learning the MAC addresses of the connected host computers and will only send data destined for a specific host through the connection associated with a unique MAC address. By routing the data stream to the intended recipient, switching creates a more efficient method for network transmission.
- Since the bridge needs to examine all data sent through it, it creates some processing overhead which slows the data transmission rate. Bridges typically support data transmission rates of 10, 100, and 1000 megabits per second (Mbs).
- The network **router** offers yet another level of technical sophistication over the network bridge. Like the network bridge, a router is capable of examining the

contents of the data passing through it and is able to discern the identity of the sender and the intended recipient. However, instead of relying on the value of the hardware NIC MAC address (which is fixed and not configurable), the router is capable of discerning data based upon a software configurable identifier known as the **Internet Protocol address (IP address)**.

- The IP address is a configurable 32-bit numeric value (e.g., 192.123.456.789) that is used to uniquely identify devices and the networks to which they belong. Using this schema, a host that is accessible globally must have a unique IP address. With 232 possible combinations (IPv4), this provides for 4.3 billion unique addresses. Under IPv6, there are 2128 possible combinations allowing for far greater unique addresses.
- The **hostname** of a computer is a human-readable unique label for a computer on a network (e.g., mycomputer145.nowhereuniversity.edu). Every device on a LAN or WAN or the public Internet has a unique hostname.
- An IP address may be designated as **fixed** (unchangeable) or **dynamic** (modifiable, reusable). Every hostname has a unique IP address associated with it.
- Network routers maintain **network routing tables** that define the topology of a network, the relationship of devices on a network, and how to reach them.
- With the billions of computers in use today connected to the public Internet, there are not enough unique public IP addresses for each computer to have its own unique address.
- A computer that is hidden within a **private network** need not have a globally unique address (it only needs to be unique on the local network). This scheme allows for conservation of unique IP addresses. That is, two internal networks can use the same IP subaddresses, as long as those computers are not exposed to the rest of the Internet.
- A **subnetwork** is a small network of computers that is connected to a larger network through a **router**.
- The typical **broadband network router** used in home networking has additional features such as **DHCP (dynamic host configuration protocol)**, **NAT (network address translation)**, and a network **firewall**. These additional features provide a secure connection between the home LAN and the ISP WAN.
- **DHCP** is used to orchestrate how devices are automatically configured on a network whereby individual devices "negotiate" with the network controller or router to establish a path for communication.
- The router using **NAT** serves as a proxy that allows multiple computers to share a single public Internet IP address. The broadband network router assigns each computer in the home network its own IP address that is *only unique within the home network*.
- It is through this mechanism that a LAN with dozens or hundreds of computers can share a single IP address to the public Internet.
- The network **firewall** is primarily a security device (hardware and software) that filters traffic between the network, adjacent networks (WAN or LAN), and public networks. Multiple firewalls can exist within an organization to protect for unauthorized access.

6.4.3 Network Processes and Protocols

- To communicate effectively, each device must adhere to a specific set of rules for communication called **network protocols**. Networks are usually comprised of a heterogeneous group of devices of different make, model, vintage, and performance. The most ubiquitous network protocol over Ethernet is the **Internet protocol suite (IPS)** or **Transmission Control Protocol/Internet Protocol (TCP/IP)**.
- TCP/IP is a software abstraction of protocols and services necessary for the establishment of communication between two computers on a network. This network abstraction was set down by **the International Organization for Standardization (ISO)** and is referred to as the **ISO network model**. The model describes five to seven **information layers** that link computer software applications to the hardware that must perform the actual transmission and receipt of data.
- The layers in the network ISO model rely upon protocols to regulate how information is passed up through and down the ISO stack.
- The Internet protocol suite defines a number of rules for establishment of communication between computers. In most instances, the connection is a one-to-one relationship. Two computers go through a **negotiation process** prior to making a connection. The negotiations include request and acceptance of an initial connection, the type of connection, the rate of transmission, data packet size, data acknowledgement, as well as when and how to transmit missing data.

6.4.4 Data Packets

- Data transmitted over a network is broken up into multiple small discrete chunks or **packets** before being sent over the network by the NIC. Packet size is variable and is part of the "negotiations" when establishing a network connection with another computer.

> **KEY CONCEPT: Data Packets**
>
> Since each packet is self-contained and auto-routable, different packets from a single message can travel over completely different routes to arrive at the same destination. This offers redundancy to networks.

- Since a network segment can only be used by a single computer at any one instant and the physical parts of the network (i.e., cabling and switches) are shared by many computers, splitting data streams up into smaller parcels in a shared network model improves network efficiency dramatically.
- Switching and assigning resources on a shared network is a complex process – one which needs to occur in microseconds to maintain efficient communication between thousands of devices that are potentially competing for these resources. This is a precisely managed and timed process whereby unique data packets are

embedded into network traffic in shared routes and redirected based upon prede-termined routing rules.

- Despite the refined sophistication of the system, there are instances where two or more computers attempt to send data along the same segment simultaneously. This phenomenon is termed a **collision**. Optimum network design mandates minimizing collisions and maximizing **collision detection** to maintain fidelity of data transmission. In these instances, the controller may request the originating site to resend the lost packet(s).
- Additional metadata is automatically married to each data packet based upon protocols specified in IPS and contains information such as the data type, packet number, total number of packets, as well as the IP address of the sender and receiver. This is analogous to placing a letter (packet) in an envelope with deliv-ery information (sender and return address). Data packets with this additional data **wrapper** are referred to as **data frames**.
- Since each frame of transmitted data contains information about where it origi-nated and where it is supposed to go, routers can then examine each packet and forward it through the relevant pathway that is pre-configured to reach the recipient network. *Moreover, since each packet is self-contained and auto-routable, packets from a single message can travel over completely different routes to arrive at the same destination.* Routers instantaneously analyze and balance network traffic and will route packets over segments that are currently under a lighter load.
- At the receiving end, the ISO model also details how to reassemble the individual packets back into the original file.
- Each packet bears both an identifier and sequential number that tell what part of the original file each packet contains. The destination computer uses this infor-mation to re-create the original file.
- If packets are lost during the transmission process, TCP/IP also has methods for requesting retransmission of missing or corrupt packets.

6.4.5 Bandwidth and Latency

- **Network bandwidth** is defined as the rate at which information can be transmitted per second (bits/sec) through a network. In the par-lance, a wider "pipe" can provide greater bandwidth. This can vary tremendously depending upon the type of physical connection, switches, and medium (i.e., cabling versus fiber versus wireless).

KEY CONCEPT: Theoretical Bandwidth

In general, actual bandwidth is approx-imately one-half of theoretical values. Other infrastructure factors that can reduce bandwidth include use of a firewall.

- Theoretical bandwidth of Ethernet, for example, varies from 10 to 1000 megabits per second and is generally twice that of actual bandwidth due to infrastructure constraints (e.g., use of a firewall) and network load.
- Another technology, known as asynchronous transfer mode (**ATM**), can support bandwidths ranging from 155 Mb/sec to 2488 Mb/sec.
- **Latency** is another network parameter that is often used to gauge performance of a connection. It describes the time for a data packet to take a round trip from sender to receiver and back to the sender expressed in milliseconds (ms).
- Under optimal circumstances a network should achieve high bandwidth and low latency.

CHECKLIST: Theoretical Bandwidths

- Wired bandwidths
  - Ethernet   10 Mbps
  - Ethernet   100 Mbps
  - ATM (OC3)   155 Mbps
  - ATM (OC12)   622 Mbps
  - Ethernet   1000 Mbps
  - ATM (OC48)   2488 Mbps
- Wireless bandwidths
  - 802.11b   11 Mbps
  - 802.11g   54 Mbps
  - 802.11n   600 Mbps
  - 802.11ac   600 Mbps
- Cellular bandwidths
  - 3G - HSPA   7.2 Mbps
  - 3G - HSPA+   21 Mbps
  - 3G - DC-HSPA+   42 Mbps
  - 4G - LTE   100 Mbps
  - 5G   20,000 Mbps

- The term **broadband** is often used to describe high-speed Internet access with a minimum of 25 Mbps download and 3 Mbps upload speed. This type of network performance is achievable today through a number of mechanisms (e.g., Wi-Fi, cable, satellite, and cellular).
- Current **wireless (Wi-Fi)** bandwidth speeds rival many hardwired network protocols allowing for streaming media to handheld devices without performance degradation.
- It is important to recognize that there can be a substantial difference between the values of a theoretical bandwidth and **actual** achieved bandwidth. While packets of data move at the speed of light, other factors such as quality of cabling and efficiency of network switches and firewall contribute to **network overhead** that can impede actual performance.

6.5 Client-Server Architecture

- The **client-server computing model** is one of interdependency between two or more computers where one computer provides data or services to the other.
- Early networks were used primarily to back up data to a central

DEFINTION: Server-Client

A server is a computer that provides application services or data. A client is a computer or software application that receives those services and data.

location during off-hours. Each user kept complete versions data and the applications used to create that data on their local devices. This model is expensive to deploy and maintain.

- Cost to deploy and maintain applications and data on separate computers in a large organization has become prohibitive.
- Centralized **data center** with redundant servers that provide services to thousands of remote clients has become the standard architecture in most healthcare systems, largely due to the improvements in network speeds. This allows for data and applications to be centrally managed.

6.5.1 Cloud Computing

- Current considerations include a shift to a **cloud computing** infrastructure whereupon an organization leases computing resources from large, redundant, and geographically disparate locations to obtain access to servers, storage, databases, software, and business intelligence resources.
- The primary advantages of cloud computing are **scalability** and low maintenance costs since an organization is not required to support a physical data center.

6.5.1.1   SaaS, PaaS, and IaaS

- The three types of cloud computing services are **software as a service (SaaS), platform as a service (PaaS), and infrastructure as a service (IaaS)**. Each has variable local maintenance and management requirements. SaaS, for example, is characterized by all management maintained by the cloud provider.
- **SaaS** provides access to software that runs on client computers without installing the software locally. Examples include Google apps, Dropbox, DocuSign, etc.
- **PaaS** provides a development platform in the cloud to create applications, databases, and services as a replacement for local development servers in a data center. Examples include Google Cloud Platform (GCP) and Amazon Web Services (AWS).
- **IaaS** consists of infrastructure such as storage, networking, and virtualization services in the Cloud. Examples include Amazon Elastic Cloud Services (EC2).

6.5.2 Web Services

- As technology has continued to evolve, there has been a growing convergence of desktop computing and network computing. In the past, maximizing computing efficiency required application software and data to reside on the client computer.

- A **fat client** (thick or rich client) is a host application that performs the bulk of data processing operations for the user with minimal to no reliance on network resources. It is typically installed on each local computer.
- By leveraging the power of faster network services, real-time transfer of data and application resources to the client desktop computer is afforded. The client makes requests from a dedicated, powerful networked computer (a server) which stands ready to provide application services or data to the client over the network.
- While any computer can be configured to act as a server, most servers have additional hardware capacity to support the increased demands of multiple simultaneous users (i.e., faster multicore CPUs, large memory stores, and larger hard drives).
- This close interrelationship of multiple clients and a server is known as **client-server architecture**. Almost all of the structure of the Internet is based upon the client-server model. This infrastructure supports delivery of web pages over the World Wide Web and email.

> **KEY CONCEPT: Client-Server Architecture**
>
> In its purest form, client-server architecture concentrates on maximizing virtually all of the computational power on the server while minimizing the computational requirements of the client stations. This affords great economies of scale without loss of functionality.

- The most basic client application is the web browser, which interacts directly with the server to render data, images, or advanced visualizations. Any application that is accessed via a web browser over a network that is coded in a browser-supported language (i.e., JavaScript, Java, HTML5, CSS, etc.) is called **web application or web app**.
- A **thin client** (lean or slim client) is an application that relies primarily on the server for processing and focuses principally on conveying input and output between the user and the server.

> **DEFINITION: Thin Client**
>
> A software application that does not depend upon any local software components and does not perform any processing on the local host.

- The term thin-client application is often misused by industry to refer to any function or application that runs within a web browser – however, this is an incomplete definition. Even if the application is used inside of a web browser, if additional software or browser plug-ins are required or local data processing occurs, the term **hybrid client** is more appropriate. Most PACS client viewing software that runs within a web browser is classified as hybrid client; there is a local installation of viewer software, but there are tight interdependencies with servers to render the images. Similar relationships exist for post-processing platforms.
- Modern PACS systems are designed to leverage this configuration where the majority of the image management is controlled by a powerful central server which responds to multiple simultaneous requests for image data from relatively inexpensive, less-powerful client viewing stations.

- Software applications that are designed to operate principally over a network in a client-server configuration are grouped collectively into something known as **web services**. There are established profiles and specifications which define how these services are supposed to interoperate with service providers and service requesters. Web services differ from web applications in that web services need **not** run inside of a browser or be constructed with web elements.

6.5.3 Protocols

- Clients and servers rely on mutually agreed upon **protocols** for the exchange of information. These are set up by international standards bodies such as the Internet Engineering Task Force and the World Wide Web Consortium (W3C).
- In addition to specifying the ubiquitous medical imaging format, the **DICOM** protocols specify how to discover and exchange images between a PACS client and an archive (see **Chap. 12**).
- There are many protocols in use for the exchange of information. The most common is **Hypertext Transfer Protocol (HTTP)** which is the basis for data exchange on the Internet and in web browsers.
- The **Simple Mail Transfer Protocol (SMTP)** is a standard for email clients to negotiate, transmit, and receive email messages.
- **Simple Object Access Protocol (SOAP)** is used to exchange structured information and is often used to negotiate PACS clients with servers.
- **Representational State Transfer (REST)** is a client-server architecture that promotes stateless retrieval of information from a server by a client. **Statelessness** refers to the condition where each data exchange has no dependencies on the prior exchanges of information; they are all independent.
- **Application Programming Interfaces (API)** allow other software to send commands to the application and are often built using REST transactions between the client and server.

6.6 Database Applications

- Many useful web services and web applications provide direct access to databases.
- There are a number of **database models**; however, the **relational model** is used most often. In the relational model, data is abstracted into **tables** with rows and columns. Each row is an individual

DEFINITION: Database

A structured collection of data. Data which is housed in a database is more amenable to analysis and organization. Databases are ubiquitous and are the essential component of nearly every computer application that manages information.

record, and each column is a separate **attribute or field** for each record. One or more tables are linked logically by a common attribute (e.g., an order number, serial number, accession number, etc.).

- Databases also support an **indexing** mechanism which confers greater speed to the system when accessing or updating data. Indexing comes at some cost since it adds some processing overhead to the system.
- The most common programmatic operations on a relational database include reading or selecting records for analysis, adding records, updating records, and deleting records.
- **Structured query language (SQL)** is a database-specific computer language designed to retrieve and manage data in **relational database management systems (RDMS)**. SQL provides a programmatic interface to databases from virtually any development platform.
- Databases are integral to the infrastructure of most business systems including information systems in radiology. Virtually every aspect of radiology services is tied to relational database functions from patient scheduling to transcription.
- For more information on databases, see **Chap. 11**.

PEARLS

- Although the microprocessor is frequently personified as the "brain" of the computer, it has no innate "intelligence" or inherent ability to make decisions. The microprocessor's strength is in its ability to process instructions and manipulate data at amazing speeds.
- All application software runs *on top of* the operating system, and the operating system, in turn, is directly integrated with the hardware. In general, application software cannot interact directly with the hardware; all interactions are brokered by the operating system.
- A computer that is accessible globally must have a unique IP address; however, a computer that is *hidden* within a private network need not have a globally unique address (it only needs to be unique on the local network). This scheme allows for conservation of unique IP addresses.
- A thin client (lean or slim client) is an application that relies primarily on the server for processing and focuses principally on conveying input and output between the user and the server.
- Software applications that are designed to operate principally over a network in a client-server configuration are grouped collectively into the term "web services."

Self-Assessment Questions

1. The core hardware components of a digital computer include everything **except**:

   (a) Microprocessor
   (b) Memory
   (c) Bus
   (d) Keyboard
   (e) Operating system

2. Volatile memory is distinguished from nonvolatile memory by:

   (a) Poorer performance of volatile memory
   (b) Flammability of volatile memory
   (c) Inability of volatile memory to retain data with power loss
   (d) Greater expense of volatile memory
   (e) None of the above

3. Which is **not** true about storage?

   (a) Online storage is readily available.
   (b) Near-line storage requires human intervention.
   (c) Off-line storage is not accessible by robotic devices.
   (d) Data is stored on media such as tape, compact disk, and DVD.
   (e) None of the above.

4. Which statement is true regarding virtual machines (VMs)?

   (a) A VM doesn't really exist.
   (b) A VM is a software representation of computing hardware.
   (c) Using a VM is not the same as working with a real computer.
   (d) A VM is more difficult to control and maintain.
   (e) None of the above.

5. How does a container differ from a virtual machine?

   (a) Containers are more isolated than VMs.
   (b) Containers only allow one user, whereas VMs allow many.
   (c) A container is an abstraction of a software layer, whereas a VM is an abstraction of the hardware components.
   (d) Containers are more stable than VMs.
   (e) None of the above.

6. Which is the best statement regarding the motherboard data bus?

   (a) It connects to the keyboard.
   (b) It connects to the power supply.
   (c) It interconnects the components on the motherboard.
   (d) It connects to the disk drive.
   (e) None of the above.

7. What is the fundamental distinction between software and hardware?

   (a) Price.
   (b) Hardware is a physical entity.
   (c) Packaging.
   (d) Complexity.
   (e) None of the above.

8. The purpose of the operating system (OS) is:

   (a) To manage memory allocations
   (b) To copy files to disk
   (c) To manage the user interface
   (d) To manage computer resources
   (e) All of the above

9. Computer drivers are:

   (a) Names for a specific type of golf club
   (b) Large programs that take control of the operating system
   (c) Small programs that provide a bridge or interface between hardware and software
   (d) Similar to computer viruses
   (e) None of the above

10. Low-level programming languages are:

    (a) Fairly simple to learn and use
    (b) Are primarily used by human computer programmers to create applications
    (c) Are not as costly as high-level programming languages
    (d) Are used primarily by the CPU
    (e) All of the above

11. The most complex network switch is the:

    (a) Network hub.
    (b) Network router.
    (c) Network bridge.
    (d) They are all similar in complexity.
    (e) Not listed.

12. What statement is true regarding networking addresses (IP)?

    (a) All IP addresses are a fixed unique number.
    (b) We are running out of unique IP addresses.
    (c) IP addresses can by dynamic or fixed in value.
    (d) The computer MAC address is the same as the IP address.
    (e) IP addresses are recognizable names and places.

13. Which is true of thin-client applications?

    (a) They require a third-party web browser to run.
    (b) They do not need software.
    (c) They require a networked server.
    (d) They require an internal database.
    (e) All of the above.

Chapter 7
Data Storage

Edward M. Smith, Thomas Jay Crawford, and Katherine P. Andriole

Contents

E. M. Smith (Deceased)

T. J. Crawford (✉)
University of North Carolina School of Medicine, Department of Radiology,
Chapel Hill, NC, USA
e-mail: jay_crawford@med.unc.edu

K. P. Andriole
Brigham and Women's Hospital, Harvard Medical School, MGH & BWH
Center for Clinical Data Science, Boston, MA, USA
e-mail: kandriole@bwh.harvard.edu

© The Author(s), under exclusive license to Springer Science+Business Media,
LLC, part of Springer Nature 2021
B. F. Branstetter IV (ed.), *Practical Imaging Informatics*,
https://doi.org/10.1007/978-1-0716-1756-4_7

7.1 Philosophy of Storing Electronic Protected Health Information (ePHI)

- The storage and retrieval of ePHI is a multifaceted function ranging from archival of data within the healthcare facility and related off-site practices, to the referring physician's office, to the patient and to regional, national, and international repositories.
- Requires the purchasing of and adherence to interoperability standards for all hardware, software, and applications that touch the institution's digital environment.
- Image objects consume 95% or more of the storage requirements versus 5% or less for non-pixel data.
- This includes not only radiologic data but visible light images, digitized pathology slides, and some genomic data.
- Estimating storage requirements is at best an educated guess due to new innovations generating increasingly larger amounts of information and the expanding digital imaging environment in health care.
- Storage management components should be purchased separately from the clinical and administrative applications to reduce cost and ensure vendor independence (**vendor-neutral archives**) while requiring interoperability between all components in the digital environment.

7.1.1 Enterprise Storage Versus Departmental Silos of Storage

- Isolated independent silos of departmental storage are difficult to manage.
- Divorcing storage components from administrative and clinical applications:
  - Allows administrative and clinical departments to acquire applications that optimize workflow and productivity.
  - Creates independence from application vendors by eliminating proprietary storage formats, thus minimizing future cost of data migration and costs due to obsolescence of technology.
- Reduces cost of hardware, software, licensing, and maintenance fees as well as personnel cost.
- Provides an integrated storage and storage management system.
- Provides high availability and redundancy of information at a reduced cost.
- Satisfies state and federal retention periods for medical information and HIPAA requirements in the most cost-effective manner.
- Allows for consistent Information Lifecycle Management Policies to be enforced.
- Allows for a more complete view of the patient's imaging studies, across departments or across affiliations.

FURTHER READING: Economics of Enterprise Storage

Cecil RA. Solve the enterprise archive puzzle. Imaging Economics. 2007 Jan; 38–43.

Langer SG. Global PACS archiving. Enterprise Imaging and Therapeutic Radiology Management. 2008 Sep; 61–7.

Smith EM. Integrated implementation revamps information storage. Diagnostic Imaging. 2005 Jan; 39–43.

Smith EM. Storage management: one solution doesn't fit all. Imaging Technology News. 2004 Nov/Dec; 80–3.

7.1.2 Storage Management Responsibilities

- **Information Technology (IT) Department** is primarily responsible for storage management including funding, providing necessary infrastructure, hardware, and software management and meeting administrative and clinical departmental requirements, including the following:
  - Meeting storage volume requirements.
  - Periodically upgrading hardware and software due to technological obsolescence and migrating information to new infrastructure.
  - Providing 24×7 accessibility to all information.
  - Meeting required clinical and administrative **response times** for retrieval of information.
  - Adhering to HIPAA and other mandated federal, state, and local security and retention requirements for health-related information.
  - Consistently providing required disaster recovery (DR) and business continuance (BC) processes including timely backup and replication of required information (see **Chap. 28**).
- **Administrative and Clinical Departments** are responsible for:
  - Working with IT to ensure that their applications adhere to the purchasing and interoperability standards mutually agreed upon.
  - Being realistic in their requirements for response times for information queries.
  - Estimating clinical storage requirements for a 12- to 24-month period.
- **Chief Financial Officer** understands that:
  - Storage management is an on-going cost.
  - Life cycle of many of the components is 3–5 years due to technical obsolescence.

7.1.3 Economics of Storage Management

- The cost of storage management is an operational cost that must be budgeted annually.
- Cost of storage management includes
  - Hardware, infrastructure, and software
  - Initial cost
  - Maintenance and licensing fees
  - Replacement cost due to technological obsolescence
  - Storage media cost
  - Personnel
  - Utilities
  - Physical space in a datacenter
  - Costs related to data backup and replication, business continuity, and disaster recovery
  - Data migrations due to technology obsolescence or overgrown capacity
- To minimize the cost of storage management:
  - Reduce the number of isolated silos of storage.
  - Implement a scalable storage management design, reduce the use of proprietary components, and adhere to archival and integration standards.
  - Purchase media based on projected volume and growth needs for periods of 12–24 months since **storage costs decrease** with time.
  - Purchase subsystems and associated media based on performance (e.g., data retrieval time) requirements of applications.

7.2 Datacenters

The IT department is responsible for funding, managing, and supporting the datacenter.

- Providing power and cooling for a datacenter with high-density computing resources is a significant cost.
- Healthcare facilities computing resources should reside in a secure datacenter providing a level of availability of medical information that meets or exceeds the clinical requirements of the institution.
- Clinical departments must specify the characteristics of the computing resources and availability requirements for medical information meeting the clinical requirements.

FURTHER READING: Datacenters

Updated tier classifications define infrastructure performance, www.uptimeinstitute.org.

A quick primer on data center tier rating, www.itconsultant.boblandstrom.com.

7.2.1 Tier Rating of Datacenters

- The Uptime Institute provides industry recognized and accepted standards for high-density computing and mission critical facilities in a vendor neutral manner.
- The primary attribute of the Tier rating of a datacenter is the availability of the computing resources it contains.
- Tier rating may be too expensive and rigorous for many healthcare facilities, but it does provide a guideline and may assist in selecting a datacenter for outsourcing some aspect of a center's computing resources or for choosing disaster recovery services:
  - Tier 1 datacenter has no redundant components such as on-site generator, uninterruptible power supply (UPS), fire suppression system, heating, ventilation and air conditioning (HVAC), etc. in which availability is affected regardless of whether the outage was planned or unplanned.
  - Tier 2 datacenter has redundant components, but only a single-distribution system. This provides availability for planned outages, but not for unplanned outages.
  - Tier 3 datacenter has redundant components and distribution systems plus dual public power supplies that provide the capability to operate self-sufficiently. All computer resources have two independent power sources. These features provide system availability during routine maintenance as well as for unplanned outages.
  - Tier 4 datacenter has all the features of Tier 3 plus the topology is configured such that any single component or distribution failure has no negative impact on availability (Table 7.1).

Table 7.1 Tier characteristics of data centers

Characteristics	Tier 1	Tier 2	Tier 3	Tier 4
Year first deployed	1965	1970	1985	1995
Single points of failure	Many + HE[b]	Many + HE[b]	Some + HE[b]	Fire, EPO[a] + Some HE[b]
Planned maintenance shutdowns	2 per year at 12 hours each	3 per 2 year at 12 hours each	None	None
Typical site failures	6 over 5 years	1 every year	1 every 2.5 years	1 every 5 years
Annual downtime due to site unavailability	28.8 hours	22 hours	1.6 hours	0.8 hours
Availability based on site caused downtime	99.671%	99.741%	99.982%	99.995%

[a]*EPO* emergency power off
[b]*HE* human error

7.3 Types of Medical Data

- From a storage perspective, imaging data can be divided into:
  - Data that may change after initial storage and are thus managed as a variable content file (VCF).
  - Data that will not change once stored and are thus managed as a fixed content file (FCF).

7.3.1 Variable Content Files (VCF)

- VCF or transactional data consist primarily of databases that comprise approximately 5% of the total stored image-related data.
  - Examples: radiology information system (RIS), hospital information system databases, and the demographic database of the PACS.
- The frequency of read/write commands to the database dictates the storage technology used to manage and replicate or backup the database.

7.3.2 Fixed Content Files (FCF)

- FCF imaging data consist primarily of DICOM objects such as images, structured reports, and curves that comprise approximately 95% of the total stored image-related data.
- Typical storage scenarios for image data include:
  - Storage on the acquisition modality for one or more days.
  - Forwarding of an image copy from the modality to "Tier 1 storage" (on-line storage) and possibly to one or more workstations for local storage of emergent studies.
- Tier 1 storage is managed by the PACS and is typically configured to store between 3 and 15 months or more of study volume depending on the clinical setting (e.g., outpatient, inpatient).
  - The PACS verifies the information in the DICOM header of the study against the information in the Radiology Information System (RIS) order for that study.
  - The PACS forwards a copy of the study to "Tier 2 storage" (long-term storage) where it is retained for the legal life of the study; a duplicate copy is either:
    - Forwarded to another storage system at a remote location or
    - Copied to tape or other media and manually carried off-site for "Tier 3 storage" (disaster recovery) and retained for the legal life of the study.

- Initially, four copies of a study exist until deleted from the modality
  - Then, three copies until eliminated from Tier 1 storage.
  - Finally, one copy will remain on Tier 2 and one on Tier 3 storage.
  - These Storage Tiers are different from the Datacenter Tiers discussed above.

7.4 Storage Requirements for ePHI

7.4.1 Health Information Portability and Accountability Act (HIPAA)

- The security regulations of HIPAA effective April 21, 2005 cover the confidentiality, integrity, and availability of ePHI.
- PHI has the potential to enable identification of an individual and includes: details of past, present, or future physical or mental health
  - Provision for health care or
  - Past, present, or future payment for health care

> **DEFINITION: Retention Period**
>
> Time, mandated by federal, state, or local statute, that medical information must be retained in its original and legal form.

- HIPAA covers ePHI stored on any type of storage media or through any means of information delivery including:
  - Portable computers and related devices
  - Electronic transmission via the Internet
  - Via e-mails or other related methods

Confidentiality is the assurance that ePHI is available to and viewable by only authorized persons or organizations.

- Requires that ePHI that is stored on media or transmitted electronically be encrypted to avoid access by unauthorized individuals (e.g., individuals in a facilities datacenter) or organizations.
- Both when in transit and when stored on physical media.

Availability is the assurance that systems responsible for delivering, storing, and processing ePHI are accessible in a timely manner by those who need them under both routine and emergency situations.

- HIPAA requires that two copies of ePHI must exist, so if one copy is accidentally destroyed during its legal life (retention period), a second copy will be available in a secure and accessible location.

Integrity is the assurance that ePHI is not changed unless an alteration is known, required, documented (via audit trial), validated, and authoritatively approved.

- When ePHI has been authoritatively approved, it should be stored electronically in a format that inhibits unauthorized alterations, e.g., Write Once, Read Many (WORM).

See **Chap. 30** for more information about HIPAA.

7.4.2 Storage Requirements for Clinical Studies

Typical storage requirements for radiologic studies are listed in Tables 7.2 and 7.3.
- Storage requirements vary widely depending on
  - Image size
  - Number of images
  - Slice thickness
  - Protocols
  - Sequences
  - Modality vendor

CHECKLIST: DICOM Attributes Needed to Determine Image Size

DICOM Tag	Attribute	Description
0028,0010	Rows	Number of Rows in the image (X dimension)
0028,0011	Columns	Number of Columns in the image (Y dimension)
0028,0100	Bits Allocated	Number of bits allocated for each pixel sample (Divide by 8 (for 8-bit bytes) to get bytes per pixel)
0028,0008	Number of Frames	Number of frames in a multi-frame image

Table 7.2 Representative uncompressed storage requirements for various modalities

Modality	Image size			Per study basis			
				No. of images		Uncompressed MB	
	X	Y	Bytes	Avg.	Range	Avg.	Range
CR	2,000	2,500	2	3	2–5	30	20–50
DR	3,000	3,000	2	3	2–5	54	36–90
CT	512	512	2	60	40–300	32	21–157
Multi-slice CT	512	512	2	500	250–4,000	262	131–2.1 GB
MR	256	256	2	200	80–1,000	26	11–131
Ultrasound	640	480	1[a]	30[b]	20–60	9.2	6.1–18.4
Nuc Med	256	256	2	10	4–30	1.3	0.3-3.8
Digital Fluoro	1024	1,024	1	20	10–50	20	10–50
Rad Angio	1024	1,024	1	15	10–30	15	10–30
Breast Tomosynthesis			2	50	10–100 per breast	1800	450 MB–3GB

[a]3 Bytes for color
[b]For Multi-frame Series' multiply by number of frames per series

Table 7.3 Typical uncompressed storage requirement per 100,000 studies for a general radiology practice

(Excludes CTA, 3 Tesla MR, MRA, PET/CT and mammography studies)			
Modality	% of Studies	Avg. MB/Study	GB/Year
Angiography	3	15	45
CR and DR	64	42	2,688
CT	20	52	1,040
MR	5	39	195
Nuclear Medicine	3	1.3	3.9
Ultrasound	5	18	90
Total TB per 100,000 studies			**4.1 TB**

Table 7.4 Average mammography storage requirement by type of detector

Resolution (microns)	Study type	Uncompressed storage requirement (MB)	2.5-1 Lossless compressed storage requirement (MB)
50	Screening	197	79
50	Diagnostic	296	118
70	Screening	96	38
70	Diagnostic	144	58
100	Screening	52	21
100	Diagnostic	78	31

Table 7.5 Representative storage requirement for breast MR

Views	Number of sites	Uncompressed (MB)		Mean – lossless compressed 2.5-1 (MB)
		Range	Mean	
Axial w/o contrast	5	63–132	98	39
Axial with contrast- typically, 5 sequences	5	223–336	294	118
Sagittal	5	42	42	17
Typical lossless storage requirements			174	

- Protocols requiring contrast increase storage requirements substantially.
- Tertiary care and/or specialty settings may have a greater percentage of cross-sectional modalities in their total study volume.

Breast Imaging
- CR: 50-micron resolution—storage requirement **4 times greater** than 100-micron resolution.
- Average mammography storage requirements based on 70% large cassette/paddle and 30% small cassette/paddle and 4 images for screening and 6 images for diagnostic studies (Table 7.4).
- Protocols and exam sizes vary by vendor (Table 7.5).

- Don't forget:
  - To account for outside imaging studies imported into PACS.
  - To consider growth
       Acquisition of or merger with new facilities or imaging centers
       New modality technology which may increase number of images and/or file sizes acquired (e.g., breast tomosynthesis)
       Increased volumes due to reduced scan times and efficiency improvements

7.5 Retention and Destruction Requirements for ePHI

7.5.1 Retention Requirements for ePHI

- Depending on the local, state, or federal statutes, ePHI must be retained in its original form (from which diagnosis was made) for a period of from 5 to 7 years or longer.
- Healthcare facilities should establish and document retention periods for all types of ePHI based on the requirements imposed by various statutes.
- Images stored for purposes of complying with regulatory backup (DR) requirements must be of the same quality as images used for diagnostic purposes.

KEY CONCEPT: Retention

The retention period for ePHI varies and
- Is dependent on type of ePHI
- Is dependent on the age of the individual
- Is specified by federal statute
- Varies by state and type of provider
- Complies with state's statute of limitations
- Mammography has special regulations
  - Federal Register 900.12©(4) (i),(ii)

- ePHI for minors may have to be retained until the individual reaches the age of 21 or beyond, depending on when the ePHI was acquired.
- Regulations exist (typically state statute of limitations) that require ePHI be retained for a period of 2 years after the death of a person.

7.5.2 Film Screen and Digital Mammograms

- Retained for not less than 5 years.
- Not less than ten years if no additional mammograms of patients are performed at the facility
- Longer if mandated by federal, state, or local statutes.
- Digitized film screen mammograms cannot be used for legal retention purposes (not original) but can be used for comparison with current digital mammograms.

- Recommended (but not required) that computer-assisted diagnosis (CAD) reports be retained as part of the mammography study.
- Lossy compressed mammograms cannot be used for legal retention purposes.

7.5.3 Destruction Requirements for ePHI

- ePHI must be destroyed so there is no possibility of reconstructing identifying information.
- Resulting from the complex rules governing retention of ePHI, automation of its destruction is not currently possible.
- The most cost-effective solution to manage outdated ePHI may be permanent retention.
- Destruction of ePHI must be documented including
  - Date of destruction
  - Method of destruction
  - Description of disposed records
  - Inclusive dates covered
  - Statement that the records were destroyed in the normal course of business
  - Signature of individual supervising and witnessing the destruction
- Magnetic and optical media
  - CD, DVD, and other magnetic or optical media should be shredded.
  - Degaussing is the preferred method to destroy data on magnetic disk or tape.

> **KEY CONCEPT: Digital Image Destruction**
>
> When a study is deleted from a PACS storage system, the study is deleted from the demographic database so it can no longer be located or retrieved. The actual study itself *should not be deleted* from the digital media.

7.6 Storage Technology

7.6.1 Types of Storage Media

- Parameters used to select storage media
  - Functionality—does it meet the clinical requirements for the application?
  - Response time (to read/retrieve and write information) and storage capacity.
  - Longevity—how long will the media and the components used to read and write to the media be available and be supported (technology obsolescence?),

> **FURTHER READING: Storage Media**
>
> Kerns R. Information archiving: economics and compliance. Boulder; 2012.

will there be backward compatibility, or will information have to be migrated? Information migration is expensive and can be time consuming. For most media, technical obsolescence is between 3 and 6 years depending on when it is purchased in the technology life cycle.

- Total cost of ownership (TCO) of the entire storage management system for the storage media used is the total cost of purchasing and supporting the storage management system and includes hardware, software, maintenance and licensing fees, personnel, utilities, space, and information migration costs.
- Cost—media is typically less than 5–10% of the TCO of the storage management system.
- Durability—information stored on media must be accessible for a long period of time, factors that affect durability include wear and tear from read/write components, temperature, and humidity changes, etc.
- Compliance features—HIPAA requirements regarding immutability and integrity of ePHI (e.g., storing in WORM format).
- Remove ability—media that can be removed from the read/write source; evaluate the pros and cons for the specific application.
- Storage media cabinets should have redundant power supplies and fans to minimize system failures.

- Optical Media
  - Used primarily to provide a transportable copy of individual patient study and as a low-cost, long-term storage, and disaster recovery media.
  - Inferior performance characteristics to spinning magnetic disk with respect to read/write speed capabilities and storage capacity.
  - Optical media maintains integrity of stored information for the long term if properly handled but limited useful life of 6 years due to technology obsolescence.
  - Data are typically written in Write Once Read Many (WORM) format which is advantageous for purposes of long-term storage and HIPAA requirements.
  - **Compact disk (CD)** used primarily as transportable media for an individual patient study stored in DICOM Part 10 format as WORM with a DICOM viewer. CDs are available as CD-R, WORM version, and also CD-RW, a re-writeable version that **must not** be used for storage of medical information or ePHI. Storage capacity is up to 700 MB.

> **FURTHER READING: Optical Media**
>
> www.en.wikipedia.org/wiki/computer_data_storage#optical.

  - **Digital versatile disk (DVD)**
    Available as DVD-R and DVD-RW; only the DVD-R version should be used to store medical information or ePHI.
    Single-sided, single-layer DVD will store up to 4.7 GB and the single sided, double-layer will store 8.5 GB.
    These disks are typically used for inexpensive long-term storage or DR within a robotic storage system.

- Spinning magnetic disk
  - Also known as Hard Disk Drive (HDD)
  - Most storage today uses spinning media
- Performance
  - To decrease time to access data, increase rotational speed (measured in rpm).
  - To increase throughput and storage capacity, increase media storage density (measured in Terabytes). This number is likely to rise as technology improves.
- Redundant Array of Independent Disks (RAID)
  - RAID writes parity data across the array of disks, which are organized so that the failure of one disk in the array will not result in loss of any data.
  - A failed disk can be replaced by a new one, and the data on it reconstructed from the remaining data and the parity data.

> **FURTHER READING: Hard Drives and RAID**
>
> www.en.wikipedia.org/wiki/hard_disk_drive.
> www.en.wikpedia.org/wiki/redundant_array_of_independent_disks.

  - As a result of this redundancy, less data can be stored in the array.
  - Selection of the appropriate RAID level depends upon the application, degree of protection against data loss, storage capacity, and performance (number of write/read per second).
  - RAID is not a substitute for backing up data on another media located remotely from the RAID.
  - There are several different types of RAID configuration (Table 7.6).

CHECKLIST: Commonly Used Types of RAID

RAID 0—(Striping) Data are striped across several disks to improve performance and obtain 100% storage capacity. No redundancy is provided; if one disk fails, data on that disk are lost.

RAID 1—(Mirroring) Two groups of similar disks store exactly the same data. No data will be lost as long as one group of disks survives.

RAID 5—(Striped disk with parity) Combines three or more disks in a way that protects data against loss of any one disk. Storage capacity is reduced by one disk's worth. A "hot spare" disk should be added to the array so data can be quickly and automatically restored. If an additional disk fails while data are restored, data in the entire array can still be lost.

RAID 6—(Striped disk with dual parity) Can recover if two disks in the array are lost. A "hot spare" disk should be added to the array so data can be quickly and automatically restored.

Raid 1+0 or RAID10—uses both striping and mirroring, consists of a striped set of mirrored subsets, provides fault tolerance and improved performance.

- Content-addressable storage (CAS) is a method for storing information based on its content (object-based) rather than its storage location and is used for fixed content files of ePHI to meet regulatory requirements.
- Solid state media, as used in USB flash drives, has begun to replace HDD on most computers, but is not yet inexpensive enough for mass storage.

Table 7.6 Characteristics of RAID levels in common use

Feature	RAID 0	RAID 1	RAID 5	RAID 6	RAID 1+0
Minimum number of drives	2	2	3 + hot spare	4 + hot spare	4
Data protection	None	Single drive failure	Single drive failure	Two drive failures	One drive failure in each sub-array
Read performance	High	High	High	High	High
Write performance	High	Medium	Low	Low	Medium
% Storage utilization	100	50	67–94	50–88	50
Typical applications	Not applicable for storage of ePHI	Operating systems, transactional databases	Tier 1, 2, and 3 storage of ePHI	Tier 1, 2, and 3 storage of ePHI – high availability required	Fast transactional databases, application servers

7.6.2 Storage Management Infrastructure and Hardware

- Data storage is more than just the right choice of hardware. An entire system for storage management must be built around that hardware. Considerations include
  - Capacity—amount and type of data (file level or block level) to be stored or shared
  - Performance or availability—input/output and throughput requirements
  - Scalability—long-term data growth
  - Availability and reliability—how mission-critical is the application
  - Data protection—backup and recovery requirements
  - IT staff resources and capability
  - Initial and annual budget availability
- Direct attached storage (DAS)
  - Simplest and least expensive storage technology where computer (server) is directly attached to storage device such as RAID or tape system.
  - Workstations must access server to connect with storage system.
  - Since the server must handle processing for the applications as well as servicing the storage device, availability of stored data is impacted and thus system performance, for example, queries for clinical studies are compromised.
  - Other disadvantages of DAS are scalability and the inability to automate backup and minimize planned system downtime.
- Network attached storage (NAS)
  - Developed to address the inherent weaknesses of a server-based infrastructure such as DAS.
  - NAS is a file-based storage system with management software that is 100% dedicated to serving files over a network.

- NAS eliminates the need for the server supporting storage and responding to read/write responsibilities.
- Uses industry standard IP network technology and protocols (Transmission Control Protocol/Internet Protocol [TCP/IP], Common Internet File System [CIFS], and [NFS]).
- NAS can provide:

  Simple and cost-effective ways to achieve fast data access for multiple clients at the file level.

  Performance and productivity gains over DAS.

  Data protection features such as replication and mirroring for business continuance.

  Ability to consolidate DAS resources for better utilization.

  Scalability with storage capacity in the multi-terabyte range with efficient use of datacenter space.

- Storage area network (SAN)
  - A SAN is a dedicated, high-performance storage network that transfers data between servers and storage devices, separate from the local area network.
  - SAN moves data at the block level rather than at the file level

    as does DAS and NAS, thus it is ideal when large quantities of data must be moved.
  - Since the SAN operates on a block level and workstations operate at the file level, the PACS or other application must provide a block level to file level conversion.
  - A SAN environment is more costly, complex to manage, has many components, and requires sophisticated management software than other storage management environments; however, it provides superior:
    - Performance
    - 24/7 data availability
    - Reliability, with a high degree of fault tolerance
    - Scalability
    - Data protection
    - Storage virtualization
  - In a SAN infrastructure, storage devices such as DAS, NAS, RAID arrays, or tape libraries are connected to servers using fiber channel.
  - Since a SAN provides a high-speed connection between a storage device and a server,
    - The server can respond to the computations required by the applications without supporting the storage system.
    - Copies of the server's operating system and applications can reside on the storage systems supported by the SAN and can be rapidly restored should they fail.

- Fiber channel (FC)
  - FC is a gigabit-speed network technology used primarily for storage networking.
  - FC uses special cabling to move large volumes of data without the distance and bandwidth limitations of SCSI.
  - FC has transmission rates of 1, 2, 4, 8, 10, and 20 Gbps.
  - FC is highly reliable and enables simultaneous communication between workstations, mainframes, servers, data storage systems, and other peripherals.
- Hybrid SAN/NASs
  - Adds file interface to SAN
  - Supports NAS standards
  - Leverages a common storage infrastructure
- Internet Small Computer System Interface (iSCSI) Storage system
  - iSCSI uses IP networks rather than fiber channel to transmit data.
  - Unlike FC that requires special-purpose cabling and is more expensive, iSCSI can run existing, less expensive network infrastructure.
  - iSCSI enables data storage and retrieval from remote and independent storage systems because IP networks such as LANs, WANs, and the Internet are widely available.
  - iSCSI has transmission rates of 1 Gbps and 10 Gbps but require more overhead than FC.

7.6.3 Storage Management Software

Storage management software is primarily used for data protection, including:
- File backups
  - Daily backups of entire system, with continuous data redundancy
  - Used for VCF such as RIS or demographic database
  - Make daily manual backup to tape and stored in a secure off-site location
  - Various automate backup methods available; however, secure off-site copy must have
    - Replication
    - Point-in-time (PIT) copies
    - Continuous data protection
- Archiving
  - Used for FCF such as patient studies.
  - Can be automated using hierarchical storage management (HSM) application, grid storage, or clinical information lifecycle management application (CILM).
  - Can be performed manually by copying studies acquired each day to tape or other removable media and stored in a secure remote off-site location.
- Grid storage
  - Software application used to manage Tier 2 and Tier 3 storage of FCF at multiple geographically separated locations.

- Each location may have one or more nodes of the grid software operating on off-the-shelf hardware that manages a storage resource.
- Nodes are interconnected via network links and can process DICOM store and query requests from any node.

7.6.4 Cloud Storage

Cloud technology is transforming the architecture of imaging application delivery and storage. In many cases, facilities have determined that the purchase of on-site physical storage is not a cost-effective investment. The high upfront capital costs and physical space requirements combined with rapidly increasing media capacities make the cloud solutions an attractive alternative. Furthermore, newer storage methods (e.g., magnetic tape to magneto-optical Jukeboxes to spinning disk RAIDs) have the potential to render established archives obsolete or lacking support for the clinical workflow.

- Cloud storage is service based.
  - The service is designed to serve the specific needs of a set of consumers.
  - The performance of cloud storage is based on service level agreements and response time, not on technology limitations.
- Is scalable and elastic.
  - The service can scale capacity up or down as the consumer demands.
  - This scalability is a feature of the underlying storage infrastructure.
  - Elasticity is a trait of shared pools of resources.
- Is shared.
  - The underlying infrastructure, software, and/or platforms are shared among the storage users. IT resources are used with maximum efficiency.
- Is metered by use.
- Applies the standards of Internet technologies.
- Types of Clouds
  - SaaS (Software as a Service): Cloud providers install and operate application software in the cloud and cloud users access the software from cloud clients.
  - PaaS (Platform as a Service): Cloud providers deliver a computing platform including operating system, programming language execution environment, database, and web server.
  - IaaS (Infrastructure as a Service): Cloud providers offer computers—as physical or virtual machines, raw storage, firewalls, load balancers, and networks.
- Introduces unique challenges in PHI and privacy compliance.
- Application Service Provider (ASP)
  - Many vendors now utilize cloud technologists to offer an ASP Contract Version.
  - These ASP contracts can be structured as a SaaS or an IaaS model.
  - Contract imposes a charge per study and/or a fixed monthly recurring charge.
  - May be penalties for exceeding contracted study volumes.

7.6.5 *Vendor Neutral Archive (VNA)*

Most PACS vendors would prefer to control the data storage of images. But storage technology is commoditized, so that third-party storage solutions can be appended to the PACS.

- Advantages include:
  - Provides a comprehensive imaging record for patients across an enterprise
  - Patient Centric—view of all image types from different departments
  - Scalable image and data storage with Life Cycle Management
  - Ability to query and retrieve images and related information
  - Use open standards
  - Transparent to vendor changes and upgrades
  - Does not require data migrations, conversions, or changes to data formats or interfaces
- Caveats include:
  - Must maintain patient privacy and security
  - Any viewing, acquisition, and workflow management components use compatible interfaces

7.7 Compression of Medical Images

7.7.1 *Basic Concepts*

- Reasons to compress medical images

  KEY CONCEPT:
  Compressed Storage

  The image format from which the diagnosis is made *must* be the format in which the study is stored.

  - Decrease transmission times for medical images
  - Decrease storage requirements for medical images
  - Decrease bandwidth requirements for the transmission of medical images
  - Reduce cost for storage management and infrastructure
- Caveats
  - The primary justification for compressing FCF DICOM objects is reducing the time to transmit an image from one location to another that directly affects productivity and reduces storage requirements and cost.
  - Studies interpreted based on a lossless compressed image **must** be stored in lossless compressed format.

- Studies interpreted based on a lossy compressed image MUST be stored using the same lossy compression algorithm.
- All medical images must be stored in either a lossless or lossy DICOM compliant compression format.
- Proprietary compression formats.
    Will negatively impact interoperability of images and data migration
    Can lock you into your current PACS vendor

7.7.2 Lossless Compression

- Run length encoding (RLE)
    - Uses the redundancy within the image to decrease the image size
    - Replaces sequences of the same data values within a file by a count number and a single value
- Reduces image size between 1.8 and 2.8 depending on modality and body part

> **DEFINITION: Lossless Compression**
>
> Digital data compression in which all the original data information is preserved and can be completely reconstituted.

7.7.3 Lossy Compression

- Primarily used for web distribution of images to the enterprise for review purposes rather than primary interpretation.
- Lossy compression ratios must be stated on each image of a study.
- Study can be restored without clinically significant data loss.
- Lossy compression ratios depend on body part and modality.
- Typical compression ratios used when interpreting lossy compressed images.
    - DR and CR: 20 to 1
    - CT: 10 to 1
    - MR: 5 to 1

> **DEFINITION: Lossy Compression**
>
> Methods of digital compression in which the original information cannot be completely reconstituted.

PEARLS

- Eliminate isolated silos of storage and implement an enterprise storage solution such as a vendor-neutral archive.
- There are various storage media types and storage architectures to choose from. Be aware of the major acronyms in this field.
- Estimating storage requirements is at best an educated guess. Plan for the future, not the present.
- Understand the privacy requirements that apply to stored medical data.
- Retention and destruction of medical data require well-reasoned policies and strict adherence. Do not delete data to make space—buy more space to make space.

Self-Assessment Questions

1. Which of the following is an advantage of departmental storage over enterprise storage?

   (a) Vendor independence and best-of-breed purchasing
   (b) Reduced cost of hardware and licensing fees
   (c) Ease of providing redundancy
   (d) Ease of initial setup

2. Which of the following is true about the economics of storage management?

   (a) Once storage is purchased, it is no longer an ongoing annual budget item.
   (b) Media itself accounts for approximately 50% of the total cost of storage.
   (c) Storage costs include personnel, utilities, datacenter space, and data backup.
   (d) Technological obsolescence will require upgrades approximately every 10 years.

3. Regarding datacenters, which of the following is true?

   (a) Tier 4 is the highest Tier rating for datacenters.
   (b) The IT Department is responsible for specifying the characteristics of the resources and the availability requirements.
   (c) Power and cooling represent a small cost fraction of datacenter costs.
   (d) 24/7 information availability is desirable, but not necessary.

4. The retention period for PHI depends on all of the following EXCEPT:

   (a) Age of patient
   (b) Gender of patient
   (c) Federal statues
   (d) State statutes

5. Which of the following must be documented when destroying PHI?

   (a) Method of destruction
   (b) Inclusive dates covered
   (c) Statement that the records were destroyed in the normal course of business
   (d) All of the above

6. Which of the following is an example of optical media?

   (a) DVD
   (b) Hard drive
   (c) Tape drive
   (d) Flash drive

7. Which of the following is **not** a form of network storage?

   (a) RAID
   (b) SAN
   (c) NAS
   (d) VNA
   (e) Cloud

8. A Tier 4 datacenter with a guaranteed availability of 99.995% allows for how much downtime per year?

   (a) None
   (b) 5.25 minutes/year
   (c) 26.28 minutes/year
   (d) 52.56 minutes/year

9. How frequently would you schedule an event to remove imaging data that was due for deletion?

Chapter 8
Data Security and Patient Privacy

James Whitfill

Contents

8.1 Background

8.1.1 Definitions

8.1.1.1 Patient Privacy

- Patient privacy refers to the right of patients to determine when, how, and to what extent their health information is shared with others.
- It includes maintaining confidentiality while sharing identifying data or protected health information (PHI), only with those healthcare providers and related professionals who need to know in the course of caring for the patient.

J. Whitfill (✉)
Internal Medicine and Biomedical Informatics, University of Arizona College of Medicine
Phoenix, Phoenix, AZ, USA
e-mail: JWhitfill@honorhealth.com

© The Author(s), under exclusive license to Springer Science+Business Media, LLC, part of Springer Nature 2021
B. F. Branstetter IV (ed.), *Practical Imaging Informatics*,
https://doi.org/10.1007/978-1-0716-1756-4_8

8.1.1.2   Data Security

- Information security includes the measures healthcare providers must take to protect patients' PHI from unauthorized access or breaches.
- Security also refers to maintaining the integrity of electronic medical information and ensuring availability to those who need access and are authorized to view such clinical data, including images, for the purposes of patient care.
- Research and educational activities are not exempt from the privacy and security requirements for PHI.
- Institutional policies protect the privacy of individually identifiable health information while allowing reasonable access to medical information by the researcher, educator, or trainee.
  The basic techniques involved include:
- Physical safeguards: include device isolation, allowing direct physical access only to authorized personnel; backing up of data and maintaining copies and emergency contingency protocols; and proper device disposal
- Technical safeguards: include firewalls and secure transmission modes for communication such as virtual private networks (VPN) or secure sockets layer (SSL) and encryption techniques.
- Administrative safeguards: include requirements for documenting departmental security policies, training staff about these policies, maintaining audit trails of all system logs by user identification and activity, enforcing policies for storage and retention of electronic data and backup of all systems, adhering to specific methods for incident reporting and resolution of security issues, and clearly documenting accountability, sanctions, and disciplinary actions for violation of policies and procedures.

> **FURTHER READING:**
> **Patient Privacy**
>
> Andriole KP, Khorasani R. Patient Privacy and Security of Electronic Medical Information for Radiologists: The Basics. JACR. 2010; 7(6):397–9

PACS and other image management systems must incorporate the following components within their system security policies and procedures:
- Authorization
- Authentication
- Availability
- Confidentiality
- Data integrity
- Nonrepudiation

8.1.2 History

Cybercrime generally follows a simple economic formula. If the rewards of the crime are greater than the risks and costs of the attack, then an attack is likely. Conversely, if one raises the barriers to attack, by raising either the risks or the cost, then the odds of an attack fall.

- Rewards can come in many different forms, but the two dominant types are **financial and political**. Financial rewards can be either **direct or indirect**:
  - Examples of direct financial rewards: stealing someone's identity in order to take out debt in their name; stealing credit card information; and black market sale of PHI.
  - In the late 2010s, indirect forms of financial rewards became more prevalent. In this case the data affected by the crime is not sold but held for ransom, and the owner of the data is extorted to pay money to get that data back.

> **KEY CONCEPT: Stolen PHI**
>
> Because health information has so much personal information attached to it, black market prices for a stolen medical record are 10 times that of an email account and 50 times that of a social security number. This value difference highlights the attractiveness of a target like protected health information. E-commerce sites on the dark web have databases of PHI that are available for hundreds of thousands of dollars.

> **DEFINITION: Ransomware**
>
> A form of cybercrime with indirect financial rewards. Critical data is encrypted, and payment is demanded in exchange for the de-encryption key. The healthcare industry has become a major target of ransomware attacks.
>
> Ransomware is the greatest threat most health systems face. When activated, it usually renders all computer systems inoperable. Recovery can take days to weeks.

- The amount of financial return from ransomware caused a rapid shift in the cybercrime economy. Between 2016 and 2017, the revenue from ransomware rose from $24 million per year to $1 billion in just 12 months. At the time, a "do it yourself" ransomware kit is sold for only $10 US, showing that the ease of entry for new criminals was very low.
- Initially the rise of ransomware did not impact healthcare, but the global attack by the WannaCry malware in May 2017 impacted multiple industries:
  - Most notably, the United Kingdom's National Health Service had multiple systems taken offline, including phone systems and EHR systems.

- As clinical workflows fell back to paper, the throughput in emergency departments plummeted to 10% of normal capability.
- Equally concerning, OR cases had to be cancelled including cardiothoracic surgeries for patients with life-threatening conditions.
- WannaCry revealed that healthcare enterprises were inviting targets, and attacks on health systems spiked across the globe. In the first half of 2019 alone, healthcare was the #3 target for ransomware globally, and 491 institutions were attacked.
- 99% of the time, ransom was demanded in bitcoin.
- While cyber insurance generally covered these ransoms, the skyrocketing cost of premiums has led some municipal systems to stop paying ransoms.
- The city of Baltimore famously spent $18 million to avoid a $76 K ransom, and Atlanta spent $17 million to avoid a $52 K ransom. The reason for this approach was the escalating cost of ransomware payments.

> **KEY CONCEPT: Targeted vs. Untargeted Attacks**
>
> A cyberattack may be targeted at a specific healthcare entity either for financial or personal reasons. There may be a specific individual at the institution who is vulnerable to extortion or in league with the cybercriminals. Most attacks, however, are untargeted – infiltration attempts are directed at many institutions in the hopes of getting one or two hits.

> **FURTHER READING: The Cost of Cyberinsurance**
>
> https://www.cpomagazine.com/cyber-security/ransomware-attacks-are-causing-cyber-insurance-rates-to-go-through-the-roof-premiums-up-as-much-as-25-percent/

8.1.3 Regulations

- Information Security Regulatory Laws are covered more completely in **Chap. 30**:
  1. HIPPA (Health Insurance Portability and Accountability Act)
     (a) US-based
     (b) Enforced by office of civil rights
     (c) Focused on privacy and security of health information
     (d) Gives guidance on topics but does not call for standards:
        (i) For example, health information in transit should be encrypted, but the law does not specify what kind of encryption.
  2. HITECH (Health Information Technology for Economic and Clinical Health Act)
     (a) US-based
     (b) Expanded protections for information systems with a focus on EMRs

        (c) Attached to Federal "Meaningful Use" policies
- 3. GDPR (General Data Protection Regulation)
  - (a) EU-based
  - (b) Focuses on privacy of data more than security
- Compliance vs. cyberthreat mitigation
  - Early efforts at cybersecurity were focused on regulatory compliance with the above rules.
  - In the last 5–8 years, the rise of attacks on health systems has required more than just a focus on regulatory compliance.

8.1.4 Targets and Adversaries

Healthcare systems are in inviting target for cybercriminals. Most attacks focus on obtaining financially valuable information such as PHI. But some attacks escalate to directly threaten patient health.

Cybercriminals have varied motivations that may affect the type of attack or the target of the attack.

CHECKLIST: Healthcare Targets for Cybercriminals

Listed in order of threat level to patients:

1. Personally identifiable information
2. Personal health information
3. Patient health
4. Healthcare infrastructure

CHECKLIST: Types of Cybercriminals

- **Individuals**
  - Motivated by profit and fame
- **Political groups/paparazzi**
  - Motivated by political and commercial advantage
- **Organized crime**
  - Motivated by money or extortion
- **Terrorism**
  - Motivated to cause fear and harm
- **Nation-states**
  - May target individuals, state leaders, or entire companies and countries

8.2 Attacks on Patient Health

While traditional cyberattacks pose a threat to patients' information, researchers have grown increasingly worried about threats to patient health itself. This may take the form of direct attacks on a particular patient or an attack on the healthcare infrastructure.

FURTHER READING: Attacks on Patient Health

"Securing Hospitals". Independent Security Evaluators https://www.ise.io/wpcontent/uploads/2017/07/securing_hospitals.pdf www.securityevaluators.com

CHECKLIST: Potential Targets of Patient Health Attacks

- Active medical devices
  - Interrupt lifesaving action or modify to deliver lethal results
- Medicines
  - Destroy inventory, change allergy records, and change dosage delivery
- Surgery
  - Change work order and medical records, disrupt remote access, disrupt environment, and disrupt equipment
- Clinicians
  - Misdirection or misinformation

- One important vector of attack on patient health comes from medical devices. The software systems in these items often have multiple vendors or sources, and the device often is used for years longer than the software code is maintained. This results in multiple vulnerabilities that can allow a malicious actor to take over the device:
  - The first example of this was the Hospira PCA3 infusion pump, which received the first FDA safety communication for a software security vulnerability.
- Medical devices open up an entire new front in the cyberwar that threatens patient health. Common issues with devices include:
  - Failure to provide timely security patches and updates to medical devices and address vulnerabilities related to legacy devices

FURTHER READING: Health Care Industry Cybersecurity Task Force: Improving Cybersecurity in the Health Care Industry

https://www.phe.gov/preparedness/planning/cybertf/documents/report2017.pdf

  - Malware
  - Unauthorized access to the network
  - Device reprogramming caused by malware or unauthorized access to the network
  - Denial of service attacks
  - Poor password management

- Poorly designed software security features for off-the-shelf products
- Poor configuration of networks and security practices
- Failure to close unused ports
- By 2018 the US Food and Drug Administration responded to this growing threat of medical devices and created a Safety Action Plan with the following areas of focus:
  - Establishment of a robust medical device patient safety net in the USA.
  - Exploration of regulatory options to streamline and modernize timely implementation of post-market mitigations
  - Innovation toward safer medical devices
  - Advancement of medical device cybersecurity
  - Integration of CDRH's (the FDA's Center for Devices and Radiological Health) pre-market and post-market offices and activities to advance the use of a Total Product Life Cycle (TPLC) approach to device safety
- In response to this growing concern, the National Electrical Manufacturers Association created the Manufacturer Disclosure Statement for Medical Device Security or MDS2:
  - A vendor document that should be available on every healthcare device sold
  - Contains a list of the software systems embedded in the device and the known vulnerabilities

8.3 Network Attacks

Early networks allowed any connected device to communicate with any other connected device. Services like DHCP (Dynamic Host Configuration Protocol) were created to make adding items to a network easier. However, due to the need to secure internal networks, most networks use Network Access Control systems to assign and manage permissions of devices.

DEFINITION: Promiscuous Mode

A DICOM receiver can be set to accept data from any network device (promiscuous) or can be set to only accept data from pre-defined, known senders (non-promiscuous). These settings can be useful when troubleshooting errors.

SYNONYMS: Network Access Control

- Client Validation
- Node Validation
- Network Admission Control
- Network Access Control
- Network Access Protection
- Secured Networking
- Assured Networking

> **KEY CONCEPT: Network Access Control**
>
> A new modality needs to be defined within the Network Access Control system and within the DICOM objects in order to function correctly.

This extends into DICOM devices, which can be set to be either promiscuous, which means they will accept a DICOM object from any other network node, or non-promiscuous, which means a DICOM object has to be defined in the receiving system before being allowed to send information.

Chapter 6 contains more detailed information about computer networks.

8.4 Social Engineering

Cybercriminals can gain access to your computer network in several ways. With robust digital security measures in place, the weak link in cybersecurity is usually an unsuspecting authorized computer user in your enterprise. Taking advantage of these human weaknesses to gain illicit access to a computer network is called social engineering.

> **FURTHER READING: Social Engineering**
>
> Mores, Julio. Social Engineering in the Modern World. Harcourt Brace 2006.

8.4.1 Phishing

- Phishing
  - Fake emails used to obtain passwords.
  - Usually mimics a familiar website such as payment systems, banks, or software companies.
  - Benign-appearing links in the email may allow malicious software onto the network.

> **DEFINITION: Phishing**
>
> A form of social engineering in which an email is sent that mimics a legitimate business communication. The goal is to trick the recipient into revealing passwords or accidentally accepting malicious code into the network.

- Phone
  - Calling user and convincing them to share username and passwords or to go to a website and click on an item in order to execute code on their system. Common examples include claiming to be for the user's IT department and doing a security audit.
- Spear phishing
  - Targeted email at a user and which contains content that is specific to that user so as to gain trust
- Altruism exploits
  - Pretending to be a family member to obtain protected health information

8.4.2 Protection Systems

- Intrusion detection system
  - Computer systems which contain both logging (to track attempts at attack) and also "honeypots" which are directories or systems which appear attractive to hackers and entice them to break in, which activates logging and additional security.
- Regularly test your users with safe but authentic-appearing phishing attempts, and use the results of these campaigns for education.
- Prevent unknown USB devices from connecting to the network.
- Review your vendor's code vulnerabilities.

> **DEFINITION: Physical Security**
>
> The physical environment around a computer system that prevents unauthorized access to equipment. Examples include locks, security guards, video cameras, and biometric devices. Hospitals are notoriously weak at physical security because they want to appear welcoming to patients and families.

> **DEFINITION: Trojan Horse**
>
> Malicious code that accompanies useful code onto the system during a download or routine maintenance

OUR EXPERIENCE: Network Viruses

In July 2003, our academic medical center was infected with the FunLove4099 virus. The initial vector of infection was our corporate Intranet web server, which was missing one critical security patch. Once the server was infected, it infected client desktops whenever they viewed an infected web page. Infected clients quickly infected other desktops, network drives, servers, and individual files. Overall network performance dropped to a standstill.

We were forced to disconnect our network from the Internet for 2 days because our firewalls couldn't handle the virus attack traffic. The first night was spent working closely with our antivirus vendor to get virus signature data files. These were quickly distributed to all machines on our network.

It took us 2 weeks to locate and clean infected files across the network. We had to shut down many ports if the owners didn't have up-to-date contact info. We tightened access controls to virtually all network files.

KEY LESSONS LEARNED

- Keep critical patches up-to-date.
- Have an incident handling process in place before trouble arrives.
- Assign proper permissions; not every user should be an admin on their desktop.
- Have IDS or IPS at key locations throughout the network.
- Critical alerts must be communicated by pager 24/7.

- Ask for your vendor's MDS2 (Manufacturer Disclosure Statement for Medical Device Security).
- Be wary of a product with "zero" vulnerabilities. It means no testing has been done.
- Use the 80/20 principle; you don't have to scan or segment every piece of equipment but should assess and prioritize areas that have the most critical vulnerabilities and the most dangerous impact.

8.5 Future Threats

Most attacks on healthcare systems were thought to be largely untargeted. While encryption would render their data unusable until a ransom was paid, the clinical findings and data itself were not altered. However, by 2018, new forms of vulnerability in both HL7 and DICOM data transmission showed that these systems were vulnerable to man-in-the-middle attacks.

> **DEFINITION: Man in the Middle**
>
> A cyberattack in which the attacker places a device on the network within an institution and is able to intercept or modify the traffic from a sending system to a receiving system

- A malicious tool called Pestilence is able to intercept lab values from a laboratory information system being sent to an electronic medical care record:
    - Serum potassium levels and blood type are two examples of records that if altered in transit could cause lethal consequences for patients assuming subsequent treatment decisions were based on these incorrect data.
- For IIPs, a terrifying development occurred in mid-2019 when researchers were able to show how a DICOM object could be intercepted in a similar man-in-the-middle attack and pathology could be added or removed from the image by use of a type of deep learning called an adversarial network:
    - When nodules were introduced that were not actually present, 99% of radiologists and AI systems diagnosed the patient as having a malignant finding.
    - When malignant findings were actually present but were removed, 94% of the time a diagnosis of no disease present was given.
    - Even when the readers were told that the images had been tampered with, 60–90% of the time, they were still fooled.
- Deep learning techniques and artificial intelligence introduce another potential vulnerability:
    - One famous example is a deep learning algorithm that was trained to diagnose pandas, but with the introduction of noise into the image, which did not affect the image to the human eye, the diagnostic algorithm thought the image was a gibbon (https://arxiv.org/abs/1412.6572).
    - Similar techniques might wreak havoc in AI interpretations without leaving any evidence that can be identified by humans.

PEARLS

- Threats in the cyberlandscape are evolving rapidly.
- Threats previously targeted personal information and then protected health information, but the latest threats target patient health.
- Cybersecurity has had to pivot from a compliance-based activity to focus on continued threat response and counterattack models.
- Ransomware is the primary area of growth, but nation-state activity is a looming threat.
- Phishing and other forms of social engineering are important tools in the cybercriminal's toolkit.

Self-Assessment Questions

1. Social engineering is:

   A. A type of phishing
   B. A form of physical security
   C. A way to prevent cyberattacks
   D. A less-intensive type of graduate engineering degree
   E. A means of obtaining illicit access to a computer network

2. Ransomware is:

   A. A cyberattack that results in direct financial rewards
   B. Less important to healthcare than to other industries
   C. A type of cybercrime that has been around for decades
   D. A threat to patient health
   E. A countermeasure employed by hospital security teams

3. Which of these is most valuable to a cybercriminal?

   A. Social security number
   B. Email address
   C. Protected health information
   D. Medical record number
   E. Telephone number

4. Which of these is immune to cyberattack?

   A. Medications
   B. Medical devices
   C. Laboratory results
   D. CT images
   E. None of the above

5. A hacker posing as a member of the IT team to obtain passwords is an example of:

   A. Sniffing
   B. Social engineering
   C. Intrusion detection
   D. Probing
   E. Log analysis

6. Place these potential targets in order from least dangerous to most dangerous:

   A. Patient health
   B. Personal health information
   C. Healthcare infrastructure
   D. Personally identifiable information

7. List several reasons for the increasing frequency and complexity of network security attacks.

Chapter 9
PACS and Other Image Management Systems

Nikki Fennell, Matthew D. Ralston, and Robert M. Coleman

Contents

9.1 Introduction: What Is PACS?

Picture Archiving and Communications System (PACS) is the core technological infrastructure for enabling the management of digital medical imaging. The primary functions of a PACS are storage, distribution, and

> **DEFINITION 9.1: PACS**
>
> Picture Archiving and Communications Systems store, distribute, and display digital medical images.

display of images. PACS functionality is further strengthened when integrated with other clinical application infrastructure, such as the hospital information system (HIS), the electronic medical record (EMR) or electronic health record (EHR), the

N. Fennell (✉)
Radiology Partners, El Segundo, CA, USA
e-mail: Nfennell2170@gmail.com

M. D. Ralston · R. M. Coleman
Maine Medical Center, Portland, ME, USA

© The Author(s), under exclusive license to Springer Science+Business Media, LLC, part of Springer Nature 2021
B. F. Branstetter IV (ed.), *Practical Imaging Informatics*,
https://doi.org/10.1007/978-1-0716-1756-4_9

radiology information system (RIS), and dictation or voice recognition (VR) report generation systems.

KEY CONCEPT 9.2: CIIP

A Certified Imaging Informatics Professional (CIIP) earns and maintains a nationally recognized credential demonstrating a commitment to and understanding of clinical healthcare and information technology in the field of imaging informatics. The American Board of Imaging Informatics (ABII) is the credentialing organization for the IIP certification and was founded in 2007 as a collaborative effort between the Society for Imaging Informatics in Medicine (SIIM) and the American Registry of Radiologic Technologists (ARRT).

Management of PACS is complex and requires skilled personnel both for the initial deployment and for ongoing system and application support. Ensuring that PACS is administered by qualified imaging informatics professionals is imperative to the overall success of a PACS program.

A new or replacement PACS implementation typically involves a combination of expenses for system hardware, software, and services. This is fundamentally different from traditional large imaging department purchases, like a CT or MRI scanner, in that PACS is not regarded as a revenue generator. It can be a challenge to quantify; however, the real value of a modern PACS comes in the improvements to diagnostic capabilities and operational efficiencies. Given the volume of medical imaging examinations and the number of images generated per study, it is difficult to imagine operating a modern radiology department without a PACS.

FURTHER READING: Return on Investment

Chan L, Trambert M, Kywi A, Hartzman S. PACS in private practice-effect on profits and productivity. J Digit Imaging. 2002;15 Suppl 1:131–6.

9.2 History of PACS

- The initial concept of PACS can be traced back to Dr. Richard Steckel in 1972.
- The first large-scale PACS was implemented at the University of Kansas in 1982.
- First-generation PACS adopters encountered many challenges with the review and archival of imaging studies across disparate platforms due to proprietary formats:
  - This gave rise to a concerted effort to create an interoperability standard.
  - In the early 1980s, the American College of Radiology (ACR) and the National Electrical Manufacturers Association (NEMA) initiated work on the formation of what is now known as the DICOM (Digital Imaging and Communications in Medicine) standard.

The **DICOM Standard** has evolved to be the primary source that defines the formats for medical images that can be exchanged with the data and quality consistency necessary for clinical use.

> **KEY CONCEPT 9.4: DICOM**
>
> Digital Imaging and Communications in Medicine is *the* international standard to transmit, store, retrieve, print, process, and display medical imaging information (see **Chap. 12**).

9.3 Core Components of Traditional PACS Architecture

Traditional PACS architecture contains a variety of components, and each organization's environment will be different based on numerous factors. Figure 9.1 depicts one example.

9.3.1 Acquisition Devices

- **Modalities** are the machines that acquire patient imaging, such as an MRI, CT, or US scanner.
- **Specialized workstations** are image post-processing systems that are generally a component of a modality like a CT scanner, but can also refer to standalone computers that deliver access to third-party software for advanced image processing.

> **DEFINITION: Modality**
>
> The word "modality" may refer to a technology used to create images (e.g., CT) or to a specific machine that is producing images (e.g., CT scanner #3 in the emergency department).

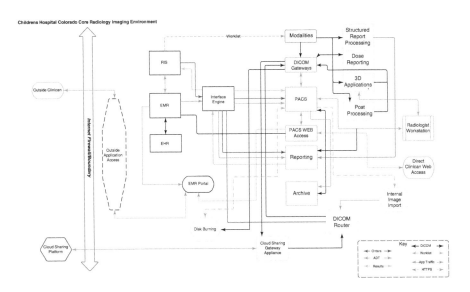

Fig. 9.1 Example of an integrated PACS environment

- The reading stations where radiologists view images are another type of special-ized workstation. Although these workstations do not always produce new con-tent for the PACS, there may be annotations or post-processing built into these workstations that need to be permanently stored.

9.3.2 Network

Network design plays a very important role in PACS architecture (see **Chap. 6**). Ideally the network is configured to process PACS traffic on a VLAN (virtual local area network) that is segregated from other enterprise data traffic for increased performance, through-put, and high reliability. This is also important for information security to enable protec-tions on patient health information (PHI) in the event of a security breach.

9.3.3 Archive

A PACS image archive may be hosted in a variety of locations including on-premise in either a designated or shared storage capacity, off-site data centers, and off-site storage within the cloud. The archive should be structurally redundant and physi-cally reside in at least two locations to meet business continuity and disaster recov-ery needs. Most data archives are built upon various **tiers of storage** determined by organizational structure and needs:

- **Short-term storage** is designed to make data quickly accessible. In an image archive, this is typi-cally where current exam data is housed as well as recently acquired exam data. The informa-tion lifecycle management (ILM)

> **SYNONYMS 9.8: Storage Tiers**
>
> Short-term storage = online, near-line, hot, and active
> Long-term storage = offline, passive, and cold

  timeframe is generally defined by physician requirements. Short-term archives are smaller in size due to the higher costs associated with specified fast-perform-ing storage media.
- **Long-term storage** is generally inactive or infrequently altered. A long-term archive is typically used for older exam data or historical reference data that will seldom be recalled for comparison review. Long-term archives are larger in size due to the lower costs of assigned storage media that offers less performance capability.
- For a more complete discussion of data storage, see **Chap. 7**.

> **KEY CONCEPT 9.6: Network Terms**
>
> **LAN** is a local area network that connects local devices to each other.
> **WAN** is a wide area network that connects LANs to each other.
> **Gateways** are the point of entry for devices external to a defined network, and they act as the protocol convertor which allows data to flow between networks.
> **Switches** connect devices on the network using packet switching to receive and forward data to network destinations.
> **Routers** are devices that analyze the contents of packets transmitted within the network and determine the best route for information to travel.

9.3.4 Database

The database is the heart of a PACS and responsible for the organization and management of images and their associated information within the system. Pertinent data elements included within the database are:

> **KEY CONCEPT: Thin vs. Thick Clients**
>
> Thick clients are software that is installed on a workstation with strict hardware dependencies. Thin clients generally work through a web browser and do not require specific installation on the workstation.

- Patient demographics
- Associated reports
- Study or exam descriptions
- Where the images were obtained
- Where the images are stored in the archive

High-volume PACS environments can benefit from the use of DICOM routers or gateways to evenly distribute image ingestion and export from the archive, and to assist with balancing the workload of the database.

9.3.5 Image Viewers

While the design and means of distribution for PACS image viewing software continues to evolve, this software generally falls under two distinct models:

> **FURTHER READING 9.10: PACS Clients**
>
> Toland, C., Meenan, C., Toland, M. *et al.* A Suggested Classification Guide for PACS Client Applications: The Five Degrees of Thickness. *J Digit Imaging* 19, 78–83 (2006). https://doi.org/10.1007/s10278-006-0930-z

- Web-based and thin client viewers, often called "clinical" viewers, utilize existing web technologies to render image data for display and are easy to access and manage. Zero-footprint viewers are included here.

- Web-deployable or designated workstation thick clients, often called "diagnostic" viewers, have direct licensing and increased hardware dependencies and require more overall support.

9.3.6 Radiology Information System (RIS)

- The RIS is the application that technologists, radiology administrators, and other department staff utilize for most of their daily workflow activities. Staff can enter, edit, and update patient order and exam information in the RIS.

> **SYNONYMS: Thin Client**
>
> Web-based viewer
> Zero-footprint viewer
> Clinical viewer

- In an integrated clinical systems environment, the RIS receives and processes initial patient and order information from a HIS, EMR, or EHR.
- The RIS is responsible for generating the unique exam **accession numbers** that are necessary for tracking studies in PACS.

> **DEFINITION: Accession Number**
>
> A unique identifier for a single billable examination. From an accession number, your PACS database can determine which patient, what date, and what type of exam was performed. Sometimes, a single examination is coded with multiple accession numbers, only some of which have associated images.

- RIS functionality has been incorporated as a direct module or component of most large medical record systems eliminating the need for a separate system.
- The RIS may also be configured to receive results information from a third-party VR system.
- The protocol the RIS uses for communicating with other systems is Health Level 7 (HL7; see **Chap. 12**).

> **FURTHER READING 9.13: Enterprise Imaging**
>
> Enterprise Imaging White Papers (2020). Society for Imaging Informatics in Medicine.   https://siim.org/general/custom.asp?page=himss_siim_white_pap. Accessed 10 Sep 2020.

9.3.7 Interface Engine/PACS Broker

- An interface engine or PACS broker is responsible for processing messaging between PACS and other connected systems such as the RIS, HIS, EMR, EHR, and VR.
- The engine/broker is the bridge that converts HL7 messages into DICOM format, and vice versa.

9.4 Other Image Management Systems

- **EMR/EHR integrated storage**: It is common for EMR/EHR vendors to offer a form of integrated storage, which can also be referred to as **enterprise content management (ECM)**. While primarily used for medical document management, photos like those captured in dermatology or surgical wound care often find a storage home here.

> **KEY CONCEPT 9.11: HL7**
>
> Health Level 7 is a comprehensive framework and related standards for the exchange, integration, sharing, and retrieval of electronic health information that supports clinical practice and the management, delivery, and evaluation of health services (see **Chap. 12**).

- **Departmental or specialty image storage (mini-PACS)**: Different departments or specialties, such as cardiology and ophthalmology, may have their own PACS which are sometimes referred to as "mini-PACS." These systems offer clinicians targeted image review tools, typically with limited capabilities for integrating with the HIS, EMR, or EHR. Alternatively, other departments may piggyback on the full radiology PACS, and store and view their imaging studies there.

- **Point-of-care ultrasound (POCUS)**: POCUS vendors offer focused application software with associated storage configurations designed for use in conjunction with their devices. Elements of the POCUS image-capture workflow differ greatly from traditional PACS workflow, and may require added functions like data entry, reporting, image storage, billing, credentialing, and quality assurance for specialty programs to achieve optimal clinical use.

> **DEFINITION: POCUS**
>
> Ultrasound machines have become small, inexpensive, and safe for non-radiology personnel to use. These machines may be scattered around the hospital and used by other healthcare providers to augment their physical examinations. This is referred to as point-of-care ultrasound.

Enterprise archive or vendor-neutral archive (VNA): Enterprise Imaging strategies have been the driving force behind the increased adoption of enterprise
archives and vendor-neutral archives. These repositories are capable of ingesting and storing data objects in both DICOM and non-DICOM formats, allowing
for integrated image storage at the enterprise level. Architected to be the core
infrastructure of an Enterprise Imaging platform, they enable standards-based
services for enterprise-level image management (see **Chap. 7**).

9.5 Imaging Workflow Elements of PACS and Other Image Management Systems

The basic imaging workflow elements that PACS and other image
management systems facilitate
include:

- Acquisition and storage of studies
- Validation of DICOM and HL7 data
- Retrieval and display of studies and reports by image consumers (i.e., radiologists, other physicians, clinical staff)
- Automated retrieval and display of pertinent comparison studies
- Added support for additional image consumer needs, such as technologist quality assurance or the production of discs for distribution by a digital librarian

DEFINITION 9.14: Nighthawk

Preliminary interpretations provided
for studies performed overnight and on
weekends. A nighthawk radiologist or
reading service is tasked with interpreting studies within a few minutes of
receipt, and then sending back preliminary reports. This is a service used by
many healthcare organizations, particularly those that do not have radiologists available to provide 24×7 onsite
support.

9.6 Valuable Imaging Workflow Advances Made Possible by PACS and Other Image Management Systems

- Integrated programmable peer review
- Asynchronous communication tools, such as those used with ED physicians
- Inclusion of nighthawk reads
- Feedback mechanisms for over-reading of studies, as with resident workflows
- Digital teaching files
- Shared conference or interdisciplinary learning files

OUR EXPERIENCE: Redesigning the Outside Imaging Workflow

At Children's Hospital Colorado, we treat patients from all over the world, and those patients come with prior imaging performed at other institutions. This imaging arrives via various methods including cloud sharing, optical discs, VPNs, and even occasionally physical film. The volume and diversity of outside imaging has warranted an entire team of staff members dedicated to ensuring the studies get ingested and tracked into PACS appropriately. Historically this work was all performed manually, leaving a lot of room for improvement.

Last year a representative from the imaging informatics team was selected to lead a Green Belt process improvement project, with the focus on streamlining the outside imaging workflow. The top complaints being received about the existing workflow came from our physicians and included (1) the need to enter an order for every outside exam upload request and (2) the overall length of time it took from the exam arriving at our door to its availability for review in PACS. The Green Belt project was subsequently designed to solve these two key challenges.

Using a DICOM router and corresponding HL7 tools, a process was created to automate order creation in the EMR/RIS upon receipt of a study, and then appropriately edit and route the updated study directly into production PACS. After extensive assessment, testing, and optimization, the new and improved process was launched this March. There were many positive changes that occurred as a result of this work, but the key areas of impact are below:

1. We eliminated the need for physicians/staff to place an order for any reference study.
2. We reduced the amount of time from exam arrival to review availability in PACS by 94%.

- Incorporated advanced visualization technologies
- Electronic transfer of DICOM imaging with other organizations
- Teleradiology
- Image-based data mining and research

FURTHER READING 9.15:
Teaching Files

Siddiqui, KM., Branstetter, BF.: Digital Teaching Files and Education. In: Dreyer, KJ., Hirschorn, DS., Thrall, JH., Mehta, A. (eds.) PACS: A Guide to the Digital Revolution, pp. 495–522. Springer, New York (2006)

PEARLS

- PACS as a concept has been around since the early 1970s, but practical systems were first put in place in the 1990s.
- The core components of a traditional PACS include:
  - Acquisition devices
  - The network
  - The archive
  - The database
  - Image viewers
  - The interface engine/broker
  - Other connected clinical systems like RIS and SR
- Other examples of systems where image management occurs include:
  - EMR/EHR integrated storage (ECM)
  - Departmental or specialty image storage (mini-PACS)
  - Point-of-care ultrasound (POCUS) systems
  - Enterprise archives or vendor-neutral archive (VNA)
- PACS and other image systems have enabled advanced imaging workflows such as:
  - Programmable peer review
  - Asynchronous communication
  - Inclusion of nighthawk interpretations
  - Feedback mechanisms for over-reads
  - Digital teaching files and shared conference files
  - Advanced visualization technology integration
  - Teleradiology
  - Image data mining for research

Self-Assessment Questions

1. The primary functions of PACS are storage, _____, and display of images.

   A. Integration
   B. Distribution
   C. Quality assurance
   D. Interpretation

2. The ACR and _____ are responsible for the creation of the DICOM standard.

   A. SIIM
   B. HIMSS
   C. NEMA
   D. ASNR

3. PACS acquisition devices include modalities such as CT, MR, US, and _____.

   A. Card scanners
   B. Microphones
   C. Keyboards
   D. PET

4. The primary protocol for transmitting medical images from modalities to PACS is:

   A. HL7
   B. IHE
   C. DICOM
   D. HIPAA

5. Which credential is the designated industry-recognized standard for professionals working in the field of imaging informatics?

   A. CISO
   B. DO
   C. CIIP
   D. MCSE

6. The PACS database is responsible for managing which pertinent data elements? Select all that apply:

   A. Patient demographics
   B. Associated reports
   C. Where the images are stored in the archive
   D. Where the images should be sent

7. Though technology continues to evolve, most PACS image viewers can be classified as web-based, thin client, _____, or thick clients.

   A. Browser
   B. Web-deployable
   C. HTML
   D. Solid state

8. Other systems that manage images besides PACS include:

   A. VNA
   B. RIS
   C. VR
   D. CDS

9. PACS provides basic imaging workflow elements such as:

   A. Acquisition and storage of studies
   B. Validation of DICOM and HL7 data
   C. Automated retrieval and display of pertinent comparison studies
   D. All of the above

10. Which of the following advances, when part of PACS or other image management systems, gives attending radiologists the ability to share important or interesting cases with residents for future review?

   A. Integrated programmed peer review
   B. Digital teaching files
   C. Incorporated advanced visualization technologies
   D. Teleradiology

Chapter 10
Ancillary Software

Tessa S. Cook

Contents

10.1 Introduction

In addition to PACS, RIS, and the EMR, there are a number of software applications used in an imaging department. Depending on the structure of the department and the organization in which it exists (e.g., academic teaching hospital, standalone community hospital, private practice, etc.), ancillary software is necessary to support a number of operational, educational, and quality improvement initiatives. In this chapter, we discuss some of those applications and the infrastructure that is typically needed to support them.

T. S. Cook (✉)
University of Pennsylvania School of Medicine, Philadelphia, PA, USA
e-mail: Tessa.Cook@pennmedicine.upenn.edu

© The Author(s), under exclusive license to Springer Science+Business Media, LLC, part of Springer Nature 2021
B. F. Branstetter IV (ed.), *Practical Imaging Informatics*,
https://doi.org/10.1007/978-1-0716-1756-4_10

10.2 Build Versus Buy

- The **build versus buy** question arises when an imaging practice has to decide whether the software solution they need exists and can be purchased or will have to be developed in-house.
- Commonly used software in a radiology practice, such as the PACS, RIS, and EMR, are most often purchased. However, some of the ancillary software applications discussed in this chapter are not available on the market, and imaging departments and practices have chosen to custom-build these solutions for their own use.

> **HYPOTHETICAL SCENARIO: Build Versus Buy**
>
> Suppose your imaging practice needs a software solution that would cost $100,000 to buy and support, but only $50,000 to build. While the home-built solution may seem less expensive at face value, this cost doesn't account for the support and maintenance, which can sometimes consume a substantial amount of a valuable employee's time.

- Advantages of **home-built** solutions include the potential for **customization** to the environment, greater knowledge of necessary data streams and interfaces, better **integration** into the clinical workflow, and easier navigation of any **governance approvals** or security clearances that may be required.
- Advantages of **commercial** solutions include **service contracts** that will provide application maintenance and updates, which would free up internal resources that might otherwise be consumed in the maintenance of a home-built solution.
- An organization that has chosen to build their own internal application may eventually have to decide whether to continue as is or **pivot** and invest in a commercial solution. Multiple factors will contribute to the decision, including the cost of maintenance, the frequency of updates, the short-term disruption associated with the transition, and the long-term return on investment.

10.3 Results Management

10.3.1 Critical Results

- Radiologists are required to notify ordering physicians/advanced practice providers (APPs) of **critical results** identified on imaging.
- This notification typically consists of a **nonroutine communication** (e.g., a phone call or electronic message, rather than

> **DEFINITION: Critical Result**
>
> According to the National Patient Safety Goals set forth by the Joint Commission, a critical result represents a finding that could threaten a patient's life.

solely relying on a note in the radiology report) soon after the study is interpreted. The ACR Practice Parameter for Communication of Diagnostic Imaging Findings provides guidelines on how to correctly document the communication of an imaging result.

- **Standardized documentation** of critical results is necessary for compliance with the National Patient Safety Goals established by the Joint Commission (TJC), and particularly for NPSG.02.03.01: "report critical results of tests and diagnostic procedures on a timely basis."

- Critical test results management (CTRM) systems can connect to the various software applications that the radiologist uses (PACS/RIS, EMR, report generation system, paging system) as well as alert the referring physician/APP, in an effort to establish **closed-loop communication** and provide options for escalation where necessary.

- Depending on the CTRM system, alerts may take the form of phone calls, electronic pages, or text messages. The CTRM system will continue to attempt to reach the ordering physician/APP until they **acknowledge receipt** of the message or the number of attempts reaches some prescribed threshold. At that point, the system can follow a prescribed **escalation protocol** to reach another designated individual, for example, a service line chief. If no one acknowledges receipt of the message, these systems are designed to alert someone in radiology to attempt a phone call or in-person message delivery.

- CTRMs can also audit the alerts and communications for a radiology practice to assess **compliance** with guidelines set forth by TJC or hospitals served by the practice.

> **DEFINITION: The Joint Commission**
>
> The Joint Commission (TJC) accredits and certifies hospitals and other healthcare organizations. TJC conducts periodic on-site surveys, applying strict criteria across numerous metrics. These site visits typically require substantial preparation from hospital personnel.

> **FURTHER READING: Results Communication**
>
> ACR Practice Parameter for Communication of Diagnostic Imaging Findings (https://www.acr.org/-/media/ACR/Files/Practice-Parameters/CommunicationDiag.pdf)

> **DEFINITION: Advanced Practice Providers**
>
> APPs (also called physician extenders) are healthcare providers with degrees such as physician assistant or registered nurse practitioner who can provide independent care to patients with indirect physician supervision.

10.3.2 Noncritical Actionable Findings

- Unlike critical findings, which could harm a patient within minutes to hours, noncritical or unexpected actionable findings have the **potential to harm patients** in the future and are still important to follow up.
- Individual practices may have **different policies** on whether and how radiologists should notify ordering physicians/APPs about the need for follow-up of such findings.
- There are **multiple challenges in identifying and tracking** these findings, including variability in the language radiologists use to document the need for follow-up, longer timelines for follow-up completion (months to years), incomplete/unavailable patient records that may not reflect prior workup of the same finding, and other aspects of the patient's medical history that may impact the need for follow-up.
- Some CTRM systems can be configured to handle noncritical actionable findings in addition to critical test results. However, because noncritical findings are typically more common than critical results in radiology, the CTRM system needs to be able to **automatically detect** these follow-up recommendations. A system that requires the radiologist to both dictate the report and then manually identify each recommendation would be time-consuming and risk missing some of the recommendations.
- A **recommendation-tracking system** will typically need access to the radiology report stream, either within the report generation system or the RIS/EMR. Ideally, the system would identify each finding of interest, the recommended follow-up, and the timing, and notify the ordering physician/APP in a closed-loop fashion that the recommenda-

> **FURTHER READING: Structured Reporting for Follow-Up Monitoring**
>
> Cook, TS et al. "Implementation of an Automated Radiology Recommendation-Tracking Engine for Abdominal Imaging Findings of Possible Cancer." *J Am Coll Radiol* 14 (5): 629–36; 2017.

tion has been issued and received. A strong system would facilitate communication between the radiology practice and the ordering physician/APP in case the recommendation is not actionable due to other clinical factors (e.g., imaging follow-up on a terminal patient). Assuming that the recommendation was appropriate, the system would then monitor the patient's record for evidence of a completed follow-up and alert the ordering physician/APP in the absence of that evidence.
- Many radiology practices use **structured reporting** as a hybrid solution for identification of noncritical actionable findings. Follow-up recommendations that are reported using a structured template can more easily be extracted from the radiology reports and used in a recommendation-tracking system. They typ-

> **VIEW TO THE FUTURE: Notifying Patients of Noncritical Actionable Findings**
>
> Although the need for follow-up is typically communicated to the ordering physician/APP rather than directly to the patient, may the time come when patients are directly notified about the need for follow-up?

ically require the radiologist to discretely specify the recommended downstream follow-up (imaging exam, laboratory test, or office visit) and its timing within the template. These data can be mined from radiology reports and imported into the system. However, the success of these types of systems hinges on the radiologists being willing to take the additional step of codifying their recommendation within the provided structured template. Some systems include compliance modules that review radiology reports for missed or unintelligible recommendations and request this information of the interpreting radiologists in order to track the recommended follow-up to completion.

- The **IHE Radiology Results Distribution** (RD) profile guides the transmission of radiology reports between systems via an HL7 version 2 Observation Results (ORU) message. This serves as a precursor to a future IHE profile intended to address the specific challenges of following up these findings.

> **FURTHER READING: IHE Results Distribution (RD) Profile**
>
> https://www.ihe.net/uploadedFiles/ Documents/Radiology/IHE_RAD_ Suppl_RD.pdf

OUR EXPERIENCE: Pennsylvania Act 112

Beginning in December 2018, Pennsylvania Act 112 (The Patient Test Results Information Act) required radiology practices to notify patients of imaging results that "would cause a reasonably prudent person to seek additional or follow-up medical care within 3 months" (https://www.legis.state.pa.us/cfdocs/legis/li/uconsCheck.cfm?yr=2018&sessInd=0&act=112). Radiology practices took different approaches to implementing solutions to meet the requirements of the state legislature, including prompting radiologists to add an Act 112 flag if appropriate before signing every report, including specific text tags in reports which met the Act 112 requirement, and using natural language processing to identify follow-up recommended within 3 months in reports. Some practices had to try different approaches, driven by the RIS or the report generation system, until finding one that fit into their workflow without significant disruption.

A review of 1 month's worth of reports flagged for patient notification showed that fewer than 1% of physician/APP discussions with patients around follow-up were directly linked to their receipt of the letter mandated by Act 112. A statewide analysis of data from multiple practices may yield more data on the impact of this intervention.

KEY LESSONS LEARNED

- Legislation can lead to the need for novel informatics solutions on an abbreviated timeline.
- Informatics can play a significant role in quality and safety initiatives at the practice, hospital, health system, or even geographic level.

10.4 Radiation Exposure Management

- **Radiation exposure monitoring** (REM) tools are an essential component of a radiology practice's informatics and quality improvement initiatives. REM tools enable a radiology practice to monitor radiation dose indices for different modalities that use ionizing radiation. It is important to note that some of the values collected by REM tools do not represent the actual dose delivered to the patient and absorbed by their organs, but rather a surrogate, such as the amount of radiation emitted by the scanner to produce the images. For this reason, the values are referred to as "dose indices" rather than "doses."

- Modalities that use **ionizing radiation** (such as CT, projection X-ray) can cause either deterministic (dose-based) or stochastic (probabilistic) tissue damage in patients. In particular, pediatric patients and pregnant patients are at increased risk for potential adverse effects of ionizing radiation. For this reason, it is important to monitor radiation dose indices for both diagnostic examinations and interventional procedures in *all patients*, to identify unexpected modifications to protocols or examinations with a higher-than-expected radiation exposure to the patient.

- There are a number of relevant **dose indices** for each modality that uses ionizing radiation. For CT, the volume CT dose index ($CTDI_{vol}$) and dose-length product (DLP) are most commonly used. In addition, there is the size-specific dose estimate (SSDE), a scaling factor for $CTDI_{vol}$ developed by a task group of the American Association of Physicists in Medicine (AAPM). For radiography and fluoroscopy, the dose-area product (DAP) or kerma-air product (KAP) and cumulative air kerma (CAK) are relevant, as are the calculated peak skin dose (PSD) and the fluoroscopy time. In mammography, the average glandular dose (AGD) is often monitored. As mentioned earlier, none of these values represent the actual radiation dose delivered to the patient.

> **FURTHER READING: DICOM RDSR**
>
> The DICOM standard contains templates for radiation dose indices for CT, X-ray, and nuclear medicine examinations.
> https://www.dicomstandard.org/using/radiation

- Dose indices can be generated and stored by the modality in one of two ways: in a legacy dose sheet or a DICOM Radiation Dose Structured Report (RDSR) object. The **legacy dose sheet** is typically a DICOM Secondary Capture object, with the numeric data burned into the pixels of the image. Early REM efforts were hampered by storage of essential dose indices in this fashion. By comparison, modern imaging equipment rarely uses this as the only means to record dose indices. The **DICOM RDSR** is a DICOM object that provides a structured format for storage of radiation dose indices. Most CT scanners manufactured after 2012 either natively support the DICOM RDSR (as a result of the **MITA XR-29** Dose Check standard) or can do so after a firmware upgrade. However, older equipment may not have this functionality.

- Developing a **radiation exposure monitoring program** requires more than a software tool. Although there are many technical decisions that need to be made to implement the tool in a radiology practice, it will only be effective if there are individuals designated to review and act upon the data collected by the tool. For this reason, it is important to also assemble a **multidisciplinary review committee**, consisting of radiologists, physicists, and technologists, among others, who will periodically review reports from the REM tool and identify areas for improvement. Separately, a smaller group of individuals should be designated who will be responsible for receiving and promptly acting on alerts for higher-than-expected radiation outputs by scanner equipment.

- The **IHE radiation exposure monitoring** (REM) profile specifies how imaging modalities should communicate radiation dose indices to other systems, such as dose index registries, dose information reporters, and dose information consumers. Figure 10.1 illustrates the actors and transactions in the REM profile. It is important to note that the dose information reporter, which in practical terms represents the REM software,

> **FURTHER READING: IHE REM**
>
> https://wiki.ihe.net/index.php/Radiation_Exposure_Monitoring

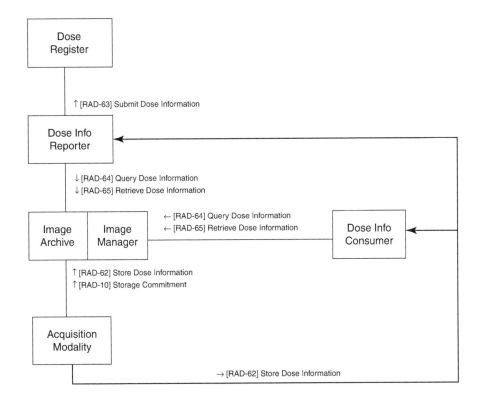

Fig. 10.1 The IHE REM profile. (© IHE® International; used with permission)

should be able to retrieve dose information from the image archive and transmit it to a dose registry, such as the **Dose Index Registry** maintained by the ACR (https://nrdr.acr.org/Portal/DIR/Main/page.aspx). Also important is the fact that the profile allows for a dose information consumer that is separate from the dose information reporter, although in reality these may be functions performed by the same application.

- **Diagnostic reference levels** (DRLs) can help imaging facilities determine if the radiation exposure from a particular imaging examination or procedure is unusually high. They are typically established at the 75th percentile for radiation dose indices across a wide range of practice types. However, they do not represent a firm upper limit of

> **INTERNATIONAL CONSIDERATIONS: DRLs**
>
> Diagnostic reference levels for radiation exposure from medical imaging, image-guided procedures, or radiation therapy can vary on a national or regional level.

exposure, because the radiation dose indices from which they are derived can vary according to patient factors. Instead, they are intended as a guide to encourage imaging facilities to review protocols and exams that exceed the specified DRLs. A REM tool should allow users to set thresholds for specific dose indices which will trigger alerts; DRLs can be used as these thresholds until enough data are collected to customize the thresholds.

CHECKLIST: Choosing a REM Software Tool

Modality-Specific Questions
- Which modalities are you going to monitor – CT? Projection X-ray? Radiopharmaceutical administration?
- How do these modalities currently store radiation dose indices?
- Can they generate DICOM RDSRs? If not, can the firmware be updated to enable this functionality?
- Can the modalities send radiation dose indices to a DICOM destination, either in the form of a legacy dose sheet or a DICOM RDSR?

REM Software-Specific Questions
- Can the software act as a DICOM listener/receiver?
- Can the software ingest dose indices from the modality directly or only from the archive?
- Can the software ingest legacy dose sheets?
- What modalities does the software support?
- Will the software send alerts if dose indices exceed prescribed thresholds, such as DRLs? Can the thresholds be customized?
- Can the software generate radiation exposure monitoring reports with specific levels of focus, including but not limited to site, equipment, operator, examination, and patient?

10.5 Decision Support

10.5.1 Clinical Decision Support

- The Protecting Access to Medicare Act (PAMA) of 2014 included legislation that required ordering physicians/APPs to use a qualified **clinical decision support mechanism** (CDSM) when ordering certain types of advanced imaging examinations (including CT, MRI, PET, and nuclear medicine exams).

> **DEFINITION: Clinical Decision Support (CDS)**
>
> A tool consulted by an ordering physician/APP that applies appropriate use criteria to determine if an imaging order is the best choice of test in light of a patient's symptoms.

- The goal of this requirement is to decrease inappropriate use of medical imaging in Medicare beneficiaries. Ordering physicians/APPs who are deemed to be outliers will be required to obtain **pre-authorization** for their patients' imaging examinations.
- The most well-known appropriate use criteria (AUC) for radiology are the ACR's Appropriateness Criteria (https://www.acr.org/Clinical-Resources/ACR-Appropriateness-Criteria).
- Under PAMA, CMS will only **reimburse** radiologists for the interpretation of advanced imaging that is ordered using a qualified CDSM, either one incorporated into the EMR or a freestanding online resource.
- If the CDSM is integrated into the EMR, it will generate the **numeric appropriateness score** (ranging from 0 for least appropriate to 9 for most appropriate) based on the ordered exam and the indication chosen from a picklist of options. If a free-text indication is entered, some CDSMs attempt to map the text to an option on the list. If a freestanding online CDSM is used, the ordering physician/APP must enter the appropriateness score into the order comments to receive credit for using the tool.
- It is important to be able to mine appropriateness scores whether they are generated by the EMR or entered in the order comments. All appropriateness scores can be monitored to better understand physician/APP ordering patterns, the number and nature of outliers among physicians/APPs ordering

> **FURTHER READING: Radiology Clinical Decision Support**
>
> Huber TC et al. "Impact of a Commercially Available Clinical Decision Support Program on Provider Ordering Habits". *J Am Coll Radiol* 15 (7): 951–57, 2018.

advanced imaging, and potential opportunities for a radiology practice to counsel its referring population about **appropriate imaging utilization**.
- Although clinical decision support is currently being implemented for Medicare beneficiaries, private payors may soon institute a similar requirement.
- Although the legislation was passed in 2014, its implementation was postponed multiple times. Voluntary participation and reporting began in January 2018, and

the Educational and Operations Testing Period commenced on January 1, 2020. **Full implementation** with penalties for noncompliance is slated to begin on January 1, 2022.

CHECKLIST: Factors Affecting Adoption of Clinical Decision Support

1. Seamless integration into the EMR and clinical workflow
2. Sufficient education of end-user physicians/APPs
3. Customization of the CDSM to the clinical context
4. Level of experience of the CDS vendor

Marcial LH et al. "A qualitative framework-based evaluation of radiology clinical decision support initiatives: eliciting key factors to physician adoption in implementation". *JAMIA Open* 2(1): 187–96, 2019.

10.5.2 Radiologist Decision Support

- While clinical decision support in radiology typically refers to guidance around ordering imaging, radiologists can also benefit from guidance during the interpretation process. This guidance may help radiologists craft more consistent and evidence-based follow-up recommendations, provide differential diagnoses based on findings identified on the images, or standardize the language used to report particular findings. These functions are sometimes referred to as **radiologist decision support**.
- **Report generation systems** sometimes contain radiologist decision support modules, but their adoption depends on whether the radiologists in the practice agree with the guidance offered by the system. Some commercial systems do offer the option to customize the recommendations that are produced.
- **CAR/DS** is an open framework for computer-assisted reporting and decision support. It is an eXtensible Markup Language (XML)-based system that can be used to encode follow-up guidelines in a radiologist's report generation system, to make clinical guidelines accessible at the point of care.

> **FURTHER READING: CAR/DS**
>
> Alkasab TK et al. "Creation of an Open Framework for Point-of-Care Computer-Assisted Reporting and Decision Support Tools for Radiologists". *J Am Coll Radiol* 14(9): 1184–89, 2017.

- Modules implemented using CAR/DS can prompt the radiologist for specific **data elements** (e.g., the size of a pulmonary nodule; whether the nodule is solid, subsolid, or ground glass; and whether or not the patient has a smoking history) and compute the appropriate time interval for follow-up chest CT. In turn, they can generate the appropriate language to be inserted into the radiology report to communicate the follow-up recommendation to the ordering physician/APP.

- The **ACR Assist** modules have been developed using the CAR/DS framework, and provide a vendor-neutral implementation of a number of reporting and data systems supported by the ACR (including BI-RADS for breast

imaging, LI-RADS for liver mass reporting on MRI, and Lung-RADS for CT lung cancer screening), as well as the incidental findings management algorithms published in the *Journal of the American College of Radiology*.

- **MARVAL** is an authoring tool developed by the American College of Radiology (https://assist.acr.org/marval/) that enables users to review and test CAR/DS modules.

- Another type of radiologist decision support focuses on assisting radiologists with differential diagnoses based on a set of findings. **Bayesian networks**, which are built using a set of conditional probabilities, can be used to implement point-of-care decision support for radiologists who have identified the characteristics of an imaging abnormality but are unsure what it represents. As with CAR/DS modules, the radiologist can manually enter the features

into the decision support tool, which will generate a list of differential diagnoses based on the conditional probabilities in its database. Alternatively, **deep learning** can be used to identify and analyze the imaging findings, and itself serve as input to the Bayesian network decision support tool.

- For these tools to successfully function in the clinical workflow, they need to be integrated with either PACS or the imaging modality to process the images as they become available, and generate a result that can be injected to the radiologist's developing report in the report generation system. This often requires middleware that can translate the output of the decision support tool into report text, for example, by consuming a DICOM SR object from the decision support system and correctly mapping it to custom fields in a report template.

10.6 Education

10.6.1 Teaching Files

- In the PACS era, teaching files have taken many forms. The simplest version mimicked the physical film-based teaching file, by creating multiple **folders in PACS** into which interesting cases were filed. However, these were difficult to organize and search. For that reason, they were sometimes only made available to radiologists organizing multidisciplinary conferences or teaching rounds.
- However, this often left individual radiologists to their own devices to organize and curate their interesting cases. As a result, a handful of standalone teaching file software applications entered the market. Images for cases could be saved from PACS and uploaded into these applications, some of which were web-based. This put the burden of proper de-identification of the images on the radiologist building the teaching cases.
- Some applications could be configured as **DICOM destinations** on PACS to enable users to send cases into the teaching file system. However, these applications were required to reside behind the organizational firewall, which limited consumption of the cases to trainees at that institution. To address this limitation, some commercial teaching files provided the option to create both public and private versions of a teaching case, and restrict any fields that might contain PHI to the private version. This allowed users to more easily share cases outside their institution or even access them after leaving the institution.
- Today, many PACS vendors sell an **integrated teaching file module** that may offer functionality ranging from tagging cases with searchable keywords to a full set of fields containing patient history, presentation, findings, diagnosis, and discussion. The advantage of these modules is seamless use and access during the clinical workday. However, exporting cases from these systems may be more challenging.
- Some residency programs also developed their own in-house teaching file applications and incorporated useful features such as the ability to flag cases for follow-up.
- The **IHE Teaching File and Clinical Export** (TCE) profile enables users to more efficiently create teaching file cases from PACS directly. **MIRC TFS** (https://mircwiki.rsna.org/index.php?title=MIRC_TFS), the RSNA Medical Imaging Resource Center's teaching file system, is a community-supported, open-source teaching file that uses IHE TCE. MIRC TFS has the ability to receive DICOM from PACS, de-identify it, and create draft teaching file cases for users to populate later. Publicly shared cases are also available at http://mirc.rsna.org/query.

> **FURTHER READING: IHE TCE**
>
> Kamauu AW, Whipple JJ, DuVall SL, et al. "IHE Teaching File and Clinical Trial Export Integration Profile: Functional Examples". *RadioGraphics* 28 (4): 933–45, 2008.

- The ACR also has a teaching file system: the Radiology Case Management System, **RCMS** (https://www.acr.org/Practice-Management-Quality-Informatics/Imaging-3/Case-Studies/Information-Technology/An-Educational-Ecosystem), which radiology training programs can install locally to manage their educational resources.
- Both the ACR (https://cortex.acr.org/) and the RSNA (https://cases.rsna.org) now offer **online case collections**/teaching files. However, at present they do not offer functionality to connect and push images from PACS directly.

10.6.2 Discrepancy Tracking

- Residents' off-hours workflow (on evenings, weekends, and holidays) can vary from site to site, even within the same training program.
- Residents may dictate full **preliminary reports**, which are subsequently reviewed by attending radiologists. Alternatively, they may only be required to issue an enumerated impression or a brief note in PACS or on a bidirectional communications dashboard (e.g., one that is visible to the emergency department). In the latter instances, the full dictation is issued by the attending radiologist, often the next day.

> **DEFINITION: Preliminary Report**
>
> Usually, when an examination is interpreted, a formal report is immediately generated. However, there are situations where a temporary interpretation is rendered and reviewed and finalized later (e.g., radiology residents on call, nighthawk systems). Curating discrepancies between preliminary and final reports is potentially challenging

- Independent call carries great educational value for residents, but that education is partially contingent on feedback from their faculty. For this reason, many radiology programs have some type of feedback system to alert residents of errors or discrepancies between their preliminary interpretations and the final attending reads.
- Attending feedback can be relayed back to residents in many ways. The simplest, although least convenient approach, is an email summary of changes to reports. This may not necessarily capture all the details of each report modification and is difficult for residents to meaningfully consume.

> **FURTHER READING: Discrepancy Tracking**
>
> Chen PH, Chen Y, Cook TS. "Capricorn-A Web-Based Automatic Case Log and Volume Analytics for Diagnostic Radiology Residents". *Acad Radiol* 22(10): 1242–51, 2015.

- Some residency programs have additional workflow orchestration systems that can be used to generate **exam-specific messages** to residents. In the past, these systems may have been third-party products separate from PACS, or add-on plugins developed in-house. Newer PACS products also have built-in chat functionality that can be used to send residents messages (even while offline) with links to cases and case-specific feedback.

- The most sophisticated systems are home-built platforms that leverage **structured reporting** in templates used by the attending radiologists reviewing the cases, to stratify the feedback to residents and allow them to review additions to their reports as well as major and minor **discrepancies** between the preliminary and final reports. These systems facilitate large-scale reporting and analytics, including assessment of the rates of major (typically <2% of interpreted exams) and minor discrepancies among residents.

- These systems are often web-based applications that allow residents and program directors to interact with the data while reviewing discrepancies. These systems are typically not connected to PACS, although such connections would be useful during review to immediately pull up images from an exam to better understand the discrepancy.

- Additionally, discrepancy tracking systems can sometimes also collect data on all exams interpreted by residents throughout their training. These data are important when reporting compliance with Mammography Quality Standards Act (MQSA) requirements for interpretation of mammography during residency, data to demonstrate achievement of American Council for Graduate Medical Education (ACGME) Milestones (https://www.acgme.org/Specialties/Milestones/pfcatid/23/Radiology), or exam logs for procedural competency (e.g., performance and interpretation of coronary CT angiography). Automated collection of these data is valuable not only to residents, who must collect it for individual reporting purposes, but to residency program directors, who report it for periodic program assessments and renewal of program accreditation. Residents also often need to export these data to demonstrate evidence of procedural competency for applications for fellowship or future employment.

10.7 Quality Improvement

10.7.1 Adverse Event Reporting

- The 1999 Institute of Medicine report "To Err is Human: Building a Safer Health System" suggested that as many as 98,000 patients die in the United States every year due to medical errors. This report jump-started the quality and safety movement in American medicine.

- Reason's **Swiss cheese model** can be applied to medical errors and patient safety (Fig. 10.2). The model describes the fact that medical error is rarely unifactorial and that there are multiple contributing factors that must align to result in the error. An adverse event or error occurs when a series of conditions align to produce a result that negatively affects a patient. **Near misses**, sometimes referred

Fig. 10.2 The Swiss
cheese model of
medical error

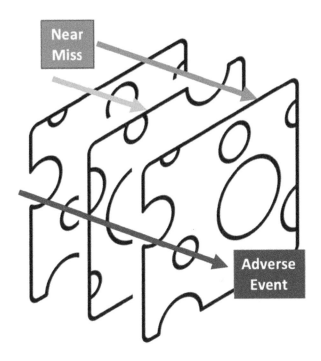

to as close calls, bring to light conditions that can contribute to potential adverse events, but have not yet impacted the patient directly.

- Most hospitals today have **adverse event reporting systems** that aim to collect data about the incident that occurred, in an effort to learn more about the contributing factors and strategies to avoid the incident in the future. These systems are typically sophisticated, web-based applications that are accessible throughout a health system or hospital and allow users to file incident reports either anonymously or associated with their identities. Such systems often prompt the user for very specific information about the patient location and other factors related to the incident.

- However, while a great deal of data is collected in each report, it is often transmitted directly to the hospital's risk management office. As a result, individuals who file incident reports may not always get feedback unless the event is severe enough to warrant a **root cause analysis** (RCA). In some cases, the feedback will only acknowledge the report and inform the reporter that the incident has been reviewed and acted upon.

> **DEFINITION: Root Cause Analysis**
>
> A formal review of a medical error or near miss that looks at all the factors contributing to the error. The RCA uses just culture techniques to avoid blaming individuals and seeks to address systemic issues that can result in global changes to avoid future errors.

10.7.2 Opportunities for Improvement

- While adverse event reporting systems typically collect data on near misses and adverse events, they may not as frequently be used to collect data on opportunities for improvement.

FURTHER READING: Radiology Event Reporting

Schultz SR, Watson Jr. RE, Prescott SL, et al. "Patient Safety Event Reporting in a Large Radiology Department". *Am J Roentgenol* 197: 684–88, 2011.

- As a result, radiology departments and practices may seek other ways to collect this data, and some may even develop home-built applications to collect and review these data. One advantage of such applications is the flexibility to collect data that is:

  1. Specific to the different locations that may make up a department or practice
  2. Revealing workarounds in workflow that should be addressed with direct solutions
  3. Identifying a specific exam or care of a specific patient that brought the opportunity to light

- As with hospital- or health system-level adverse event reporting systems, these are often web-based applications accessible throughout the radiology practice. Although they will likely collect more radiology-specific data (such as study accession numbers and imaging locations) than the enterprise-level systems, they rarely require connections to the PACS.

10.8 Consultation Tools

- Technological advances in radiology have made it possible for radiologists to render exam interpretations without being in the same building as the imaging equipment. As a result, **teleradiology** practices exist that provide radiology coverage for multiple different imaging centers without requiring a radiologist to be physically on-site.
- Additionally, during the COVID-19 pandemic, radiologists who normally worked on-site suddenly found themselves reading remotely more frequently or, sometimes, permanently. As a result, the need for tools to facilitate **virtual consultations** with ordering physicians/APPs grew quickly and unexpectedly.
- Multiple approaches can be considered to implement virtual consultations. For a simple, point-of-care solution that does not require web conferencing software,

a **smartphone camera** pointed at the PACS monitor would enable the consulting physician/APP to see the screen and hear the radiologist as they are reviewing the images. This could even be used to allow a radiologist to guide a technologist during a complicated imaging examination, if the technologist points the camera at the scanner console.

- However, while this is a feasible solution for brief consultations between radiologists and their clinical colleagues, it does not **scale** well beyond a one-on-one interaction. Radiologists often participate in multidisciplinary conferences and tumor boards, where they consult on a number of different imaging examinations with multiple other members of the care team.

- A more sophisticated solution can be achieved by using a **web conferencing** software that allows the radiologist to share their PACS viewer screen while speaking to the consulting physician/APP. Some web conferencing apps even allow participants to request control of the screen, to enable the consultant to take the mouse and scroll through an imaging exam to the area of interest or question, which can improve the quality and yield of the consultation. While this is a viable option for sharing a single PACS workstation display, it does not effectively replicate the experience of viewing the exam as if standing with the radiologist at the workstation.

- To truly mimic the experience of viewing an examination on PACS in a collaborative environment, customized viewing software is necessary. Multiple PACS vendors are working on developing truly **collaborative image viewing** tools. Similar technology could also be used for remote readouts with residents whose faculty may not be in the same reading room or on the same campus.

> **FURTHER READING:**
> **Consultation Tools**
>
> Matalon SA et al. "Trainee and Attending Perspectives on Remote Radiology Readouts in the Era of the COVID-19 Pandemic". *Acad Radiol* 27: 1147–53; 2020.

- One challenge in creating these collaborative environments is **security considerations** around displaying protected health information on a screen that is then shared, potentially to someone who is located outside the organizational firewall but is still allowed to access the information. Having a collaborative platform that requires both parties to be behind the organizational firewall, e.g., one that is provided by the PACS vendor, adds a level of security over using external web conferencing software.

- Collaboration software can also be used to enable radiologists to communicate with patients, to discuss imaging findings and management steps, as well as to counsel patients prior to image-guided procedures.

PEARLS

- When it comes to ancillary software, solutions that fit the requirements may not always be commercially available. This leads radiology practices to the build-versus-buy decision: purchase a product that doesn't quite fit the need or invest resources to build and maintain a solution in-house.
- The success and adoption of applications such as CTRM systems and CDS tools hinges greatly on their integration into the existing clinical workflow.
- There are few education-related informatics tools on the market, leading many programs to independently build tools that meet this need.
- The COVID-19 pandemic created new opportunity for virtual collaboration between radiologists and ordering physicians, especially as more radiologists began to work remotely.
- There is significant overlap between informatics and quality improvement initiatives. Much of quality improvement is data-driven, which is why informatics can play a major role in both sourcing the data and supplying the intervention.
- There are IHE integration profiles for the development and interoperability of ancillary software, including REM, TCE, and RD.

References

1. Larson PA, Berland LL, Griffith B, et al. Actionable findings and the role of IT support: report of the ACR actionable reporting workgroup. J Am Coll Radiol. 2014;11(6):552–8.
2. Wandtke B, Gallagher S. Reducing delay in diagnosis: multistage recommendation tracking. Am J Roentgenol. 2017;209(5):970–5.
3. Mattay GS, Mittl GS, Zafar HM, et al. Early impact of Pennsylvania act 112 on follow-up of abnormal imaging findings. J Am Coll Radiol. 2020; https://doi.org/10.1016/j.jacr.2020.05.014.
4. Kanal KM, Butler PF, Sengupta D, et al. U.S. diagnostic reference levels and achievable doses for 10 adult CT examinations. Radiology. 2017;284(1):120–33.
5. Berland LL, Silverman SG, Gore RM, et al. Managing incidental findings on abdominal CT: white paper of the ACR incidental findings committee. J Am Coll Radiol. 2010;7:754–73.
6. Rauschecker AM, Rudie JD, Xie L, et al. Artificial intelligence system approaching neuroradiologist-level differential diagnosis accuracy at brain MRI. Radiology. 2020;295(3):626–37.
7. Schmitt JE, Scanlon MH, Servaes S, et al. Milestones on a shoestring: a cost-effective, semi-automated Implementation of the new ACGME requirements for radiology. Acad Radiol. 2015;22(10):1287–93.
8. Milch CE, Salem DN, Pauker SG, et al. Voluntary electronic reporting of medical errors and adverse events. An analysis of 92,547 reports from 26 acute care hospitals. J Gen Intern Med. 2006;21(2):165–70.

Self-Assessment Questions

1. Which of these costs of home-built software applications is often overlooked during the build-versus-buy decision-making process?

   A. Up-front financial expenditure
   B. Maintenance and support cost
   C. Hardware infrastructure
   D. User training

2. Which of the following features of a recommendation-tracking system is important for decreasing the likelihood of an adverse patient outcome?

   A. Asynchronous messaging
   B. Message logging
   C. Text paging
   D. Closed-loop communication

3. What is the most salient difference between a critical imaging test result and a noncritical actionable finding?

   A. Timeline during which patient harm may occur
   B. Size of the detected abnormality
   C. Modality on which the finding was identified
   D. Location where the patient was imaged

4. Which actor in the IHE REM profile transaction diagram would be expected to collect dose indices from exams sent to PACS?

   A. Acquisition modality
   B. Image archive
   C. Dose information consumer
   D. Dose register

5. What output does a CDS system generate in response to the selection of an imaging exam and associated indication for the study?

   A. Pre-authorization
   B. Appropriateness score
   C. Peer-to-peer authorization
   D. Explanation of benefits

6. What is the major advantage of using radiologist decision support to generate follow-up recommendations?

   A. Standardization of recommendation language across a practice
   B. Increased revenue from follow-up imaging
   C. Increased need for structured reporting templates
   D. Decreased cost to the department or practice

7. Which of the following is a potential pitfall of teaching file systems that ingest DICOM image objects?

    A. Limited data storage due to larger file sizes
    B. Compromise of PHI still in the DICOM header
    C. Slower loading times for individual teaching cases
    D. Less likelihood of backward compatibility

8. Which of the following systems is *least* likely to need connections to PACS?

    A. Teaching file
    B. Radiation exposure monitoring
    C. Discrepancy tracking
    D. Clinical decision support

9. Which of the following systems requires the *least* integration with the PACS, RIS, or EMR?

    A. Critical test results management
    B. Radiologist decision support
    C. Recommendation tracking
    D. Incident reporting

10. Which important feature do web conferencing applications generally *lack*?

    A. Interactivity via chat or question/answer box
    B. Simultaneous audio and video sharing
    C. Multi-monitor display to replicate PACS viewer functionality
    D. Collaboration features, e.g., sharing mouse control

Part III
Imaging Informatics

Chapter 11
Databases and Data Retrieval

Andrea G. Rockall

Contents

11.1 Introduction

Developing a good database for imaging research is an essential task that should not be underestimated. One of the main aims of developing an accurate and user-friendly database is to support high-quality research for discovery of imaging biomarkers, biological validation of existing and novel imaging biomarkers, and model development in the machine learning domain [1]. Quality data curation is at the foundation of reliable research findings and the avoidance of false discovery. Imaging databases may range from relatively small study-specific datasets to much larger population biobanks.

> **DEFINITION: Imaging Biobank**
>
> Organized database of medical images and associated imaging biomarkers (radiologic and clinical) shared among multiple researchers and linked to other biorepositories.

A. G. Rockall (✉)
Department of Cancer and Surgery, Imperial College London, London, UK
e-mail: a.rockall@imperial.ac.uk

FURTHER READING: Imaging Biobanks

ESR Position Paper: Imaging Biobanks 2015. https://www.ncbi.nlm.nih.gov/pmc/articles/PMC4519817/
Whole-Body MR Imaging in the German National Cohort: Rationale, Design, and Technical Background 2015. https://pubmed.ncbi.nlm.nih.gov/25989618/

Regardless of the size of the database, there are some overarching principles:

1. Protection of patient privacy is fundamental: avoidance of disclosure of protected healthcare information (PHI) must be assured while retaining the scientific integrity of the data collected.
2. Common standards are important for data sharing and reuse of data, which are often expensive and time-consuming to collect. Each database should have a standardized structured model using common data elements ensuring that all data are clearly defined and categorized. This will ensure sustainability and best use of the research investment [2, 3].
3. It is important to define the storage software and the available analysis tools. Ideally, the database should be flexible enough to allow additions in the future as new tools are developed.
4. Data security, data access, and data sharing need to be managed according to information governance principles.

Scalability of high-quality image data curation, while ensuring data integrity, remains a big challenge that needs to be met in order to harness the true research potential of medical images.

11.2 Developing a Database for Imaging Research

11.2.1 Planning What Data Need to Be Collected for an Imaging Research Protocol

- Most research studies will have an ethically approved research protocol which details the research question and the outcome measures. These are usually provided in a summary table. The data points that are required for each of the outcome measures should also be detailed in the protocol. It is important to ensure that all data points required for the outcome measures are included in the database, at the outset.
- Ensure that there are clear instructions for the data collection so that the responsibilities of each party are very clear.

HYPOTHETICAL SCENARIO: Planning Data Collection

A study asks the research questions: does tumor size on CT predict progression-free survival after surgical removal of tumor?

The outcome measure of progression-free survival requires:

1. Measurement of tumor size on CT
2. Date of surgical removal
3. Definition of disease progression
   - Increase in tumor marker
   - New site of disease on CT or increase in the size of existing lesion(s) consistent with disease progression
4. Date of confirmed progression

Some examples of other questions to answer prospectively:

- Is the tumor size data point measured on original CT by reporting radiologist or will there be a central retrospective measurement?
- Is the tumor size based on maximum transverse diameter on axial image or can a sagittal or coronal reformat be used for the maximum tumor diameter?
- Is tumor size based on volume and if so how is the volume measured?
- Is the date of progression-free survival from the date of only one measure of progression (e.g., doubling of a circulating tumor maker) or are both measures required (doubling of tumor marker **and** new disease on CT)?

- Continuous review and **monitoring of data collection** is important to ensure that the data collection protocols have been understood and correctly applied. This is particularly important in multicenter data collection. It is better to discover any issues early on and to correct these than wait until the end of data collection.
- Identify ambiguity as early as possible. No protocol is perfect, and if the monitoring of data collection identifies a problem whereby there are differences in interpretation, leading to differences in data collection, then address this early on. Consider amending the data collection instructions/user manual to clarify any ambiguity and feedback to data collectors at the research sites. This may require a protocol amendment; most often this can be dealt with by clarifying data collection manual within study protocol appendices.
- Monitoring of data collection may lead to data queries which will need to be resolved throughout the course of the database development. The audit trail of data queries and data changes should be fully transparent.

DEFINITION: Audit Trail

A record of all the changes made to a database, usually with timestamps and user logs.

- It is helpful to have a database scheme which clarifies the **provenance of data** and its pathway, in order to assist with data cleaning and data queries:
  - Research site
  - Machine vendor
  - Machine version and software version
- There are major differences in imaging databases:
  - **Image repository** developed using previously acquired prospective research studies (such as in the Tumor Cancer Imaging Archive).
  - **Prospectively acquired** database such as the UK Biobank or other national imaging biobanks.
  - **Retrospective data** curated from standard of care clinical imaging. It may be curated for a disease process (e.g., breast cancer) or imaging type (e.g., mammogram or head CT). Huge unstructured datasets in imaging are currently uncommon, partly due to the large file sizes. If data mining is intended, this may take place within the clinical PACS or a large trusted research environment.

> **KEY CONCEPT: Prospective vs. Retrospective**
>
> Prospective data is acquired after the research question and protocol have been established, so that biases and missing data can be minimized.
>
> Retrospective data is mined from existing sources and is more prone to bias.

> **DEFINITION: Big Data**
>
> Extremely large datasets that are analyzed computationally to reveal unexpected patterns, trends, and associations. Data may be structured, semi-structured, or unstructured. Data may grow exponentially with time.

- Imaging protocol and potential variations should be recorded:
  - Which images? For example, non-contrast, arterial phase or portal venous phase CT?
  - Which sequences on MRI?
  - Which time points? A study could use a single time point or multiple time points over a course of treatment or disease.
  - When can we make exceptions (e.g., if a patient has an allergy to contrast)?
- Clarify whether unprocessed imaging or processed imaging should be collected:
  - For example, in whole-body MRI, should the individual stations be used or the composed volumes?
  - Should reformats or subtracted images be included?
  - Should still or video sequences be included?
- Indicate whether the original radiology report should be included, for example, for research into natural language processing. If so, the anonymization process and linkage to the image information is an important aspect of the data collection plan.
- **Clinical metadata** collection should be detailed. Items required, system for extraction, storage, and linkage to image data need to be planned. Examples include patient age, current diagnosis, and medications.

- **Missing data** is an inevitable part of healthcare databases. This will be present in both retrospective and prospective databases. It may be due to patients declining to continue in a prospective study, missing scans during the course of a study, or data becoming corrupted. In retrospective data collection, data may be quite heterogeneous due to differences in clinical practice and patient circumstances. The plan for handling missing data should be included: it may be that missing data points can be overcome by mathematical modelling, or it may be that cases with missing data will be considered unevaluable and removed from the database, perhaps being replaced by a case that is evaluable.

11.2.2 Types of Image Databases

- Not all imaging databases are planned around a specific research protocol with a specific research question and planned outcome measures. Data warehouses are an example.

> **DEFINITION: Data Warehouse**
>
> A database that collects a large amount of clinical or imaging data without a defined research question or purpose. Subsets of the data can later be mined to answer newly framed questions.

- A data warehouse aims to collect a large amount of data from one or more clinical operational system such as PACS, RIS, or EHR:
  - Data pulled from PACS or other EHR may need to undergo data cleaning and data quality check prior to being stored in the warehouse. Ideally, the data warehouse will have data integration technology and processes that harmonize and categorize data as well as applications or tools to assist researchers to use the data.
- Integration of data from multiple sources into a single database may be structured, semi-structured, or unstructured.
- **Relational database**: This is a database that stores data points that are related to one another, typically in columns and rows, e.g., image data with disease category and possibly other information such as outcome may be tabulated for each subject. An example could be a database that stores thoracic CT scan findings for multiple subjects, and also documents the presence of a lung

> **KEY CONCEPT: Structured Data vs. Unstructured Data**
>
> Structured data has well-defined relationships and can usually be stored as rows and columns. Each element has tags or descriptors that may provide additional information. Structured data is easy to query and can be stored efficiently.
>
> Unstructured data is not easily parsed. Examples include text, audio, and images themselves.
>
> Semi-structured data has some of the elements of structured data (like a DICOM header or XML tags) but is not completely categorized.

cancer, the lung cancer histopathology, and the overall survival of patient from the date of diagnosis. Examples of supporting software include Microsoft **Access** and **SQL**.

- **Open-access medical image repositories**: There are many sources of open-access medical images, most of which have associated clinical metadata. These repositories provide a variety of datasets which have varying degrees of labels or annotation,

> **FURTHER READING: Image Repositories**
>
> Many open-access repositories are listed at http://www.aylward.org/notes/open-access-medical-image-repositories.

  providing the standard of truth. In some cases, images may be unlabelled.
- **Cloud database**: This is a database that runs on a cloud computing platform. The benefits include scalability, high availability, and sustainability. Data may be stored in different ways, and most cloud database providers offer a choice of database formats, often provided as SQL or other relational databases. Using one of the main providers typically offers data protection and security, encryption, backups, and updates. These should be HIPAA/GDPR compliant for use in medical databases.
- **Hybrid cloud**: Migration of a current institutional database to the cloud may require a stepwise approach, with initial migration of some aspects or applications that may benefit most from a cloud-based provision or when a new database deployment is being planned. Some legacy or traditional on-site databases may remain in use locally, thereby resulting in a hybrid system.

11.2.3 Information Governance: Approval and Anonymization

- Prior to removing data from PACS, RIS, and/or the electronic healthcare record, it is essential that all the appropriate approvals are in place, including institutional, ethical, and information governance approvals. These will vary depending on where you work:
  - In the USA, use of data will need to comply with HIPAA.
  - In the EU, use of data will need to comply with GDPR.
- Anonymization of imaging data will require the removal of patient identifiers within both the DICOM tags and on any of the images themselves (see **Chap. 8**):
  - There are several open-source tools to assist with de-identification of images, such as clinical trials processor (CTP) or DICOM Browser.
  - A challenge may be the presence of patient name burned into the actual stored images, such as in the case of many ultrasound images or in centers where stored PDF or scanned forms include patient identifiers. A quality assurance process must be in place for detecting this.
- For anonymization of radiology reports, dedicated software should be used to remove PHI. Several automated de-identification tools are available, but they are not completely reliable.

> **DEFINITION: PHI**
>
> Protected health information is data that is legally and ethically considered private. In the USA, HIPAA legislation defines which data elements are protected; in the EU, the GDPR regulations define this. PHI must not be revealed to anyone who is not involved in treating the patient.

> **DEFINITION: Pseudoanonymization**
>
> Pseudoanonymized data contains no PHI when it is viewed in the research environment. But, behind the clinical firewall, there is a lookup table that can use a unique research identifier to deanonymize the patient and acquire more data. This is also called link anonymization.

- Data may be fully anonymized or pseudoanonymized.
- You should be able to link together all the data for one subject, even though it may come from different data sources, such as multiple time points, clinical and imaging data, and outcome data.

11.2.4 Transfer of Data from PACS and EHR: Quality Assurance

- Transfer of image data is not a trivial task due to large file sizes. Transfer from the patient record, de-identification, and deposition into an image database may require considerable network bandwidth and time.
- Check that data has fully transferred, ideally using a software tool to check equivalence of pre- and post-transfer file sizes.
- Non-image DICOM objects – plan how to handle non-image DICOM data:
  - De-identification may be problematic [4].
  - How do you integrate and structure clinical data?
  - How do you quarantine data that does not fit the data structure or fails validation?
- At what point does the anonymization step take place?
  - Need to clarify the level of de-identification and DICOM tag editing.
  - Removal of some DICOM tags can strip necessary information to reproduce the study, so careful planning is required. Poorly planned anonymization may make secondary analyses impossible.
  - Ensure integrity of linkage between the subject and new subject enrollment number as well as the study/series/date following the anonymization step. There may need to be a validation step following the anonymization procedure.

- Need to be aware of differences in DICOM conformance and application of unique identifier (UID).
- Beware DICOM inconsistencies that may result in data being quarantined, as manual repair will be time-consuming. Document changes when tracking and validating the repair.

- Use a lookup table with a uniform format of patient enrollment numbers and unique identifiers for each imaging study/series/instance. You may know what data you wish to collect but consider how best to organize the data:
  - What data should be linked?
  - What data must be blinded from other data?
  - Organization of different modalities.
  - Organization of different dates and time series.
  - Coordination of clinical metadata with imaging data.

- **Identification of duplicates**: this can be difficult in the context of de-identified data particularly if there are different instances of de-identification of the same subject.

- Recognizing and eliminating duplicates is essential to avoid bias of a dataset due to multiple instances of a particular image which could alter analysis. This can be checked using pixel-level data.

> **HYPOTHETICAL SCENARIO:**
> **Duplicate entries**
>
> You have created an anonymized research database containing imaging studies. One of your subjects gets imaged at the main hospital, and then later at an outside facility. Once the data is anonymized, how will you know it's the same patient?

- **Conformance of DICOM metadata** is important to allow interoperable use of data:
  - Remember that not all institutions use DICOM headers in the same way (especially the private tags), so it may be difficult to ensure conformity.
  - Software tools for direct manipulation of DICOM errors are available, but manual editing can be burdensome for large datasets.

11.2.5 Data Processing

- **Data formatting**
  - Following anonymization of image data, it is important to store the data according to the research study or database plan. Preservation of "raw" data from PACS may be required. During the course of a study, processed data, data labels, and annotations may be added. However, the availability of the original unprocessed data is likely to be needed and should be protected.

- Retrieval from PACS usually requires de-identification of the study by changing DICOM tags, and a copy of the DICOM data is stored. However, in addition, it may be necessary to also store other file formats such as the NIfTI format. This is an Analyze-style data format to facilitate interoperable data storage and analysis, including segmentation tasks and machine learning usage.
- Conversion of DICOM to NIfTI format may be undertaken using open-source software. However, it is important to ensure that the NIfTI conversion is uniform, as there are two versions of NIfTI, the original NIfTI-1 and NIfTI-2.

> **KEY CONCEPT: NIfTI**
>
> The Neuroimaging Informatics Technology Initiative format is one of several alternatives to DICOM for image storage, along with Minc and Analyze. Programs meant for one file type will not work well with another, and therefore file conversion is often necessary. File types are easily recognizable by their extension (.nii for NIfTI; .dcm for DICOM). The NIfTI-2 format is an update on NIfTI-1 that allows more data to be stored. Some imaging informatics tools can convert DICOM files to NIfTI format automatically.

- In research protocol databases, the type of image processing may be known ahead of time, and the file format can be planned accordingly. However, it is essential to ensure that the database has clear version control in order to distinguish the original raw data from different versions of processed, annotated, or labelled data.

- **Data cleaning**
  - Identification of corrupt files should be automated if possible, especially for large datasets.
  - Exclude unevaluable data, such as imaging artifacts:
    Contrast failure
    Metal artifacts
    Wrong body coverage
  - Some large data collections require manual visual inspection of images prior to incorporating them into the database, e.g., the National Lung Cancer Screening trial [5, 6].

- **Data harmonization**
  - **Prospective data acquisition for planned biobank**: Ideal data collection would be harmonization of image acquisition using the same machine/technology/software version by specifically trained technicians. This may be achievable in the case of strictly controlled prospective biobank collections with highly standardized imaging protocols, for example, the UK Biobank [7, 8].
  - **Prospective data acquisition in multicenter study**: This is the next level of data in which many aspects will be harmonized by the imaging manual and protocol. However, differences in machine vendor, software versions, and

day-to-day acquisition by different technicians may result in differences in images acquired.

- **Prospective data collection over long term**: In this case, an imaging manual and protocol may be applied but over the longer term, but there will inevitably be changes in technology and machines that will impact data harmonization.
- **Retrospective data curation**: Most data curation is retrospective, resulting in potentially wide variations in protocol as technology advances.
- Processing of images within a database may be required to allow similar analysis tasks to be performed. A simple example would be resampling CT volume to ensure the same slice thickness throughout a dataset. In MRI datasets, there is likely to be a need for signal intensity normalization.
- There is a balance to be struck between very harmonized data and more heterogeneous data for image analysis. Machine learning tools generated on highly harmonized data are unlikely to generalize. However, data which is too heterogeneous may not allow successful development of machine learning tools in the initial development phase. However, some degree of retrospective data harmonization is needed in most large datasets [9, 10].

11.2.6 Software for Image Databases

- Ideally, image data should be stored in an environment that allows viewing of the images, image processing, storage of unprocessed and processed image versions, as well as any version-controlled annotations and linked clinical metadata.
- Research platforms that offer such functionality include open-source platforms, including:
  - XNAT
  - Orthanc
  - Open Health Imaging Foundation Viewer [11]
- Several commercial platforms are also available.
- Ability to run on Windows, macOS, or Linux is an added advantage, although some are designed for one or another system.
- Ability to add modules such as SQL database.
- Ability to add plug-in analysis software ensures use by a variety of researchers including radiologists and computer vision scientists.

11.2.7 Security and Safety of the Database

- Need to ensure backup (cloud or institutional server).
- Data access arrangements need to be clear and transparent (see **Chap. 19**).

- Conditions and rules must be laid out for data security (see **Chap. 8**):
  - Consider the need for data encryption.
- Legal requirements depend on country:
  - GDPR compliant in the EU
  - HIPAA compliant in the USA
- Data may be held within a Trusted Research Environment or Data Safe Haven within an institution.

> **DEFINITION: Safe Haven**
>
> Data Safe Havens, a.k.a. Trusted Research Environments, are highly secure data storage environments meant for researchers who need to maintain PHI for their work. There are legal standards to ensure adequate security for these databases.

11.3 Using the Database

11.3.1 Information Governance: Data Sharing and Access

- Access to the database may be open-source or controlled. This will be part of the information governance plan for data curation.
- Sites that provide data to open-source repositories will need to have appropriate institutional approval through their information governance team, with agreed parameters.
- Some open-source databases have **data access strategies** that require researchers to request access through an access subcommittee to ensure that the application to use the data are by bona fide healthcare researchers intending to undertake viable research. Clear, transparent, and fair access policies use consistent criteria, and where there is any contentious issue, access to the biobank ethics committee should be available [4, 12].
- Image databases that are limited to approved users need a system in place for allocation of username and passwords. Access needs to be user-friendly and enable appropriate data use without requiring programming skills.
- **Data-sharing agreements** and contracts may need to be in place for use of controlled data between institutions.

11.3.2 Planning Data Usage in the Context of a Study

- Database administration should be clear and transparent. Access to certain components of the database by researchers should be appropriately restricted depending on the **user role**.

- Data access may be restricted according to allocation of data:
  - Training data for model development may be widely available.
  - Testing dataset for model performance may be restricted.
  - Allocation of training and testing data should be carefully planned. For a research protocol, this allocation should be done in partnership with the study statistician.
- In some studies, **class balance** may be important in allocation to the training and test datasets. It would not be appropriate to have all image datasets with a particular finding in one or other dataset. Stratified randomization into training and test datasets is likely to ensure unbiased class balance.
- In some studies, allocation to training and testing may be based on a very simple principle such as sequential date of the data. However, it is important to consider whether there may have been a change in machine vendor, software, and imaging protocol during the period of data collection which could result in significant differences in the images over time. This may not be of concern in relatively simple datasets, such as CXR, but could be a great significance in more complex modalities such as MRI, resulting in a failure of a model to generalize.
- Image labelling or annotation tools should ideally be available within the database, but this is not always the case. Open-source tools for image segmentation may be used, such as ITK-SNAP, 3D Slicer, or ImageJ. Online platforms for image annotation and segmentation are also available, such as MD.ai.
- Linkage of the database to processing units should be available. For example, XNAT links to NVIDIA Clara, with an automated pipeline for conversion of DICOM to NIfiTI, and then conversion back to DICOM in the model output.
- Plan for data extraction, segmentations, and results.

11.3.3 Database Merging and Sustainability

- The ability for data to be merged and integrated in the future with other data repositories is an important consideration [13].
- Tools for future sustainability are in development, such as **PRISM** for The Cancer Imaging Archive (TCIA) [14].
- There are shared software algorithms and architectures with the tools required for computing, comparing, evaluating, and disseminating predictive models [15].

> **FURTHER READING: PRISM**
>
> PRISM: A Platform for Imaging in Precision Medicine https://ascopubs.org/doi/full/10.1200/CCI.20.00001

- Archiving of unprocessed and processed data versions in clear folder structure is essential for future use or sharing of data with future collaborators.
- The enormous time invested in developing a professionally annotated dataset should be a future resource for testing external models for the benefit of healthcare research.

PEARLS

- Plan your database from the beginning with full understanding of the intended research or clinical outcomes and purposes.
- Well-defined data structure and relationships are the key to success.
- Anonymization is difficult. You have to remove protected health information from unexpected places. You might need to go back later and deanonymize.
- Validating and curating data are key elements of database creation and management.
- Databases work best when add-on software tools can access the data without manual intervention or exporting.

References

1. Fouke SJ, Benzinger TL, Milchenko M, LaMontagne P, Shimony JS, Chicoine MR, et al. The comprehensive neuro-oncology data repository (CONDR): a research infrastructure to develop and validate imaging biomarkers. Neurosurgery. 2014;74(1):88–98.
2. Prior F, Almeida J, Kathiravelu P, Kurc T, Smith K, Fitzgerald TJ, et al. Open access image repositories: high-quality data to enable machine learning research. Clin Radiol. 2020;75(1):7–12.
3. Prior F, Smith K, Sharma A, Kirby J, Tarbox L, Clark K, et al. The public cancer radiology imaging collections of The Cancer Imaging Archive. Sci Data. 2017;4:170124.
4. Rovere-Querini P, Tresoldi C, Conte C, Ruggeri A, Ghezzi S, De Lorenzo R, et al. Biobanking for COVID-19 research. Panminerva Med. 2020;
5. Armato SG 3rd, McLennan G, Bidaut L, McNitt-Gray MF, Meyer CR, Reeves AP, et al. The Lung Image Database Consortium (LIDC) and Image Database Resource Initiative (IDRI): a completed reference database of lung nodules on CT scans. Med Phys. 2011;38(2):915–31.
6. Clark KW, Gierada DS, Moore SM, Maffitt DR, Koppel P, Phillips SR, et al. Creation of a CT image library for the lung screening study of the national lung screening trial. J Digit Imaging. 2007;20(1):23–31.
7. Alfaro-Almagro F, Jenkinson M, Bangerter NK, Andersson JLR, Griffanti L, Douaud G, et al. Image processing and Quality Control for the first 10,000 brain imaging datasets from UK Biobank. NeuroImage. 2018;166:400–24.
8. Bamberg F, Kauczor HU, Weckbach S, Schlett CL, Forsting M, Ladd SC, et al. Whole-body MR imaging in the German National Cohort: rationale, design, and technical background. Radiology. 2015;277(1):206–20.
9. Basu A, Warzel D, Eftekhari A, Kirby JS, Freymann J, Knable J, et al. Call for data standardization: lessons learned and recommendations in an imaging study. JCO Clin Cancer Inform. 2019;3:1–11.
10. Bauermeister S, Orton C, Thompson S, Barker RA, Bauermeister JR, Ben-Shlomo Y, et al. The Dementias Platform UK (DPUK) Data Portal. Eur J Epidemiol. 2020;35(6):601–11.
11. Ziegler E, Urban T, Brown D, Petts J, Pieper SD, Lewis R, et al. Open health imaging foundation viewer: an extensible open-source framework for building web-based imaging applications to support cancer research. JCO Clin Cancer Inform. 2020;4:336–45.
12. Conroy M, Sellors J, Effingham M, Littlejohns TJ, Boultwood C, Gillions L, et al. The advantages of UK Biobank's open-access strategy for health research. J Intern Med. 2019;286(4):389–97.
13. Gedye C, Sachchithananthan M, Leonard R, Jeffree RL, Buckland ME, Ziegler DS, et al. Driving innovation through collaboration: development of clinical annotation datasets for brain cancer biobanking. Neurooncol Pract. 2020;7(1):31–7.

14. Sharma A, Tarbox L, Kurc T, Bona J, Smith K, Kathiravelu P, et al. PRISM: a platform for imaging in precision medicine. JCO Clin Cancer Inform. 2020;4:491–9.
15. Mattonen SA, Gude D, Echegaray S, Bakr S, Rubin DL, Napel S. Quantitative imaging feature pipeline: a web-based tool for utilizing, sharing, and building image-processing pipelines. J Med Imaging (Bellingham). 2020;7(4):042803.

Self-Assessment Questions

1. The data within an image is considered:

   (a) Structured data
   (b) Unstructured data
   (c) Semi-structured data

2. Protected health information does *not* include:

   (a) Name
   (b) Age
   (c) Date of birth
   (d) Location where images were obtained

3. Existing clinical data is considered:

   (a) Prospective
   (b) Retrospective
   (c) Introspective

4. A careful record of all changes made to the data in a database is called:

   (a) Audit trail
   (b) Governance
   (c) Warehousing
   (d) Validation
   (e) Curating

5. Unlike data use within the enterprise, data use between multiple institutions requires a:

   (a) Data access strategy
   (b) Business partnership
   (c) Audit trail
   (d) Data-sharing agreement

6. What is the difference between de-identification, anonymization, and pseudoanonymization?

7. What are the legal requirements in your country for privacy of protected health information? How could you help a researcher include PHI in a database if it was absolutely needed?

Chapter 12
Standards and Interoperability

Brad Genereaux

Contents

B. Genereaux (✉)
NVIDIA Corporation, Santa Clara, CA, USA

© The Author(s), under exclusive license to Springer Science+Business Media, LLC, part of Springer Nature 2021
B. F. Branstetter IV (ed.), *Practical Imaging Informatics*,
https://doi.org/10.1007/978-1-0716-1756-4_12

179

12.1 Introduction

There is a diverse set of hardware and software systems in a hospital, generally unique to the healthcare domain. Each of these systems contributes its own function within clinical and business workflows – but it is the harmonious integration that unlocks their true potential. These systems need to work together, resiliently and at scale.

The price of proprietary interfaces can be too high to bear. Pressures on the healthcare system result in having to do more with less and demand that operations be streamlined. Patient-centric care requires consistent access to a patient's data acquired from every institution they have been to, as clinicians require more versatile access on both desktop and mobile devices.

KEY CONCEPT: Proprietary Interface

A proprietary interface generally refers to a specification that is both defined by and solely used with a single vendor. This could be for a variety of reasons, such as an interoperable standard for such functionality was not available or in demand at the time of software development. Proprietary interfaces can increase the complexity of an integration and may increase the amount of time and resources needed to connect and support the integration through the lifetime of the solution. Proprietary interfaces should be avoided; users should demand their software providers support industry standard interfaces where possible.

Access to data has a human cost, too: if imaging studies are not readily available and accessible in interoperable systems, a patient may need to be reimaged. This may put the patient at increased risk of additional radiation and hospital-borne infections, may increase the cost to the patient and/or the healthcare system, may increase patient and caregiver discomfort and anxiety, may increase delays for the patient while reimaging takes place, and may increase the delays for other patients. Promoting interoperability can make a clinical difference.

Interoperability can help to lower the cost and barriers to healthcare, by helping to reduce delays and repeat examinations, by enabling collaboration with care teams locally and globally, and by helping to reduce medical errors through making information accessible. Standards help to enable more efficient and more effective diagnostic service delivery. This chapter will delve into healthcare Standard Delivery Organizations (SDOs); explain the standards they have created, including HL7 [1], DICOM [2], and IHE [3]; and consider why we use them.

Even as application development paradigms shift to service-oriented architectures and cloud-based services, the underlying need for interoperability remains ever-present. These versatile, dynamic environments with many systems continue to evolve, but by being able to integrate these tools deeply together, there is a direct impact on human lives. This is the promise of interoperability.

12.2 The Problem: A Dynamic Multivendor Ecosystem

12.2.1 Systems to Integrate

- For a hospital to function, many different types of systems are used to address various clinical and business needs of its staff and patients (Fig. 12.1).
- Many of these applications are created by different companies.
- Each application will have its own product lifecycle, with named versions and release dates. Hospitals may not be using the latest version for a variety of reasons.

CHECKLIST: Types of Hospital Systems

There are many types of hospital applications and services. The following list is not exhaustive.

Examples of hospital systems

Hospital information system (HIS)	Laboratory information system (LIS)
Radiology information system (RIS)	Picture archive communication systems (PACS)
Enterprise master patient index (EMPI)	Nurse call
Scheduling systems	Order entry systems
Pharmacy systems	Billing and HR systems
Diagnostic equipment	IV pumps
Drug-dispensing machines	

12.2.2 Workflows to Integrate

- Each of these systems needs to interconnect to coordinate workflow activities within the hospital.
- For example, when a patient arrives at a hospital for an ultrasound, they would first be registered via a registration system, have an order generated in a radiology information system, get images acquired on a modality, have a radiologist review these images in a PACS, have them create a report on those images in a reporting system, and ultimately share that report with the ordering physician and beyond (Fig. 12.2).
- Beyond this basic description, there are many nuanced differences to this workflow wherever implemented. Depending on the type of exam, the ordering and reporting physician, the patient condition, the patient location, the type of hospital, jurisdictional reporting and quality requirements, and remuneration requirements are just a few of the factors that might alter the specific workflow.

- Looking beyond the simple register-order-acquire-read-distribute use case, there are many other use cases to enable, including sharing studies with HIEs and VNAs, leveraging imaging acquired in other departments or in other institutions, integrating imaging into other applications (like EMRs or patient portals), advanced visualization and multimedia-enabled reports, and much more.

12.2.3 The Cost of Proprietary Integration

- The effort of developing and delivering an integration interface is not light by any means. An API (application programmatic interface) takes requirements, development, validation, post-release support, and ongoing maintenance.
- Proprietary interfaces from one system need to be mapped into another system to work properly; that takes additional effort.
- Developers also must take great care to not break interfaces when making updates – being both forward-compatible (newer integrations should work with legacy software) and backward-compatible (legacy integrations should work with new software).

> **DEFINITION: API**
>
> An application programmatic interface is a set of commands that a software vendor exposes to third-party programmers for the purpose of customizing the software and integrating it with other systems. APIs carry potential security risks and are difficult to maintain across software versions.

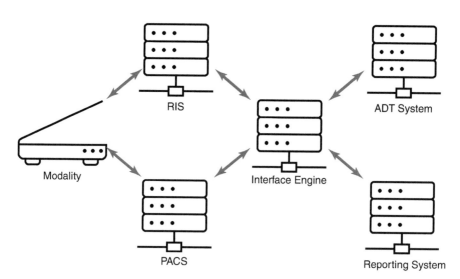

Fig. 12.1 General Radiology Systems Architecture. Each arrow represents a need for interoperability

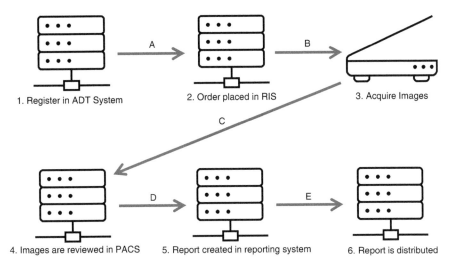

Fig. 12.2 General Radiology Imaging Workflow. A typical radiology department workflow, where each of these individual systems would need to communicate data with other systems to achieve a desired outcome (see **Chap. 16**)

- A **hospital integration team** within an IT department may manage all the interfaces for all the software that integrates together. There is a web of permutations of different vendors, software, and versions that need to be validated each time any part of the ecosystem is under maintenance. A breaking change could stop entire workflows from functioning.

12.2.4 Final Word

- Interoperability is intended to address the problems introduced by a multivendor IT ecosystem. By defining a standard that all clinical software can conform to, the resource impact on the entire ecosystem can be minimized.

12.3 HL7, the Health Data Standard

12.3.1 Overview

- HL7 is a set of international standards for transfer of clinical and administrative information between healthcare applications [4].

DEFINITION: HL7

An industry standard for the format of messages sent from one medical software system to another.

- It is used for information-centric activities by applications like EMRs to communicate clinical events, like patient registration, diagnostic orders, results, and billing information (Fig. 12.3).
- HL7 specifies both the structure of messages and the transportation protocol of the messages.
- There are two versions in common use today: v2 (version 2 messaging) and FHIR (Fast Healthcare Interoperability Resources).

> **KEY CONCEPT: HL7 versions**
>
> There are two versions of HL7 in common use: v2 and FHIR. Make sure your IT systems are using the same version, and the same subversion!

12.3.2 HL7 v2

- The v2 structure is a normative standard commonly used today.
- There are specific versions of v2 (e.g., v2.3, v.2.5.1) that have slight differences in the structure of data captured. It is important that systems that want to integrate between one another support the same version level of HL7 message.
- Each HL7 message is based on a trigger event. There are over a hundred types of trigger events; some of the most common include ADT (admission, discharge, and transfer) messages, ORM (order messages), and ORU (order results).
- The structure of an HL7 message is multiline ASCII text, with each line corresponding to a module, and each module separating its metadata using components (pipes) and sub-components (carats), generally referred to as **Pipehat notation**.
- Examples of modules include the PID (patient identification), the PV1 (patient visit), and IN1 (insurance details).
- HL7 data is transmitted using the MLLP protocol, a socket-based connection to send trigger messages. When messages are sent to a destination, an ACK (acknowledgment) message is generated. A NACK message (negative acknowledgment) is returned if the destination system was unable or unwilling to process the message.
- Order matters! Because HL7 messages are triggers for real-time events, it can be confusing to downstream systems if messages appear out of order (e.g., a patient discharge message is received before the patient admission message is received; this could happen if messages are held in queues when system downtime is occurring). Problems can also occur when clocks change – in particular, when they turn back an hour.

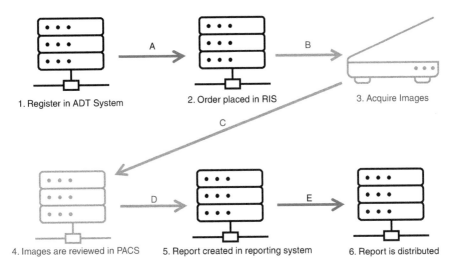

Fig. 12.3 Example HL7 v2 Workflow. Arrow A: When a patient arrives in hospital, an admission ADT message is generated, and sent to all clinical systems. System 2: When a physician orders an exam, an order ORM message is generated, and may be sent to RIS/PACS systems. Arrow E: When a radiologist completes a report, a report ORU message is generated, and sent to the EMR for the referring physician to review

12.3.3 FHIR

- FHIR is an emerging HL7 standard to describe and transmit healthcare information and, at the time of writing, has partially become normative [5].
- It is built on modular components, called resources (like "Patient" and "ImagingStudy") that can be assembled to document and communicate healthcare information and workflow.
- FHIR supports multiple exchange methods, including a RESTful variant which enables constructing new integrations that are not bound to trigger messages.
- FHIR supports multiple specifications like JSON and XML.
- A FHIR resource definition contains the attributes, data types, and cardinality to describe a particular instantiation of that object. For example, an observation (an object that conveys, for example, a hemoglobin laboratory result for a patient) would generally contain an attribute for the subject, referring to the patient.

> **KEY CONCEPT: XML and JSON**
>
> The specification of healthcare data can be done in many ways. In recent years, formats based on XML (eXtensible Markup Language) and JSON (JavaScript Object Notation) have become more prevalent, to both convey and describe the data, in condensed formats readable by both humans and machines. Both FHIR and DICOMweb use XML and JSON formats.

- In imaging workflows, the most relevant FHIR resources include ServiceRequest (the order), ImagingStudy (a representation of a DICOM study), and DiagnosticReport (the resulting report). There are many resources that support these three, including patient, practitioner, and procedure.

HYPOTHETICAL SCENARIO

It is early November, and daylight savings time is ending. At 3 a.m., the clocks are turned back, so there are two different time periods, both of which are nominally 2 a.m.–3 a.m. How will you prevent HL7 errors during this period? What systems will need to be shut down or placed on backup? How will you reconcile the data once everything is turned back on? How long will the physicians need to be on workflow continuity systems?

- An ImagingStudy representation may include endpoints, which define the ways in which the imaging study can be retrieved, using DICOM or other means.
- FHIR addresses many of the needs for interoperability in today's healthcare software ecosystem, but it is not yet universally deployed.

DEFINITION: REST

REST (REpresentational State Transfer) is an architectural programming style that ensures interoperability between computer systems on the Internet, and is used for defining APIs [17]. Made popular in many web-based applications outside of healthcare, it is becoming more and more prevalent in healthcare APIs like FHIR and DICOMweb.

12.4 DICOM, the Imaging Standard

12.4.1 Overview

- DICOM (Digital Imaging and COmmunications in Medicine) is the standard for handling, storing, printing, and transmitting information in medical imaging [6].
- It is used for imaging-centric activities (e.g., PACS, post-processing), retrieval of imaging, conveying raw data with metadata, as well as providing rendered versions of images.
- Like HL7, it includes both a file structure and communication protocol. HL7 and DICOM work together, with HL7 focusing on non-imaging-centric activities.
- DICOM is administered and published under NEMA (National Electrical Manufacturers Association) by MITA (Medical Imaging and Technology Alliance) [2].

- Vendors claim conformance to the DICOM standard through publication of a DICOM conformance statement document. This provides key insights on the capabilities of the system and how it works within an imaging ecosystem.

12.4.2 DICOM Structure

- DICOM defines the formats for images, waveforms, and derived structured data, providing the quality and metadata necessary for clinical use.
- It additionally provides some imaging workflow management, media exchange and printing, and service-based network protocols over TCP/IP and HTTP (Fig. 12.4).
- DICOM stores images and raw data from a variety of modalities, including X-ray, CT, MRI, ultrasound, mammography, angiography, PET, and dental, ophthalmology, and digital pathology.

DEFINITION: DICOM

An industry standard for the format of digital medical images and the communication of images from one software system to another.

DEFINITION: DICOM Conformance Statement

This document, provided by a system manufacturer, describes the DICOM services and structures that the system supports. Be sure to read this to gain key insights into your systems when integrating.

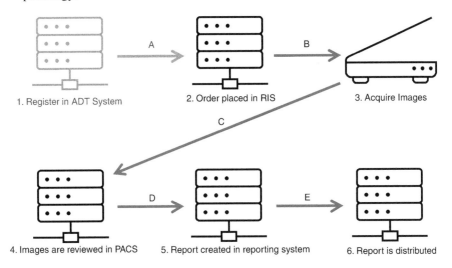

1. Register in ADT System   2. Order placed in RIS   3. Acquire Images

4. Images are reviewed in PACS   5. Report created in reporting system   6. Report is distributed

Fig. 12.4 Example DICOM Workflow. Arrow B: DICOM MWL is used by technicians acquiring images to select the right patient and order. Arrow C: Images that are acquired are transformed into DICOM objects and stored to a PACS. Arrow D: DICOM is retrieved by PACS workstations for display. Arrow E: DICOM (web versions in particular) may be viewed as part of the report review process

- The types of images stored can vary greatly; they could be single images or a stack of related images. Stacks of images could relate to multiple slices in the body (e.g., a CT stack), or it could refer to specific points of time (e.g., an ultrasound of a heart beating).
- DICOM stores more than images; it could be waveforms (such as ECG data), structured reports (such as sets of measurements), CAD or AI findings, videos captured by surgical equipment, collections of images (called KOS, or **key object selection**) organized for presentation, or image markup (called GSPS, or **grayscale presentation state**).

12.4.3 DICOM Information Object Definitions

KEY CONCEPT: Hierarchy of DICOM Objects

DICOM object hierarchy

Level	Description	Example
Subject	A patient (human or animal) who has one or more studies	Jane Smith
Study	A collection of imaging sets relating to a specific diagnostic request, with one or more series	CT abdomen W W/O contrast
Series	A collection of instances bound by the type of imaging and the general point of time, with one or more instances	CT abdomen W contrast
Instance	A specific binary payload, which may contain individual frames	Multi-frame CT instance
Frame	An optional single image that's part of an image set	Slice 236 of 1200
NPO	Various non-patient-related information, like color profiles or protocols	Routine adult abdomen CT protocol

- Besides the binary payload, DICOM captures significant metadata in the DICOM header relating to instances, such as patient identification, order details, acquisition details, protocol details, and much more.
- DICOM uses a **paired hexadecimal structure** for representing metadata. The first part of the pair represents the grouping of data; (0010) represents patient-related data, for example. The second part of the pair represents a specific attribute in that group. For example, patient name is described in tag (0010,0010), whereas the referring physician name is described in (0008, 0090).
- Each metadata attribute has a data type (such as ST for short text, or PN for person name), referred to as value representation (VR). Each attribute also has a value multiplicity, which indicates the number of values that can be encoded in this field. Lastly, each attribute will have a type which indicates its optionality (e.g., mandatory, optional, or conditional).
- Each DICOM study, series, and instance is identified by a unique identifier (UID). These numbers are globally unique, meaning that nowhere in the world

should two numbers be the same. This is done using an OID (object identifier) root, which is a string of numbers assigned to a particular institution. After the OID root, numbers are appended to make the UID unique. For example, a base OID might be "3.1.2.41.117.23," and the institution might then assign a department number, an equipment number, a study number, a series number, and an instance number.

- Patient identifiers and accession numbers are not guaranteed to be globally unique, and thus should be paired with an appropriate issuer.
- **DICOM files are not edited**; if it undergoes major changes (e.g., changes to the binary payload), it gets assigned a new unique instance number.

INTERNATIONAL CONSIDERATIONS

Various fields are represented differently throughout the world. Consider person name, which may include specific character sets, as well as ideographic and phonetic representations, as described in PS3.5 6.2 of the DICOM standard.

12.4.4 DICOM Workflow and Transport

- Aside from specifying the structure of data, DICOM also supports **transmission of data** through C-MOVE and C-STORE, discovery of data through C-FIND, connectivity checking through C-ECHO, workflows like modality worklists (MWL), modality-performed procedure steps (MPPS), storage commitment, and unified procedure step (UPS).

KEY CONCEPT: DICOM Information Object Definition (IOD)

A DICOM IOD defines a set of attributes for key concepts in a DICOM object. The following is just some of the attributes found in the Patient Module IOD [18].

Selected attributes in the Patient Module IOD

Attribute name	Tag	Type	Description
Patient's name	(0010,0010)	2	Patient's full name
Patient ID	(0010,0020)	2	Primary identifier for the patient
Patient's birth date	(0010,0030)	2	Birth date of the patient
Patient's birth time	(0010,0032)	3	Birth time of the patient
Patient's sex	(0010,0040)	2	Sex of the named patient
...	...	...	...

This table details the fields that compromise the information module. The "type" denotes whether the field is mandatory (type 1), conditionally mandatory (type 1C), mandatory with empty values permitted (type 2), and optional elements (type 3)

- Sharing DICOM content can be done using network transport and media transfer (via CD, DVD, or USB), as e-mail attachments, or via the web.
- As DICOM instances can contain patient-sensitive confidential information, transmission is secured through a variety of mechanisms including encryption, audit trails, and de-identification.
- To transmit DICOM, a **Service-Object Pair** (SOP) is constructed, which defines the specific action being performed. For example, a service "Image Storage" plus an object "MRI" would equate to an "MRI Image Storage" as the SOP Class.
- When communicating DICOM from one computer to another, there is a client, called the **SCU** (service class user), and a server, called the **SCP** (service class provider). Each of these actors is referenced by their application entity (*AE*) name and distinguished by the calling **AE** (the SCU name) and the called AE (the SCP name).

TROUBLESHOOTING: DICOM

- When troubleshooting network connectivity, first check the configuration, and that the right IP addresses, ports, and AE titles are being used for both the SCU and the SCP. Test the connection using a C-ECHO.
- Do a "telnet" test. First, be sure that a telnet command is installed on the client machine. From the command line, telnet to the IP address and port number. If the connection is denied, there is likely a network issue (with the firewall, router, or path to the destination). If the screen goes blank, it is likely not a network issue; rather, the issue is more likely at the application level.
- Verify the conformance statements of both the SCU and SCP to ensure they support the services that each needs to offer for the desired workflow.

12.4.5 DICOMweb

- DICOMweb is a collection of HTTP-driven services for access to DICOM services, in the style of REST (representational state transfer) [7].
- DICOMweb can provide incremental capability enhancements for DICOM-enabled systems, by layering HTTP-based services for discovery, retrieval, and storage.

KEY CONCEPT: DICOMweb Services

Types of DICOMweb services

Query	Discover studies and their structure, lists studies for a patient, for a procedure, for a modality, and more. Also known as QIDO-RS
Retrieve	Retrieve DICOM objects and their components; download full DICOM, headers, rendered images, and other data. Also known as WADO-RS
Store	Upload new instances into an image manager for storage; add to existing studies or add new ones. Also known as STOW-RS
Tasks	Unified procedure step to create work items and manage them through the lifecycle
Server info	Capability service that lists what a DICOMweb server is capable of

- There are five core services DICOMweb services: query (QIDO-RS), retrieve (WADO-RS), store (STOW-RS), tasks (UPS-RS), and server info.
- Querying for studies can include passing specific filter criteria and provide the ability to return additional metadata in the response. Servers may or may not support these requests. Querying can occur at the study level, at the series level, or at the instance level.
- Similarly, retrieving studies can be done at the study, series, or instance level. Retrieval could be for the raw DICOM instances, for rendered images (suitable for presentation for display in a web application), for just metadata, for thumbnails, or in other formats (like bulk data).
- DICOMweb supports both an XML and a JSON representation of the metadata.

FURTHER READING: DICOMweb Cheat Sheet

https://www.dicomstandard.org/dicomweb/dicomweb-cheatsheet

12.5 Coding Systems

12.5.1 SNOMED-CT

- SNOMED-CT [8] is a comprehensive and precise multilingual health terminology system to describe and relate concepts in the healthcare space to assist with the electronic exchange of clinical health information.
- It is developed collaboratively to ensure it meets the diverse needs and expectations of the worldwide medical profession.
- SNOMED-CT is used within HL7 [9] and DICOM [10] for anatomy, clinical findings, procedures, pharmaceutical/biologic products (including contrast agents), and other clinical terms.

12.5.2 LOINC

- LOINC [11] is a common language (set of identifiers, names, and codes) for identifying health measurements, observations, and documents.
- It is used in both HL7 and DICOM as an external vocabulary and extensively used in value sets and structured report templates.

12.5.3 ICD

- The International Classification of Diseases (ICD) [12] describes the reasons why patients seek medical care.
- These are used by health agencies around the world to produce normalized statistics and for billing.

12.6 Integrating the Healthcare Enterprise (IHE)

12.6.1 Introduction

- Having standards that define how to structure and transmit information is a tremendous step forward, but it does not go far enough.
- Just because two systems speak the same standard does not mean that they interoperate. For example, two ultrasound carts on the same network that use DICOM do not necessarily work together.
- To provide meaningful interoperable services, use cases can be identified, and broken down into individual steps. **Actors** can be identified who participate in these steps in **specific roles**. This is defined as an **integration profile**.
- **IHE International** [3] is the organization that manages these profiles and works with professional societies, academic centers, and industry to author them.
- IHE specifies a common framework for harmonizing and implementing existing standards, resulting in profiles to address specific use cases in healthcare. It promotes unbiased selection and coordinated use of established healthcare and IT standards to address these needs.
- IHE profiles enable seamless health information movement within and between enterprises, regions, and nations.

> **KEY CONCEPT: IHE Integration Statement**
>
> This document, provided by the manufacturer, describes the way a product transacts in a profile as an actor.

- At the time of writing, there are profiles in 11 clinical domains, including radiology and IT infrastructure.
- Integration profiles describe workflow use cases, standards, and the overall relationships to achieve transparent interoperability.
- Integration statements tell customers the IHE Profiles supported by a specific release of a specific product. This is an important document to review to understand a product's capabilities.
- **Technical frameworks** are the documents for each domain that specify the integration profiles and the associated actors and transactions.
- **Connectathons** are neutral testing events with multiple vendors in one room, including developers and testers, to promote rapid and robust interoperability testing.

> **FURTHER READING: IHE Frequently Asked Questions**
>
> https://www.ihe.net/about_ihe/FAQ/

12.6.2 Key IHE Profiles for Radiology

- The following profiles are important in the IHE radiology domain [13]. Review the profiles, and associated actors and transactions in the radiology technical framework.
- Scheduled Workflow (SWF) describes the basic radiology workflow, including ordering, scheduling, acquisition, storing, and viewing.
- Consistent Presentation of Images (CPI) guides the digital display of medical images, along with their presentation states.
- Cross-Enterprise Document Sharing for Imaging (XDS-I) specifies the approach to sharing imaging content between institutions, using the notion of a registry and repository.
- Encounter-Based Imaging Workflow (EBIW) describes the non-order-based workflow, typically used in enterprise imaging or ad hoc acquisition use cases.
- Invoke Image Display (IID) profile (in trial implementation at the time of writing) describes how applications can invoke a medical imaging viewer for integration into clinical applications.
- Web-Based Image Access (WIA) and Web-Based Image Capture (WIC) profiles (in trial implementation at the time of writing) describe DICOMweb extensions for accessing medical imaging.
- AI Results (AIR) and AI Workflow for Imaging (AIW-I) profiles (in trial implementation at the time of writing) describe the payloads and inference request/response pattern for artificial intelligence models.

12.6.3 Key IHE Profiles for IT Infrastructure

- The following profiles are important in the IHE IT infrastructure domain [14]. IT infrastructure focuses on interoperability problems that generally exist horizontally across all clinical domains.
- Audit Trail and Node Authentication (ATNA) defines the basis for a secure system on the network, including security and auditing requirements.
- Enterprise User Authentication (EUA), Cross-Enterprise User Assertion (XUA), and Internet User Authorization (IUA) provide important security protocols for identifying users and services for a variety of situations.
- Patient Identifier Cross-Referencing (PIX) and Patient Demographics Query (PDQ) provide services for unique identification of patients.

12.7 Bringing It All Together

12.7.1 Building an Integration

- There are many ways to integrate two applications together – whether it uses HL7 v2 or DICOM DIMSE services or the web-enabled workflows of FHIR and DICOMweb.
- Image-enabling applications can be far-reaching, including enabling patient portals, medical rounds reviews, artificial intelligence, and computer-aided detection.
- There are many open-source libraries that can be used with DICOM; this includes Orthanc (https://www.orthanc-server. com/), DCM4CHEE (https:// www.dcm4che.org/), and OHIF (http://ohif.org/). There are also great open-source HL7 tools, like HAPI (https://hapifhir.io/).
- Often, integration engines, like HAPI, are used to connect two

CHECKLIST: Healthcare Software Integrations

- Set specific goals and use cases to be addressed.
- Create architecture and flow diagrams on which systems need to talk to one another.
- Understand the depth to which each system can be integrated.
- Engage the right people from each stakeholder group.
- Include the right hardware, software, network, and security configurations.
- Create execution plan detailing milestones and go/no-go criteria.
- Include sufficient testing of both core and edge use cases.
- Ensure that there are different environments for development, testing, and production.

different systems together. These engines allow for enhanced customization of the healthcare data, by allowing it to be intercepted, adjusted, and sent to other destinations.

CHECKLIST: System Integration Details

When integrating two systems together, information about the endpoints need to be collected. These are the commonly-needed attributes.

System integration details

General	DICOM specific
Hostname	Calling AE (DICOM)
IP address	Called AE (DICOM)
Manufacturer	Modality type
Model	SOP Class
Connection time-outs	Storage commit
	Transfer Syntax
	Max associations

- Web technologies in the standards (FHIR, DICOMweb) enable integrations beyond prescribed data flows, by providing extensible building blocks to meet evolving needs and novel, unique use cases.
- Making too many API requests, regardless of interoperable or proprietary interface, may negatively impact system performance. Consider the impact of making such requests into a taxed software ecosystem: adding additional queries, requests, and storage of content will have an impact on the performance of these systems for existing users. Load should be simulated in test environments before moving to production.

12.7.2 Identity

- Identity of data is of critical importance – every patient, order, study, series, and instance will have an identifier. That allows systems to succinctly guarantee retrieval of records the user has requested.
- Maintaining identity across systems is important, but also challenging. Patient and order identifiers may collide when shared with other applications, creating dangerous combinations.
- For example, consider two hospitals, who both started numbering charts from "1" and increasing from there; patient 1001 at each hospital is a different patient. If these two systems are combined, those records could merge, creating dangerous results.

TROUBLESHOOTING: Integrations

- Test for special characters, field length restrictions, and blank fields. See https://cheatsheetseries.owasp. org/cheatsheets/Input_Validation_ Cheat_Sheet.html.
- Understand what is globally unique and what is not: issuer of patient ID and issuer of accession number are important to include when considering how applications can interoperate.
- When designing systems, account for system downtime, understand what happens when the data flow has stopped; clinical workflows should continue to function.

- To identify records using fields that are not globally unique, like patient or order number, **identity issuer fields** exist in both HL7 and DICOM that provide an organization identifier in which the identity is defined. In the previous example, "HOSPA" and "HOSPB" could be patient issuer labels, and "HOSPA:1001" and "HOSPB:1001" would thus identify the distinction between these two records.
- Aside from identity of the patient and study, there are other fields where identity could be problematic, e.g., a "chest CT study" performed at two different institutions may be quite different depending on the typical acquisition protocol at each site.

12.7.3 Security

- This chapter does not go into depth on general healthcare security requirements. The focus is on where security and interoperability collide.

- Security is about protecting data against unauthorized access, protecting data integrity against unauthorized changes, protecting data loss against unauthorized deletions, and protecting data availability against denial of service. Each of these comes into play with interoperability, with inbound requests to download, upload, and interact with sensitive data.

- Authentication focuses on identity of the client. Institutions may use LDAP-based services to authenticate a domain client or service. Applications may also provide their own user and service directories.

- Authorization focuses on understanding what a named identity has access to. It is critical to respect patient privacy regulations (PIPEDA, HIPAA, GDPR) when responding to requests.

CHECKLIST: Integration Security Considerations

This list is not exhaustive:
- Use DICOM-TLS and HTTPS for DICOMweb.
- Use appropriate authentication and authorization measures, such as strong password policies.
- Do not put usernames and passwords in URLs.
- Be aware that using user-based authentication integrations may have passwords expire and cause services to fail.
- Use appropriate at-rest encryption mechanisms.
- Control access via managed environments, strong identity management, and firewalls.
- Consider security throughout your project lifecycle, not at the end.

- Authorization models may rely on mechanisms for opt-in (granted to specific users) or opt-out (VIP patients), which typically fall under EMR jurisdiction, and may offer "break the glass" functionality when access is disallowed but it is an emergency situation.

- Authorization also controls what the user can do, including amending and sign-off on diagnostic reports, adding new markup, or viewing final and/or preliminary reports. These actions are applicable to API calls, too.

- Encryption ensures that communication between points in interoperability is protected. This includes the use of HTTPS, DICOM-TLS, and VPN technology.

- When interoperability events occur, they should be audited in a secured log, with the named service/user accounts, and timestamps. Some examples of events to be audited include authentication, query, access, transfer, import/export, and deletion.

DEFINITION: Pseudoanonymization

Anonymization is replacing patient-specific information with blanks.

Pseudoanonymization is replacing patient-specific information with fake data of a similar format (e.g., replace the patient's name with "Mickey Mouse").

- Nodes themselves should be verified. In IHE IT infrastructure, the ATNA profile [15] describes this functionality.
- **Anonymization** may be needed for specific integrations, such as for clinical trials, teaching files, and cloud processing of artificial intelligence applications. Anonymization is described in DICOM PS3.15 section E [16], which addresses removal and replacement of DICOM attributes that may reveal protected health information.

PEARLS

- Interoperability in healthcare describes how distinct clinical systems can work together to meet clinical and operational use cases.
- Done right, interoperability magnifies overall system efficiency and effectiveness, by ensuring connected systems have access to the clinical data and workflows needed to optimally deliver care.
- Standards enable software to offer a consistent, version-agnostic API that other software in the ecosystem can integrate with, without having to create last-mile customization.
- HL7 is a set of international standards for transfer of clinical and administrative information between healthcare applications (you use HL7 to send a message when an event happens).
- DICOM is the standard for handling, storing, printing, and transmitting information in medical imaging (you use DICOM to convey important metadata along with an image).
- IHE profiles are used to create workflows that are meaningful to the healthcare system and the people who work within it (you use IHE to ensure that each actor in the ecosystem knows how to play its role).
- Coding systems encode clinical concepts that are universally recognized to trigger and react to data in the workflow (you use coding systems to make sure that everyone is using the same term in the same way).
- Even with standards, a lot of work needs to happen to ensure connected systems are secure, data can be properly identified, and connected workflows truly meet the demands of the healthcare system.

References

1. HL7.org, [Online]. Available: http://www.hl7.org/. Accessed 29 Sept 2020.
2. DICOM, [Online]. Available: https://www.dicomstandard.org/. Accessed 29 Sept 2020.
3. IHE, [Online]. Available: https://www.ihe.net/. Accessed 29 Sept 2020.
4. Wikipedia definition of HL7, [Online]. Available: https://en.wikipedia.org/wiki/Health_Level_7. Accessed 29 Sept 2020.
5. HL7 FHIR, [Online]. Available: https://www.hl7.org/fhir/. Accessed 29 Sept 2020.
6. Wikipedia definition of DICOM, 30 September 2020. [Online]. Available: https://en.wikipedia.org/wiki/DICOM.

7. Genereaux BW, Dennison DK, Ho K, Horn R, Silver EL, O'Donnell K, Kahn CE Jr. DICOMweb™: background and application of the web standard for medical imaging. J Digit Imaging. 2018;31(3):321–6.
8. SNOMED-CT, [Online]. Available: https://www.snomed.org/snomed-ct/why-snomed-ct. Accessed 29 Sept 2020.
9. SNOMED-CT and FHIR, [Online]. Available: https://www.hl7.org/fhir/snomedct.html. Accessed 29 Sept 2020.
10. DICOM use of SNOMED, [Online]. Available: http://dicom.nema.org/medical/dicom/current/output/chtml/part16/chapter_2.html#biblio_SNOMED. Accessed 29 Sept 2020.
11. LOINC Homepage, [Online]. Available: https://loinc.org/. Accessed 29 Sept 2020.
12. ICD Factsheet, [Online]. Available: https://www.who.int/classifications/icd/factsheet/en/. Accessed 29 Sept 2020.
13. IHE Radiology Domain, [Online]. Available: https://www.ihe.net/ihe_domains/radiology/. Accessed 29 Sept 2020.
14. IHE IT Infrastructure, [Online]. Available: https://www.ihe.net/ihe_domains/it_infrastructure/. Accessed 29 Sept 2020.
15. Audit Trail and Node Authentication (ATNA). IHE IT Infrastructure Technical Framework, vol. 1. IHE International; 2020.
16. Attribute Confidentiality Profiles, [Online]. Available: http://dicom.nema.org/medical/dicom/current/output/chtml/part15/chapter_E.html. Accessed 29 Sept 2020.
17. Wikipedia definition of REST, [Online]. Available: https://en.wikipedia.org/wiki/Representational_state_transfer. Accessed 29 Sept 2020.
18. Table C.7-1. Patient module attributes, [Online]. Available: http://dicom.nema.org/medical/dicom/current/output/chtml/part03/sect_C.7.html#table_C.7-1. Accessed 29 Sept 2020.

Notices

HL7, CDA, FHIR, and the FHIR [FLAME DESIGN] are the registered trademarks of Health Level Seven International, and the use does not constitute endorsement by HL7.

DICOM is the registered trademark of the National Electrical Manufacturers Association (NEMA) for its standards publications relating to digital communications of medical information.

IHE International is the copyright holder for IHE materials.

The author graciously acknowledges the contributions of all those involved in the interoperability community, including those who have given so much to DICOM, HL7, and IHE for the betterment of humanity. The author also wishes to recognize the works of David Clunie, Don Dennison, Kevin O'Donnell, Chris Hafey, Kinson Ho, Rob Horn, Mohannad Hussain, Chris Lindop, Jeroen Medema, David Mendelson, John Moehrke, Jim Philbin, Chris Roth, Elliot Silver, Harry Solomon, Lawrence Tarbox, and Jonathan Whitby.

Self-Assessment Questions

1. What document do you refer to when you need to know what your new CT modality supports for interoperability?

2. What is the difference between a DICOM study and a DICOM series?

3. Where would you go to reference which standards would go into a Scheduled Workflow profile?

4. What standard would you use to discover a patient ID if you know the patient name?

5. What standard would you use to discover additional available images for a particular imaging study?

6. What are some security considerations when connecting two systems together?

7. Why would a hospital want to use healthcare standards in their IT infrastructure?

8. You just purchased a new ultrasound modality for your department. What do you need to know to connect it to your network?

9. When incorporating DICOM data from outside your institution into your PACS, what are some concerns around ingesting this data?

Chapter 13
Billing and Coding

Douglas S. Griffin

Contents

13.1 Introduction

In financially contracting environments, tighter margins compel leadership to look for innovative ways to increase profits and lower expenses. IIPs must monitor vital interfaces that transmit essential information used by many other systems such as billing and coding systems. The constricting payment model associated with bundled charges and additional payer requirements requires an adaptive team. Procedure documentation is more important than ever to guard against retrospective audits that threaten to repeal payments previously received.

13.2 Revenue Cycle

The reimbursement environment has become burdensome to healthcare providers and facilities, making electronic efficiencies essential in systems development. To appreciate the importance of this workflow, one must first understand what occurs at each stage of the revenue cycle to safeguard reimbursement (Fig. 13.1).

D. S. Griffin (✉)
Oncology Services, Southeast Health, Dothan, AL, USA
e-mail: dsgriffin@southeasthealth.org

© The Author(s), under exclusive license to Springer Science+Business Media, LLC, part of Springer Nature 2021
B. F. Branstetter IV (ed.), *Practical Imaging Informatics*,
https://doi.org/10.1007/978-1-0716-1756-4_13

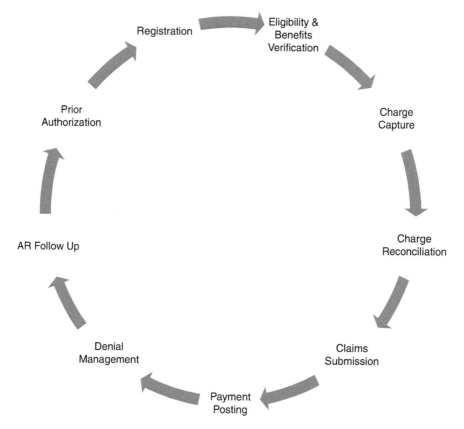

Fig. 13.1 The reimbursement cycle

A. *Registration*

During patient registration, acquiring accurate patient information is vital for downstream processes. Deficits in health literacy pose a significant obstacle to obtaining accurate information [1]. Only 4–14% of Americans have a basic understanding of health insurance, making information gathering at registration a challenge which directly affects the entire revenue cycle [2].

> **DEFINITION: Health Literacy**
>
> "The degree to which individuals have the capacity to obtain, process, and understand basic health information and services needed to make appropriate health decisions" [3].

After the patient information has been entered, verification of eligibility is initiated to assess the status of the patient's policy and associated contract benefits.

CHECKLIST: Data Elements Gathered at Registration

- Patient name
- Date of birth
- Address
- Phone number
- Referring physician
- Primary/secondary insurance
- Policy and group number
- Diagnosis code
- Ordered procedures (ICD-10 and CPT codes – see below)

B. *Prior Authorization*

After initial information is gathered from the patient, authorization from the payer is requested to perform the ordered procedure, service, or medication. In most cases, when authorization is provided, the authorization number is entered into the EMR for future reference.

C. *Order Appropriateness/Utilization*

Order appropriateness and utilization have been used for many years and are the focus of new efforts to control medical cost and lower radiation exposure. Introduced in 2014, the **Protecting Access to Medicare Act** (PAMA) ensures the appropriateness of diagnostic imaging services provided for Medicare beneficiaries. Under this program, ordering providers are expected to consult a qualified clinical decision support mechanism (CDSM). Appropriate use criteria (AUC) were developed to assist the provider in choosing the most appropriate test for the individual based on their specific condition. Various modifiers (MA-MH) are applied to the order to reflect the results generated from the CDSM [4].

> **DEFINITION: Decision Support**
>
> An interactive software tool that assists providers in making care decisions. In the context of radiology, clinical decision support is software that guides referring physicians to choose the optimal imaging technique for a given clinical situation.

> **FURTHER READINGS: Appropriate Use**
>
> Appropriate Use Criteria (AUC) for Advanced Diagnostic Imaging – Educational and Operations Testing Period - Claims Processing Requirements (https://www.cms.gov/Outreach-and-Education/Medicare-Learning-Network-MLN/MLNMattersArticles/Downloads/MM11268.pdf)
>
> Appropriate Use Criteria for Advanced Diagnostic Imaging – MLN Fact Sheet (https://www.cms.gov/Outreach-and-Education/Medicare-Learning-Network-MLN/MLNProducts/Downloasds/AUCDiagnosticImaging-909377.pdf)
>
> Clinical Decision Support – Tipsheet (https://www.healthit.gov/sites/default/files/clinicaldecisionsupport_tipsheet.pdf)

D. *Order Entry*

After the registration steps have been completed, the order must be entered into the EMR to link all subsequent charges and results. Once the order entry has occurred, future services rendered are linked via various identifying information such as medical record number (MRN), account number, and accession number.

E. *Charge Capture*

Charges are associated based on the charge description master (CDM) and Healthcare Common Procedure Coding System (HCPCS) codes. Based on the current procedural terminology (CPT), HCPCS codes represent specific procedures and services and help facilitate health insurance claims. Once a procedure has been performed, **medical coders** review the procedures that were performed and check them for accuracy against CPT and HCPCS codes. These coding systems are described in greater detail below. On charge capture, the association between relevant codes and the CDM must be accurate – this is an essential function of system build and maintenance.

F. *Charge Reconciliation*

Ensuring that every procedure was appropriately and accurately charged is a continuous part of daily operations. Typically, imaging departments have a daily task of charge reconciliation review whereby previous shift's procedures are reviewed and compared against charge entry. The charge reconciliation step guarantees that the work performed has been appropriately charged and ultimately billed.

13.3 Terminology and Standards

As part of the Joint Commission's National Patient Safety Goals, one of the required patient identifiers that are still used is the patient name. This is not the best method of uniquely identifying a patient, but in combination with date of birth and medical record number, the statistical likelihood of a patient being misidentified is low. These identifiers are similarly used by billing and coding systems.

When a patient arrives at a healthcare facility, they are also assigned a medical record number (MRN) as well as an account or **encounter number** that delineates which of the patient's visits the data correspond to:

DEFINITION: Medical Coding

Accurate and efficient completion of patient paperwork so that it can be submitted to the insurance carrier for reimbursement.

SYNONYMS: Medical Record Number

- MRN
- Unique patient identifier
- Patient ID
- Historically equated with social security number, but not since the advent of HIPAA

- The MRN is assigned to each patient and is unique to the patient by facility. (For enterprises with multiple facilities, a Master Patient Index is a centralized database that reconciles the MRNs at different facilities within the enterprise.) The MRN ensures that a patient is not mistaken for another patient with a similar name and is usually crossmatched with date of birth.
- The International Classification of Diseases, tenth revision (**ICD-10**), was developed internationally to **classify disease** and determine mortality statistics. The ICD-10 Clinical Modification (ICD-10-CM) is typically used by physician offices and hospitals to classify diagnostic, therapeutic, and surgical procedures.

> **FURTHER READING:**
> **Radiology Coding**
>
> Clinical Examples in Radiology: A Practical Guide to Correct Coding. (quarterly newsletter published jointly by the AMA and ACR)

  Alternatively, an ICD-10 code and current procedural terminology (CPT) code can be combined to identify the exam that has been ordered. When coding and billing representatives verify data, the patient name, CPT, and date of service are vital in assuring that reimbursement will be granted by the carrier.
- CPT or current procedural terminology is utilized to ensure that the correct test or procedure is performed in conjunction with medical necessity.
- The Healthcare Common Procedure Coding System (HCPCS; commonly pronounced "hicks picks") may also be used to describe services rendered to a patient.

In some practices, the interpreting radiologist provides suggested CPT and ICD-10 coding during dictation. In others, the professional billing personnel must gather and provide this information from what is included in the radiologist's report:

- Type of study
- Body part
- Number of views or sequences
- Administration of contrast
- Patient history
- Comparative data from other exams
- Diagnosis

In these cases, it is vital that complete and correct information be included in the information sent to the coders to ensure that billing is accurate and complete. Newer software such as computerized physician order entry (CPOE), and some radiology reporting systems assist in proper coding at the time of order entry and report creation.

13.4 Required Practices

Coding and billing representatives may identify improper correlation between the requested study and the study that was actually performed. This may have a negative effect on reimbursement. For example, a two-view chest X-ray has been ordered (in error) to verify line placement rather than a single-view portable chest X-ray. In other situations, the coding and billing representatives may recognize that the radiologist's report mentions one body part and the bill or charge has been created to reflect another. This happens frequently in healthcare with the use of correct or incorrect sides of the body (i.e., right vs. left). The implications of this common occurrence on reimbursement will be a denial of payment and a delay while the error is corrected.

KEY CONCEPT: Professional vs. Technical Charges

Doctors and other providers generate professional charges when they care for patients. The professional fees are generally collected by the department or physician group.

Technical charges arise from the equipment and personnel provided by the hospital or care facility. These are billed and collected by the administration of the facility itself.

If the healthcare facility is owned by the treating physicians, or there is a joint billing agreement, this may be the same billing department, but the technical and professional charges are still submitted separately.

For example, when a patient gets an MRI, the hospital submits a technical charge to pay for the MRI machine, the surrounding building, and the technologist who obtained the images. The radiologist submits a professional charge for overseeing the imaging, ensuring image quality, and interpreting the examination.

Charges are often separated into components: technical, which is usually billed and collected by the healthcare facility, and professional, which is usually billed and collected by the radiologist practice. The division of billing between the technical and the professional services is complex and requires expert (and often legal) input to determine which bills are submitted by whom.

13.4.1 CPT Codes

An understanding of the American Medical Association's CPT Codebook is an absolute requirement for coders. The Standard Edition of the CPT Codebook is comprised of the following different categories of codes:

DEFINITION: CPT

Current procedural terminology codes are used to precisely classify medical, surgical, and diagnostic services and procedures.

1. Evaluation and management
2. Anesthesia
3. Surgery

4. Radiology
5. Pathology and laboratory
6. Medicine

Radiology is further subdivided into the following sections consisting of their own numerical scheme:

1. Aorta and arteries
2. Veins and lymphatics
3. Transcatheter procedures
4. Diagnostic ultrasound
5. Abdomen and retroperitoneum
6. Obstetrical
7. Nonobstetrical
8. Radiation oncology
9. Clinical treatment planning
10. Radiation treatment
11. Management
12. Proton beam therapy
13. Delivery
14. Hyperthermia
15. Clinical brachytherapy
16. Nuclear medicine
17. Musculoskeletal system
18. Cardiovascular system
19. Therapeutic

> **FURTHER READING: CPT and ICD-10 Codes**
>
> The AMA online bookstore has numerous publications regarding proper CPT and ICD-10 coding, including many books specific to radiology.

- There are additional subsets such as results/testing/reports, special reports, supervision and interpretation, administration of contrast material(s), and written reports.
- The **format of CPT codes** is five alphanumeric characters:
  - Category I codes consist of five numbers and describe a reimbursable procedure that is part of accepted medical practice.
  - Category II codes consist of four numbers and one letter and are used for tracking performance. They are not reimbursable.
  - Category III codes consist of four numbers and one letter and are used for experimental procedures. They are not reimbursable.
- In many cases, specific **modifiers** are used to ensure proper reimbursement is achieved.
- More than one CPT code may be assigned to a single examination. This may or may not necessitate a separate radiology report or a separate section of a report.

> **DEFINITION: ICD-10**
>
> ICD-10 codes are used to classify medical diseases and a wide variety of signs, symptoms, abnormal findings, complaints, social circumstances, and external causes of injury or disease.

- **Medicare reimbursement rates** depend on CPT code and geographic area.
- The AMA has an online search tool for CPT codes: https://commerce.ama-assn.org/store/ui/catalog/.

13.4.2 ICD-10 Codes

ICD-10 codes are used to describe diseases and symptoms that justify the need for radiology procedures:

- The United States uses a variation of ICD-10 called the ICD-10 Clinical Modification (ICD-10-CM).
- The format of ICD-10-CM is a seven-character alphanumeric code. Each code starts with one letter followed by two numbers which indicate the category (the general type of injury or disease). Following the category, a decimal point denotes a subcategory which is followed by two subclassifications which further explain the cause, manifestation, location, severity, and type of injury or disease. Lastly, a trailing alphabetic character denotes the extension, which describes the type of patient encounter (Fig. 13.2).

> **KEY CONCEPT: CPT vs. ICD-10**
>
> A CPT code describes a procedure that was performed on a patient. Similar procedures are often grouped together, so CPT codes are imprecise. CPT codes determine reimbursement.
>
> An ICD-10 code describes the reason that a patient is being seen, such as events, symptoms, diseases, or physical findings. ICD-10 codes can be remarkably precise and detailed. They are used to justify the need for a procedure.
>
> In other words, the CPT code tells *what* was done; the ICD-10 code tells *why* it was done.

- Coders are expected to code to the highest level of specificity. This means maximizing the number of characters in the ICD-10 code, so that as much information as possible is conveyed. ICD-10-CM is a significant improvement over previous coding systems. With 55,000 additional codes from the previous ICD-9, ICD-10-CM allows for more precise coding.
- Multiple ICD-10 codes are often applied to a single examination.

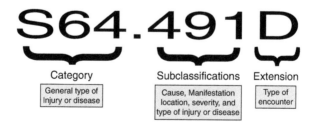

Fig. 13.2 ICD-10 format

- Unlike CPT codes (which are copyrighted by the American Medical Association), ICD-10 codes are in the public domain, so a complete list can be downloaded from several sites. Make sure that you obtain the most recent ICD-10-CM updates.

CHECKLIST: Coding and Billing Fields

To ensure quality and reduce variability, standardize information. In professional coding and billing, some fields are required to ensure proper reimbursement:
- Patient name
- Patient date of birth
- Facility name
- Date of service – date of procedure
- Department code – modality area in which the procedure was performed
- Admission date – date in which the patient was admitted to the facility
- Discharge date – date in which the patient was released from the facility

INTERNATIONAL CONSIDERATIONS

Approximately 27 countries use ICD-10 for reimbursement and resource allocation in their health system, and some have made modifications to ICD to better accommodate its utility. According to the WHO, about 70% of the world's health expenditures (USD $ 3.5 billion) are allocated using ICD for reimbursement and resource allocation.

While the WHO manages and publishes the base version of the ICD, several EU member states have modified it to better suit their needs. In the base classification, the code set allows for more than 14,000 different codes. The adapted versions may differ in multiple ways, and some national editions have expanded the code set even further, with some going so far as to add procedure codes.

For example, the German Modification (ICD-10-GM) is a direct translation into the German language of the English version of ICD-10. Since 2004, inpatient hospital services are billed based on a case-based fixed sum system, the so-called G-DRG-System (German Diagnosis-Related Groups). ICD-10-GM and the German Procedure Classification (OPS) form the basis of the G-DRG case-based fixed sum systems. The encoding of diagnoses in accordance with ICD-10-GM and of outpatient procedures in accordance with the German Procedure Classification (OPS) is a prerequisite for service remuneration in outpatient medical care.

13.5 Information Transfer

In most cases, the IIP will have more involvement in information transfer than in any other area of coding and billing:

- Most coding and billing services will make use of specialized software that imports data to be combined in coding and billing.
- Based on the software program, these applications may import flat files that may be comma delimited or fixed width in nature, or more commonly utilize HL7 interfaces.
- When successful information transfer has occurred, the software application will import the demographics file and report file into an application viewer for efficient coding review.
- If the data do not arrive simultaneously, the information may be held until its corresponding component is transferred.
- In many cases, the finalized imaging report may be delayed due to a radiologist's schedule, illness, or vacation, while the demographics file was sent upon date of discharge from the treating facility.

As with any information transfer, various approaches may be taken to ensure adequate notification when the complete data are received. Other safeguards should also be taken to ensure that the transmission may be resent in the event of disruption and that all data remain intact and available in the event of any dispute.

Radiology billing and coding, although a small component of what an imaging informatics professional needs to know, can prove to be one of the most challenging due to lack of everyday experience in this area. In most institutions, the role of the CIIP will be to ensure that timely and accurate patient demographic and billing information is available to the coding and billing team in the specific electronic format they require.

CHECKLIST: Coding and Billing Interfaces

- Interfaces to and *from* the billing system
- Data format for export from the sending facility
- Data format needed for data import of the receiving facility
- Data to be transmitted (patient demographics, reports, orders, etc.)
- Security of data transmission
- Data backup procedures should something interfere with the transmission

PEARLS

- Correct coding and billing is an essential piece of the business of medicine, and is most often the responsibility of a dedicated team of coders.
- Familiarity with the format of CPT and ICD-10 codes is needed for accurate data transfer.
- The RIS, the HIS, and the PACS all contribute elements that are needed for appropriate coding, and these data transfers must be managed individually and consolidated.
- Security and reliability of data transmission is of extreme importance.

References

1. Healthy People 2010: understanding and improving health. 2000. PsycEXTRA Dataset. https://doi.org/10.1037/e306642003-001
2. Norton M, Hamel L, Brodie M. Assessing Americans' familiarity with health insurance terms and concepts. Retrieved 24 Sept 2020., from https://www.kff.org/health-reform/poll-finding/assessing-americans-familiarity-with-health-insurance-terms-and-concepts.
3. Ratzan SC, Parker RM. Introduction. In: Selden CR, Zorn M, Ratzan SC, Parker RM, editors. National Library of Medicine current bibliographies in medicine: health literacy. Bethesda: National Institutes of Health; 2000.
4. Appropriate Use Criteria Program. n.d.. Retrieved 24 Sept 2020, from https://www.cms.gov/Medicare/Quality-Initiatives-Patient-Assessment-Instruments/Appropriate-Use-Criteria-Program

Self-Assessment Questions

1. What does MRN stand for? How does it differ from an SSN?

2. What is the difference between CPT and ICD-10 codes? Why are two different sets of codes needed?

3. What is the goal of PAMA?

4. Describe the use of CDSM and AUC.

5. Describe the format of a typical CPT code.

6. Describe the format of a typical ICD-10 code.

7. Name five data fields critical to billing and coding of radiologic procedures.

8. Where is the coding team for your imaging department physically located?

Chapter 14
Artificial Intelligence and Machine Learning

Laure Fournier and Guillaume Chassagnon

Contents

L. Fournier (✉)
Université de Paris, AP-HP, Hopital européen Georges Pompidou, PARCC UMRS 970, INSERM, Paris, France
e-mail: laure.fournier@u-paris.fr

G. Chassagnon
Université de Paris, AP-HP, Hopital Cochin, Paris, France
e-mail: guillaume.chassagnon@aphp.fr

B. F. Branstetter IV (ed.), *Practical Imaging Informatics*,
https://doi.org/10.1007/978-1-0716-1756-4_14

14.1 Introduction

Artificial intelligence encompasses a wide variety of fields. Recent developments and specifically advances in computer vision have led to a rise in interest in medical images. New machine learning strategies and neural networks (NN) are being developed to help clinical imagers detect and characterize lesions

DEFINITION: Artificial Intelligence

A field of computer science focused on creating programs that perform tasks normally assigned to human intelligence, thus simulating human intelligence.

on routine medical images. Other applications include improving image quality using NN-based reconstruction, facilitating clinical workflow, and extracting and analyzing large volumes of quantitative data from images.

OUR EXPERIENCE: The Neural Network Revolution

Huge Internet databases of pictures of animals (cats, dogs, etc.) and objects (cars, toasters, etc.) have allowed "data challenges" open to the whole world, so that teams (industrial, academic, independent "geeks") can compete to test their image recognition algorithms. The ImageNet Large Scale Visual Recognition Challenge (ILSVRC; now hosted on Kaggle), the best known challenge containing some ten million images, was shaken in 2012 by a Canadian academic team, which, thanks to a neural network, improved by 10% the performance of the best algorithms, which had plateaued at around a 25% error rate until then. These performances, which continue to improve (<5% errors in 2015), have made it possible to consider applications that until then had been science fiction, such as the self-driving car. It took only a small leap to imagine that the algorithms able to detect or recognize an object in an image could be applied to medical imaging to detect (normal/abnormal), localize, or characterize (benign/malignant) lesions.

14.2 Machine Learning and Deep Learning

Within the field of artificial intelligence, machine learning includes methods where machines automatically learn from experience and acquire information without being explicitly programmed. Briefly, an example dataset is submitted to the machine, which determines which function can best predict an output (supervised) or find structure to the data (unsupervised). It will perform the task iteratively until the best solution is found. The function learned will then be applied to new data to perform the given task. A subset of machine learning is deep learning, where neural networks are used to solve a problem instead of using human-engineered equations.

14.2.1 *"Traditional" Machine Learning*

- This term refers to machine learning methods other than deep learning. Among numerous traditional machine learning methods used for supervised learning in medical imaging, one can cite random forest, support vector machine (SVM), and LASSO (least absolute shrinkage

> **DEFINITION: Machine Learning**
>
> A field of study in which a machine learns by itself and elaborates a model from a training database.

and selection operator). Some traditional machine learning methods allow feature selection, which can be used to reduce the number of features to be included in the model. This is especially interesting for radiomics studies where a lot of features are extracted for evaluation. Unsupervised learning for cluster analysis includes methods such as k-means clustering, but unsupervised techniques are currently less used.

14.2.2 *Deep Learning and Neural Networks*

- Deep learning refers to deep neural networks, which are a subtype of NN that have recently become popular, thanks to the development of high-performance graphics processing unit (GPUs).
- The basic principle of neural networks is to mimic the functioning of the human brain by combining artificial neurons conceived on the model

> **KEY CONCEPT: Deep Learning**
>
> Deep learning is an end-to-end computer-driven approach, meaning that human-guided steps such as pre-processing and feature extraction are bypassed. The computer decides what aspects of the data are important.

of biological neurons. Deep learning is defined by the use of architectures combining several **hidden layers of artificial neurons**. Each neuron layer is composed of several neurons that combine the information transmitted by the neurons of the previous layer by assigning them different weights. During training, the weights are progressively adjusted, thanks to the backpropagation of error.
- A common approach for medical image analysis is the use of convolutional neural networks (CNN) in which artificial neurons are replaced by a series of successive **convolutions** applied to the image. During the learning phase, the algorithm progressively tweaks all the successive convolution kernels to improve the model.

> **FURTHER READING: Convolutional Neural Networks**
>
> Soffer S, Ben-Cohen A, Shimon O, Amitai MM, Greenspan H, Klang E. Convolutional Neural Networks for Radiologic Images: A Radiologist's Guide. Radiology. 2019 Mar;290(3):590–606. https://doi.org/10.1148/radiol.2018180547.

- Many different deep learning architectures are available such as encoder-decoder and atrous convolution architectures for **segmentation** with CNN.

> **DEFINITION: Segmentation**
>
> The ability to outline and identify specific anatomic structures or pathology on a radiologic image.

- Deep learning often outperforms classical machine learning methods. However, the amount of data and computing power required to train a deep learning algorithm are much greater than those required by traditional machine learning methods.
- Deep learning models behave like black boxes, which prevents their understanding by the human mind. It is important to keep in mind that deep learning does not use the same rules as the human brain for reading images, and this can result in what will be **nonsensical errors** to humans.

14.2.3 Supervised vs. Unsupervised Tasks

- **Supervised** algorithms aim to predict a given output, such as class (normal vs. abnormal, benign vs. malignant, disease 1 vs. disease 2, etc.), localization (identifying where an abnormality is located), or a continuous variable (e.g., survival). These algorithms are trained on **labeled data**, i.e., data that are already confidently attributed to a given class/localization/value. Examples of supervised machine learning are classification

> **KEY CONCEPT: Classification vs. Regression**
>
> If a deep learning model predicts real numerical values (e.g., a severity score), it is solving a regression equation.
>
> If a model predicts that an image belongs in a certain category (e.g., hematoma vs. calcification), it is solving a classification problem.

such as determining if a lesion is benign or malignant and regression such as determining a severity score.
- **Unsupervised** algorithms are trained on non-labeled data. Its aim is to identify subgroups of data sharing common characteristics such as different phenotypes of a single disease. Clustering is the most representative example of unsupervised machine learning. It can also be used in data reduction strategies. Annotated and non-annotated data can be combined in **semi-supervised methods**.
- There are different levels of **labeling** or **annotation** depending on the intended use of the data. The simplest annotation process is the labeling process in which images are classified according to their content (pneumothorax: yes/no), but the location of the anomaly is not provided within the image. These annotations can be used to build classifiers. The next level of annotation process is the use of boundary boxes to indicate the region of interest, and the most time-consuming annotation process is the delineation of the anomalies on the image. The latter is used for segmentation tasks.

14.2.4 Datasets

- The dataset is usually split into three subsets used for training, validation, and testing. The **training set** is used to build the model. The **validation set** is used to evaluate the models during the training phase and to select the best one. An alternative to this dataset splitting is the method of k-fold cross validation which allows training and validating on the same dataset. The **test set** is used at the end of the process to assess the performances of the selected model. It may be an internal test set, which is set aside before training and validation of the algorithm and is used to test the performance of an established algorithm.
- The terms "validation set" and "test set" are often used loosely, with an independent test set used to clinically validate a model.
- The final test set must not contain any of the data used to train the algorithm.
- In order to maximize model performance, it is important to have a training dataset of sufficient size and quality. As the number of available data is often limited in medical imaging, **data augmentation** methods can be used. Similarly, it is important to take into account the balance between classes in the training dataset. In case of an unbalanced dataset, **class balancing** methods should be used to properly represent the minority class, and make sure the model has "seen" enough cases of each.
- Conversely, the prevalence of each class in the test dataset must be representative of the target population in order to avoid overestimating performance of the model, especially for models used in screening.
- The quality of the dataset is essential to train the model and guarantee the capacity for the model to perform equally well on cases not seen during training (**generalizability**). It is important to have a dataset that is **representative** of the diversity of disease, the variations of normal, and the different acquisition techniques/scanners so that the algorithm has been trained to recognize the different presentations.
- In supervised models, the quality of the initial segmentation or classification must be trustworthy to produce a reliable outcome ("garbage in; garbage out").

14.2.5 Validation Metrics

- The choice of validation metrics is important to estimate the performance of the model compared to a standard of reference.
- For segmentation tasks, the Dice similarity coefficient and the Hausdorff distance are commonly used. They allow quantification of the similarity between the obtained segmentation and the ground truth.

KEY CONCEPT: Validation of AI Algorithms

Methods to validate an AI algorithm remain debated. Though accuracy and area under the ROC curve give an indication on gross performance, it may not reflect "real-life" performance when used on other datasets or when integrated in the workflow.

- For classification tasks, accuracy, sensitivity, specificity, and positive and negative predictive values are typical validation metrics for comparing binary predictions (e.g., malignant or benign) with the gold standard. However, before being binarized, the output of the algorithm is usually expressed as a probability.

FURTHER READING:
ROC Curves

Eng J. Receiver operating characteristic analysis: a primer. Acad Radiol, 12 (2005), pp. 909–916. https://pubmed.ncbi.nlm.nih.gov/16039544/

To evaluate the performance of the model in this setting, a ROC curve analysis with calculation of the AUC is the method of choice.

14.3 Applications

14.3.1 Detecting, Classifying, Localizing, and Segmenting

- Image recognition algorithms can be used on medical images for three different tasks: **detection** (is there a lesion in an image?), **classification** (is this lesion normal/abnormal, or benign/malignant?), and **localization** (where is the lesion in the image?). These tasks may be combined, for example, in a mammography CAD where lesions are detected, classified with a % chance of being cancer, and localized with a marker on the image, to be validated or invalidated by the radiologist.
- **Segmentation** (delineation of an organ/tissue/lesion of interest) is another task where deep learning-based algorithms are superior to traditional image processing methods. Applications include segmentation

DEFINITION: Registration

A single anatomic structure may appear in a different place on the image when a study is repeated, or from patient to patient. Registration is a means of identifying specific anatomic points so that two images can be "lined up" with each other and more easily compared.

FURTHER READING: Image Segmentation

Cardenas CE, Yang J, Anderson BM, Court LE, Brock KB. Advances in Auto-Segmentation. Semin Radiat Oncol. 2019;29(3):185–197. https://doi.org/10.1016/j.semradonc.2019.02.001.

of ventricles and myocardium from a dynamic cardiac MRI at the systolic and diastolic phases to calculate the ejection fraction or thickness of the myocardium. Spinal vertebrae can be automatically identified and numbered, and the loss of height of one or more vertebrae by compression fracture can be detected. The amount of pulmonary emphysema, the volume of renal parenchyma, the loss of muscle mass (sarcopenia), coronary calcifications, etc can be quantified. These segmentations enable the extraction of quantitative biomarkers that can be

used to automatically assess disease severity or health status, in addition to visual interpretation of the patient's target disease.
- Elastic registration can also be performed using deep learning methods.

14.3.2 Enhancing Image Quality

- **Image denoising** and deep learning-based reconstruction algorithms are already developed and implemented on new scanners. The algorithm reconstructs a high spatial- and/or contrast-resolution image from a noisy undersampled image. Patients could have more comfortable, less irradiating exams, and with reduced doses of contrast agent, thereby

> **KEY CONCEPT: Advantages of Deep Learning Image Reconstruction**
>
> - Reduce X-ray dose
> - Reduce volume of contrast agent injected
> - Reduce image acquisition time

decreasing potential side effects. Successful examinations could be performed even in disoriented, pediatric, and claustrophobic patients or patients in pain during the examination.
- Deep learning can be used to enhance spatial resolution of the original medical images (**super resolution**). This technique can be used to increase spatial resolution or to decrease acquisition time in MRI.
- **Real-time image quality** can also be monitored by AI. Automatic slice placement allows for reproducible image orientation. Detection of anatomical coverage allows real-time alerts in case of insufficient coverage of regions such as the lung apices. Image nonconformities such as incorrect patient position, inadequate exposure, and artifacts could be brought to the attention of the radiographer during conventional radiography acquisition.

14.3.3 Improving the Workflow

- "Intelligent" imaging **appointment management** software could allow identification of patients at risk for no-show and plan reminders or automatically reschedule an appointment when the treatment regimen is delayed, or if a patient is hospitalized. The earliest availability for scheduling could be suggested automatically taking into account the presence of the expert imager or radiographer according to the type of examination.
- The presentation of the scan for interpretation (**hanging protocol**) can be improved by automated algorithms displaying the most appropriate series according to the indication of the exam. Natural language processing software

could retrieve and display the relevant information from the patient's medical record while the exam is being read to, for example, highlight a history of surgery.

- In the emergency context, image analysis software is currently able to detect the most urgent pathologies (intracerebral bleeding, pneumoperitoneum, fracture, pulmonary embolism, etc.). They **prioritize abnormal examinations** for immediate interpretation. This will avoid diagnostic delays for patients with urgent pathologies.
- **Communication** with patients and colleagues may also be improved by AI. Alerts could be automatically sent to the referring clinical in case of life-threatening anomalies mentioned in the report. Automatic translation of report text into structured and standardized terms and format would allow both quality control of report content and further use for research or educational purposes. Communication with patients could be facilitated by translating medical terminology into lay terms and supplementing the report with schematics.

14.3.4 Guiding Interventional Radiology

- Analysis of previous procedures may allow guiding the choice of equipment and selecting the patients most likely to benefit from a procedure.
- Image segmentation and registration between two modalities will allow precise real-time identification of the organ and the lesion to be treated. Indeed, high-resolution images or images allowing visualization of the lesion, such as MRI or PET scans, can be merged with images from planar detectors or conventional radiology, to guide the radiologist during the procedure (e.g., fusion of MRI onto live ultrasound during prostate biopsy).
- Improved guidance to the target and real-time tracking should result in a reduced dose of X-rays and injected contrast agent.
- Developments in the field of **robotics** are expected with prototypes of ultrasensitive and miniaturized sensors or intravascular micro-robots allowing procedures similar to robotic surgery, which have become possible, thanks to computer-aided vision techniques and technological advances in highly reliable and latency-free communication networks to produce a signal, allowing an immersive visual and tactile experience.

14.3.5 Extracting More Information with Radiomics

- Radiomics is a high-throughput process that uses traditional machine learning or deep learning methods to extract a high number of features from images which will then be correlated to a desired outcome (when supervised). It is a process centered on discovery of new biomarkers.

DEFINITION: Radiomics

A deep learning algorithm extracts numerous features from a radiologic examination, many of which are not evident to a human observer. The resulting imaging biomarkers may provide novel diagnostic or prognostic information. The term "radiomics" is derived from the term "genomics," which is a battery of genetic biomarkers.

STEP-BY-STEP: Radiomics Process (Machine Learning)

1. Constitution of dataset representing the disease and acquisition variety of the future population on which the discovered signature is meant to be applied. The data acquisition can be prospective or (more often) retrospective.
2. Segmentation to delineate the region of interest in which the features will be extracted.
3. Pre-processing of images to prepare for quantification normalizing signal intensity.
4. Feature extraction yielding parameters quantifying or representing the signal intensity content of the image.
5. Feature reduction, an optional step which can reduce data dimensionality by eliminating nonreproducible or redundant parameters or clustering similar parameters to combine them into a single one.
6. Feature selection performed by correlating to the desired target (outcome or biological marker).
7. Validation in an independent dataset.

- Radiomics can be used to predict a biological correlate such as histological type or grade, receptor expression, gene expression or genetic mutation, etc., or an outcome such as survival or treatment response.
- The output of radiomics can be a single feature which is found to be the most correlated to the desired outcome. But more often, it will be a **radiomics signature**, i.e., a combination of features similarly to genetic signatures.
- The radiomics process can be performed using traditional machine learning methods, but deep learning can also be used, either as an end-to-end process or only for certain steps such as feature extraction and feature selection.

- In traditional machine learning radiomics, features are human-engineered. They are most often separated in three categories: **shape descriptors**, **histogram-derived parameters** describing signal intensity content of voxels, and **texture features** describing spatial distribution of signal intensities.

- Some limitations are specific to the radiomics process. The radiomics signature discovered and its performance will be impacted by choices regarding pre-processing of images, or strategies for feature extraction and feature reduction, reducing the reproducibility of findings. There is also variability in reporting of radiomics results. The same feature name may refer to different concepts in different publications, and the same concept may have different feature names according to research teams and software. Standardization of imaging across scanner manufacturers adds variability. Finally, correlation of the radiomics signature to the target does not prove a causal relationship.

> **FURTHER READING:**
> **Standardising Radiomics Metrology**
>
> Zwanenburg A et al. The Image Biomarker Standardization Initiative: Standardized Quantitative Radiomics for High-Throughput Image-based Phenotyping. Radiology. 2020 May;295(2):328–338. https://doi.org/10.1148/radiol.2020191145. Epub 2020 Mar 10. PMID: 32154773; PMCID: PMC7193906.

14.4 Limitations and Challenges

14.4.1 Data

- Large quantities of labeled data are needed to train ML/DL algorithms. According to the task, volumes of data required may range from several tens to tens of thousands. This data is both time-consuming and costly to obtain.

14.4.2 Generalizability

- Generalizability is the capacity for a model to maintain its performance when applied to new cases, unseen during training. The generalizability of a model must be evaluated on an external dataset. When a model is highly specific to the training dataset (**data overfitting**), there is a drop in performance when applied to previously unseen data.

> **KEY CONCEPT: Overfitting and Underfitting**
>
> Overfitting occurs when an algorithm fits too closely or exactly to the data in the training set, and therefore does not perform well on new data. Conversely, underfitting is when an algorithm fails to fit the data in the training dataset and therefore fails to learn.

14.4.3 Explainability or Interpretability

- A major drawback of deep learning is the **black box effect**, which precludes human understanding of the rules used by the algorithm. While the quality of the segmentations can be easily verified, reporting predictions that cannot be verified is more problematic. This is a current limit for the adoption of these tools and only partially applies to machine learning where features are human-engineered and therefore mathematically explainable. Some of these machine learning features are difficult for humans to conceptualize, such as texture features.

14.4.4 Detection of Errors

- Deep learning models have been shown to make what seems to the human mind to be **aberrant errors**. There are currently no efficient methods for DL models to integrate a detection of errors, but some of the paths pursued are the capacity for an algorithm to detect that a new image is too different from the ones included in its training and validation datasets.
- The growing popularity of using generative adversarial networks (GANs) has created **adversarial images**, a new challenge for image analysis tasks. Adversarial images are images for which the classification seems obvious to a human but cause massive failures in a deep neural network. These can be used to challenge models and improve their performance. GANs are thus contributing to the development of semi-supervised learning and possibly paving the path to future unsupervised learning.

14.4.5 Automation Bias

- When humans are placed into an environment where automated systems provide guidance, they behave as if they are in a low-risk environment and become less cautious. Thus, radiologists may become overly trustful of machine learning algorithms and interpret the examinations less carefully.

FURTHER READING

"Fundamentals of AI and Machine Learning for Healthcare". https://www.coursera.org/learn/fundamental-machine-learning-healthcare

PEARLS

- Artificial intelligence encompasses a large variety of fields, including machine learning and deep learning used for medical images.
- Convolutional neural networks are the most frequent deep learning neural network used to analyze medical images.
- Three datasets are necessary to develop AI models: training sets and validation sets, which allow the selection of the best model, and an independent test set on which the performance of the selected model can be evaluated.
- Applications include detecting and characterizing lesions in medical images, but also performing segmentation and registration, improving image quality, facilitating clinical workflow, and extracting and analyzing large volumes of quantitative data from images, or guiding interventional radiology procedures.
- Radiomics is a discovery-centered, data-driven approach for extracting large sets of complex descriptors from clinical images. It uses machine learning and/or deep learning methods to extract features and correlate them to a desired target.
- Limits of AI methods include lack of generalizability of models, the black box effect which limits the human understanding of models and results, and the lack of detection and management of errors of the models.

Further Reading

1. LeCun Y, Bengio Y, Hinton G. Deep learning. Nature. 2015;521(7553):436–44. https://doi.org/10.1038/nature14539.
2. Do S, Song KD, Chung JW. Basics of deep learning: a radiologist's guide to understanding published radiology articles on deep learning. Korean J Radiol. 2020;21(1):33–41. https://doi.org/10.3348/kjr.2019.0312.
3. Bluemke DA, Moy L, Bredella MA, Ertl-Wagner BB, Fowler KJ, Goh VJ, Halpern EF, Hess CP, Schiebler ML, Weiss CR. Assessing radiology research on artificial intelligence: a brief guide for authors, reviewers, and readers-from the radiology editorial board. Radiology. 2020;294(3):487–9. https://doi.org/10.1148/radiol.2019192515.
4. Geis JR, Brady AP, Wu CC, Spencer J, Ranschaert E, Jaremko JL, Langer SG, Borondy Kitts A, Birch J, Shields WF, van den Hoven van Genderen R, Kotter E, Wawira Gichoya J, Cook TS, Morgan MB, Tang A, Safdar NM, Kohli M. Ethics of artificial intelligence in radiology: summary of the joint European and North American Multisociety Statement. Radiology. 2019;293(2):436–40. https://doi.org/10.1148/radiol.2019191586.

Self-Assessment Questions

1. Which of the following applies to deep learning?

   A. Neural networks are used to develop deep learning models.
   B. Deep learning can only perform supervised learning.
   C. Deep learning models are complex to interpret.
   D. Deep learning extracts shape, histogram, and texture features.

2. Which of the following are required for datasets used for developing machine or deep learning models?

A. The test set is a subset of the initial data used to train the model.
B. A sufficient number of examples of each class should be present for the model in the training dataset.
C. The number of cases must reflect clinical prevalence in the test dataset.
D. Acquisition parameters need to be standardized in a dataset to train a model.

3. Which of the following steps are a part of the radiomics process?

A. Segmentation
B. Feature extraction
C. Pre-processing
D. Feature reduction
E. All of the above

4. Which of the following tasks can be improved using deep learning?

A. Lesion detection
B. Image segmentation
C. Image reconstruction
D. Increasing spatial resolution
E. All of the above

5. Which combination of machine learning approach and annotation level is the most suitable to develop a segmentation algorithm?

A. Supervised learning/labeled images
B. Supervised learning/boundary boxes drawn on images
C. Supervised learning/delineated areas on images
D. Unsupervised learning/labeled images
E. Unsupervised learning/non-annotated data

6. What are the advantages of deep learning over traditional machine learning methods?

A. It is not based on human-engineered features.
B. Models are easier to explain.
C. It often performs better.
D. Less data is required to train.
E. It does not require feature extraction.

7. Cite different fields of application of AI methods in medical imaging.

8. List some challenges to the development and adoption of AI tools in medical imaging.

9. You are installing AI decision support for your radiologists to help them identify some specific emergent diagnoses. What warnings or caveats would you give them before deployment?

Part IV
Image Interpretation and Support

Chapter 15
Roles and Relationships in Healthcare

Rasu B. Shrestha

Contents

15.1   Introduction

Healthcare is a relationship business. No amount of goodwill can create impact more than the intentional understanding and managing of these crucial relationships. This chapter describes the key elements of the evolving roles and relationships in healthcare, with an eye on the ecosystem in and around imaging informatics.

Technology is meant to be an enabler of better care but has historically often been an impediment to better care. In our zeal to roll out new technologies, we are almost always well-intentioned and correctly motivated. But our *approach* is often

R. B. Shrestha (✉)
Strategy and Transformation Office, Atrium Health, Charlotte, NC, USA

© The Author(s), under exclusive license to Springer Science+Business Media,
LLC, part of Springer Nature 2021
B. F. Branstetter IV (ed.), *Practical Imaging Informatics*,
https://doi.org/10.1007/978-1-0716-1756-4_15

misguided. Technology for the sake of technology will eventually lead to undesirable outcomes. A better approach is to understand that healthcare is a relationship business and that using technology to enhance and accentuate those relationships can lead to better outcomes.

Clarity in roles and relationships is critical to achieve aligned goals and outcomes. We are operating in an ever more VUCA (volatile, uncertain, complex, and ambiguous) environment, and clarity in roles and relationships provides the train tracks to achieving desired outcomes. It is also important to comprehend that in the ever-evolving landscape of healthcare, these roles are often evolving, with newer roles that often need to be put in place to account for newer realities and newer strategic pursuits. The evolution of different roles gives way to changing relationships which are important to comprehend – both internally within an organization and externally outside of the core organization.

15.2 Imaging – Widening the Aperture

15.2.1 Embracing the Enterprise

For over 120 years ago, radiology has been fundamental to diagnostics and integral to the science of medicine. Many new techniques have been introduced, and digital technology has transformed clinical practice

> **DEFINITION: Enterprise**
>
> An entire system of healthcare delivery that encompasses hospitals, outpatient services, and business administration.

beyond recognition. Today, the mantra of "any image, anywhere, anytime" is expected as the norm:

- Radiology IT has grown from being a departmental solution to an **enterprise asset**.
- Previously, decision-making for radiology-related services lays squarely within the department, and often within specific divisions within the department – from budgetary, operational, staffing, quality, and purchasing decisions to even decisions related to information technology.
- **Purchasing power** has often shifted to the enterprise, as health systems attempt to garner broader financial and operational efficiencies, as well as better, more coordinated clinical outcomes.
- As other specialties such as cardiology, pathology, dermatology, and otolaryngology embrace the digital environment, there is a growing need to manage these digital assets in a more coordinated manner *across the enterprise*.
- This is also an opportunity to garner efficiencies in handling these **silos of disparate imaging systems**, and enable workflows that are truly patient-centric, and not application-centric [1].

- Radiologists themselves must embrace the enterprise. Stereotypically, radiologists work in dark reading rooms, "treating" a series of images rather than the whole patient:
  - Radiologists embraced the digital norm PACS but hung on to tired ways of interpreting studies with little context around the patient, let alone access to the comprehensive longitudinal medical record.
  - To evolve the role of the radiologist, a core informatics goal is interoperability across all systems that hold pieces of the patients' data, enabling a true patient-centric approach to care.
  - Discrete data elements such as medications, allergies, problems, and diagnoses stored in disparate systems should be aggregated, organized, and semantically harmonized [2].

> **KEY CONCEPT: Silos vs. Coordinated Systems**
>
> Silos are separate areas of governance within a larger system, for example, having a separate PACS just for point-of-care ultrasound, or a separate storage system for pathology images. Coordinated systems bring similar services under a single umbrella, thus realizing efficiencies of scale. People are often loath to relinquish control of their silo, even when a coordinated system is superior.

- The role of a **medical director in imaging** is not just to manage to the best interests of the department but to manage to the broader interests and strategic pursuits of the enterprise and connect these back to the local needs [3]:
  - It is ideal to show *economic* benefits of embracing enterprise methodologies around initiatives such as enterprise storage, unified image viewing, collaborative care, and shared savings resulting from coordinated care models.
  - What may be more effective however is to show **personal** benefits in terms of improved workflow, saved time, and increased satisfaction and outcomes as a result of embracing these newer care models.

15.2.2 The Illusion of Communication

- A key adverse effect of the digital transition has been that physicians have seemingly stopped talking [4]. Many confuse the written report as the endpoint of communication. This however is an illusion. The procedure report is **one** form of communication but is hardly what is *really* needed by the ordering clinician or by the patient:
  - There should not be a "one-size-fits-all" approach to communication and collaboration, but rather an appropriate use of technologies that fit into desired workflows.
  - Encourage "critical thinking" that entails active, focused, persistent, and purposeful communication between parties in the care continuum.

- Inter-clinician communication is critical, but perhaps just as important, and often even more overlooked in imaging, is the need for better communication between the imager and the patient.
- Research has shown that patient- and family-centered care that incorporates shared decision-making can reap potential healthcare savings of $9 billion over 10 years [5].
- Consider reports that are clearer to the layperson, with key images, and links to relevant curated educational material, and a contact number for the patient to speak to if needed.

> **DEFINITION: Service Line**
>
> Service lines are a method for decentralizing administration into smaller, more manageable components. Healthcare was traditionally broken down by department, but "imaging" is now considered a service line in most hospitals. Related departments, such as neurology and neurosurgery, may combine into a single service line, ideally including neuroradiology and neuropathology.

> **HYPOTHETICAL SCENARIO: Service Lines vs. Patient-Centric Team Approach**
>
> As we refocus on the patient, there is a need to broaden the traditional concept of organization via "service lines" [6]. It is critical to take into account the patient's holistic needs (vs. just the "reason for exam") and the relationships the patient has with others across their ecosystem. In the current system, patients transfer from one service line to another, for example, from radiology to oncology, and then onto surgery and back to oncology and radiology. A team-based approach centered around the patient (e.g., in a patient with a complex cancer diagnosis) will be more in-line with an ecosystem view, where we are able to have a much more longitudinal view to the patient's journey vs. an episodic or encounter-based view. This relationship with the patient can also continue to evolve with engaging the patient more directly in their care decisions, with capabilities such as OpenNotes [7] that promote more transparent communications in healthcare and allow patients access to their own broader medical records, as well as debates and regulations around 'information-blocking' and more timely access to electronic health information (EHI).

15.2.3 Aligning with the Care Team

> **PERTINENT QUOTE: Teamwork**
>
> "The way a team plays as a whole determines its success. You may have the greatest bunch of individual stars in the world, but if they don't play together, the club won't be worth a dime." – Babe Ruth

> **KEY CONCEPT: Fee-for-Service vs. Value-Based Care**
>
> American healthcare has traditionally functioned as fee-for-service (volume-based), in which the hospital makes more money when more care is delivered, even if that care does not actually benefit the patient. For example, performing spine surgery before attempting physical therapy is very lucrative, but has not shown to improve long-term outcomes.
>
> In fee-for-value care (value-based), healthcare entities are paid based on patient outcomes or on the total number of patients being cared for.

The spiraling costs of healthcare in the USA are unsustainable, and it has been stated that "advanced imaging is the bellwether for the excesses of fee-for-service medical care" [9]. There is a definite need to shift from a volume-based fee-for-service practice of imaging to one that emphasizes **value** across the care continuum [10]. Rooted in the premise of value-based care is the notion of the care team:

- Radiologists need to partner with the ordering physicians, the care team, and patients to tip the value equation.
- Radiology as a group is facing increasing threats of commoditization. The inordinate level of focus on metrics such as report turnaround time (TAT) and fee-for-service has made the radiologist into an invisible commodity ready to be traded freely on price:
  - This is directly contradictory however to the notion of value-based imaging, and accountable care, where quality and care coordination are just as important as costs.
  - Radiologist outreach programs need to be put in place, and radiologists should be incentivized to forge meaningful relationships with their referring colleagues [10].
- An often-understated role is the medical physicist, who is the "go-to person" with regard to not only regulatory compliance but also the safety and quality of imaging [11]:
  - Patient-centric comprehensive radiation dose management is

> **DEFINITION: Commoditization**
>
> A commodity is a service or product that is interchangeable between vendors. Crude oil is a typical example, since it doesn't matter which well it is pumped from. Services like radiology interpretation can be treated like commodities if there is no discernable difference in the quality of the interpretations and no added value (such as consultations or patient interactions) from an in-house radiologist. Consultations can be provided by teleradiology organizations, but the strongest argument against commoditization is loss of the personal relationship and trust that is built over time between smaller local radiologists and doctors.

> **DEFINITION: Medical Physicist**
>
> A medical physicist is a professional who applies the principles and methods of both physics and medicine for the prevention, diagnosis, and treatment of human diseases, with a specific goal of ensuring quality services and safety to the patients exposed to radiation. The medical physics field can be divided into three main categories: radiation therapy, diagnostic imaging, and nuclear medicine.

about collaborative care, care coordination, interoperability, quality, safety, and much more.

- Optimal radiation dose management is not just mandated by legislature; it is a core issue for payers, an increasing concern for patients, and of high significance to ordering physicians.
- The medical physicist is usually hired by the radiology department and works with radiologists in each of the subspecialties.
- Flagging patients who have had an inordinate lifetime amount of radiation is good practice and requires robust IT tracking [12].
- Moving dose data upstream, to the point of order entry, is a crucial step. Appropriateness criteria become most effective when integrated with the electronic medical record's (EMR) computerized physician order entry (CPOE) system. The appropriateness criteria need to incorporate dose information, such as cumulative effective radiation dose data, and be optimized to localized protocols guided by evidence-based guidelines, clinical best practices, and contextualized patient-specific data.

15.2.4 Understanding the Imaging Value Chain

Key to understanding the roles and relationships in healthcare is in comprehending the value chain. In their book *Redefining Health Care*, Michael Porter and Elizabeth Olmsted Teisberg shed new light on why decades of reform have only worsened the problems of our

> **DEFINITION: Value Chain**
>
> The steps and processes that transform the vision and mission of an organization into products and services.

healthcare system with what they call the propagation of dysfunctional competition [13]. They argue that the root cause of the woes of our healthcare system is not a lack of competition but the sustenance of competition at the wrong level – where competition is both too broad and too narrow. Porter and Teisberg convincingly argue that competition is too broad because it currently takes place at the level of health plans, networks, hospital groups, and clinics – and not in addressing particular medical conditions. Competition is also too narrow because it takes place at the level of discrete interventions or services – and not in addressing medical conditions over the full cycle of care, including monitoring and prevention, diagnosis, treatment,and the ongoing management of the condition. Value in healthcare is created (or destroyed) at the medical condition level, not at the level of a hospital or physician practice. Their argument is a strong caution for us in radiology to take pause and re-evaluate our value chain and bring a defined set of frameworks to help capture the value that we bring to the sustainability of the healthcare delivery system at large [14]:

> **DEFINITION: Utilization Management System**
>
> A third-party service employed by an insurance company that uses independent physicians to determine whether a procedure or test is medically indicated. The insurance company will refuse to pay for tests that are not "pre-approved" by these systems.

> **DEFINITION: Clinical Decision Support**
>
> CDS systems are software add-ons to the EMR that assist referrers who are ordering imaging exams, in the hope that this will reduce inappropriate utilization of imaging. Many of these systems are based on guidelines such as the ACR Appropriateness Criteria or the ESR iGuide. They calculate appropriateness scores for the requested test, and if the test is inappropriate, the referring physician is advised (but not required) to modify the selection.

- Imaging tests are most valuable when the probability of disease is neither very high nor very low but in the moderate range [15].
- Various imaging utilization management systems have been enforced in various forms by insurance companies and radiology benefit management (RBM) companies.
- Prior authorization, prenotification, and various forms of network strategies that focus on examination costs, total quality, and practice guidelines have also had varying levels of success.
- Perhaps the most effective antidote to this trend is **intelligent personalized data** based on evidence-based medicine, presented tightly integrated into the decision support and physician order entry workflow. Ordering physicians want personalized data around image order entry appropriateness. This is difficult, but not impossible – and is a critical step toward meaningful value-based imaging [14] (Fig. 15.1).

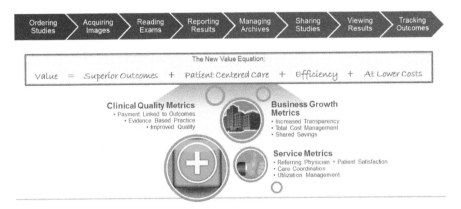

Fig. 15.1 Imaging value chain – it's more than just capturing and reading images. Adapted with input from "The Changing Radiologist Role – Adapting to New Economic Models" (The Advisory Board, 2012)

15.3 Internal Relationships

15.3.1 The Radiologist-Clinician Relationship

- The radiologist's role is evolving from diagnostician to physician-consultant.
- Radiologists are the main patient advocates for imaging appropriateness [16].
- But as healthcare organizations move from fee-for-service models to fee for value, the value needs to be quantifiable and measurable:
  - We need more data transparency, including around utilization data, appropriateness, and costs.
- The ACR's Face of Radiology campaign conveys to patients that the "radiologist is the physician expert in diagnosis, patient care, and treatment through medical imaging" [4].
- Clinicians value radiologists who are involved in interdisciplinary conferences and are available for consultation.
- IT can accentuate the humanistic elements of this relationship with a focus on better communication and collaboration.
- There is an inherent fear that radiologists will "be wasting our time manning the phone and talking instead of reading studies":
  - Technology can enable more streamlined and contextualized synchronous and asynchronous communication. We need streamlined unified communications and closed-loop, cloud-based intelligent algorithms, built into the workflow of clinicians and patients (see **Chaps. 18** and **25**).

> **FURTHER READING: The Radiologist-Clinician Relationship**
>
> Radiology in the Era of Value-based Healthcare: A MultiSociety Expert Statement from the ACR, CAR, ESR, IS3R, RANZCR, and RSNA https://doi.org/10.1148/radiol.2020209027
>
> This multi-society paper, representing the views of Radiology Societies in Europe, the USA, Canada, Australia, and New Zealand, describes the place of radiology in VBH models and the healthcare value contributions of radiology. Potential steps to objectify and quantify the value contributed by radiology to healthcare are outlined.

15.3.2 Information Technology

Radiology was among the first to embrace digital, and well before hospitals transitioned from paper charts to electronic medical records (EMRs), radiology departments had started moving from film to filmless. With the move towards a full digital workflow, roles and relationships have evolved around information technology within imaging.

- Without strong information technology (IT support), imaging's value proposition suffers dramatically:

- These can range from local workstation issues to issues with systems like PACS, RIS, HIS speech recognition, advanced visualization systems, advanced analytics toolkits, and artificial intelligence.
  - Strong IT support is also needed around cloud deployment, network adequacy, latency, and bandwidth management, as well as with information security and privacy management.
  - IT support may also be needed to help scale services to remote sites and centralized or decentralized coverage models, including for radiologists who have subspecialty expertise to offer to outlying facilities, or in dealing with coverage across all hours.
- Imaging groups often identify a director of IT who is a physician able to manage the team and liaise with enterprise leaders and other teams.
- Many groups start with an in-house PACS administrator, and perhaps a small onsite support team:
  - Growth in practices as well as a broader focus on enterprise has caused a shift to more of an enterprise IT support model. There are cost-benefit analyses that can be done to compare the in-house model to the enterprise support model, and the answer for some may lie in a hybrid model.
- Some imaging groups have IT development roles that may be critical to their goals – whether in helping with clinical, research, or academic pursuits, or other efforts that may be more focused on innovation, **technology development**, or even **commercialization**.
  - In determining the roles and responsibilities for IT development, it is important to take a broader view to staffing these positions – looking not just at a project or a principal investigator (PI) and his or her needs, but the goals and objectives of the department or the enterprise, aiming to align budgets with enterprise resources and efficiencies across cross-disciplinary bodies of work.
  - These resources should also focus on embracing innovative capabilities such as design thinking and agile development methodologies, but with a disciplined emphasis on meeting user needs, and business objectives.
- Imaging is in a position to enable true interoperability across the enterprise, not just within the imaging departments:
  - This role is often not the responsibility of one specific individual, although, arguably, it should be.
  - Imaging is no stranger to standards (see **Chap. 12**) and can act as an advisor to other IT teams.
  - The DICOM standard facilitates interoperability of medical imaging equipment by specifying protocols, transfer syntaxes and semantics of commands, information conformance standards, medical imaging services, security profiles, and content management.
  - As other specialties such as cardiology, pathology, dermatology, otolaryngology, and others embrace everything digital, there is an imperative to manage and grow these digital assets in a much more coordinated manner across the enterprise [17].

15.3.3 Alignment Models and the C-suite

- Clarity in the alignment model, and the subsequent roles and relationships with the C-suite, can be a key determinant of the success of imaging within the health system (Table 15.1 and Fig. 15.2):

> **DEFINITION: C-suite**
>
> Short for "corporate suite," C-suite colloquially refers to the roles on the business side of healthcare.

  - Physician alignment typically refers to the strength of professional, cultural, and economic relationships between physicians and hospitals. In imaging, considerations should include the degree of **coordinated integration** among radiologists, hospitals, and referring physician groups – regardless of whether radiologists are independent, employed, or otherwise affiliated with a health system.
  - These models can range from incentive-based professional services agreements (PSA) to more exclusive provider contracts and joint ventures. Additionally, there may be a management services agreement (MSA) or a clinically integrated network (CIN) arrangement.
  - These often need to be **negotiated** through with the health system chief operating officer (COO), who typically reports to the health system chief executive officer (CEO).
  - There may also be health system employment of the radiologists, either directly through an affiliated medical group or indirectly through a designated foundation.
- Models ensure optimal management of major management elements such as:
  - Clinical expectations
  - Quality assurance
  - Procurement
  - Finance
  - Operations
  - Human resources

> **KEY CONCEPT: Private Practice and Academics**
>
> Doctors who teach trainees are in academic practice. Doctors who solely care for patients are in private practice.

- Additionally, it is critical to ensure that there is an intentional focus on enterprise-level planning and strategy. There needs to be congruency among the imaging leadership and enterprise C-suite around:
  - Specific long-term goals
  - How information technology can support the clinical mission
  - Cost-effectiveness
  - All while not sacrificing quality!
- Radiologists don't just read films. Their roles have expanded to encompass a number of broader capabilities that could have strategic implications for the entire health system [18]:

- Economic gatekeeping
- Political advocacy
- Public health delivery
- Patient safety
- Quality care improvement
- Information technology

Table 15.1 The people in your neighborhood

Physician	
Student	Finished with college; now in medical school. Not quite a doctor yet
Intern	Just finished with medical school. Barely a doctor. Internship is 1 year
Resident	Finished medical school; learning a specialty, like radiology
Fellow	Finished residency; learning a subspecialty like neuroradiology. Almost done training
Attending	Full-fledged physician who has completed training
Referring (ordering)	The physician who requested that the study be performed
Clinician	A controversial term for a non-imager physician
Physician extender (nonphysician who can perform tasks like a physician)	
Physician assistant (PA)	
Certified registered nurse practitioners (CRNP)	
Technologist	
In each modality, there is one of more lead tech who supervises the other techs	
Nurse	
Nurses may have several different degrees that enable them to perform additional roles	
Medical physicist	
Exclusive to imaging departments. Improves image quality and optimizes patient safety	
Departmental administration	
Department chair	The top-ranking physician in the department
Vice-chairs	Oversee various aspects of the department
Chief administrator	Nonphysician responsible for the business side
Division chief	Oversees a subspecialty group (neuro, abdomen, musculoskeletal, etc.)
Corporate administration	
President/CEO	As in any business, someone is at the top
Chief information officer	Oversees IT; a good person for the IIP to know
VP of imaging	In large systems, a vice-president may be needed just for imaging
Medical director	Physician liaison for any internal group

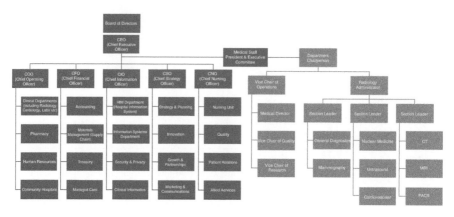

Fig. 15.2 Sample organizational chart. Orange boxes are roles within the radiology (or a similar) department. Blue boxes are corporate roles

15.4 Decision-Making

15.4.1 Organizing for Success

Healthcare needs not only the right players in the right roles, with the right levels of clarity in their responsibilities, but also the right levels of governance and structure. This increases the chances of decisions being made rapidly, with more decisive actions that are in alignment with established guidelines, policies, and mission.

> **PERTINENT QUOTE: Decision-Making**
>
> No one can whistle a symphony. It takes a whole orchestra to play it."
> –H.E. Luccock

Governance will be covered in detail in **Chap. 19**. While effective governance is essential to the growth and well-being of a practice, unfortunately, **not everyone in a practice is suited for a leadership position** [19].

- When contemplating the right leaders for the right roles, it is important to ensure **diversity** in every aspect of the word:
    - Not just race and ethnicity
    - Backgrounds
    - Experiences
    - Personalities
    - Approaches
- Look for leadership force multipliers.

Getting new voices and fresh perspectives can be essential. But there are two leadership positions in a practice that benefits greatly from longevity:

> **DEFINITION: Leadership Force Multipliers**
>
> These individuals, when placed in the right roles, and given the right levels of empowerment, can dramatically increase the effectiveness of a group – creating a team and a series of outcomes that is more than the sum of its parts.

1. The chair of the hospital radiology department, who usually sits on the executive committee of the medical staff and becomes the official voice of the group in that venue
2. The physician CEO of the group, and a small executive committee, with an active group of shareholders who are required to serve on one of the three committees (finance, operations, and new business and marketing) that are vital to the governance of the practice

15.4.2 A Seat at the Table

Radiologists should be more visible across the care continuum, as well as in strategic decisions being made across healthcare institutions and across state and federal bodies [20].

The era of accountable care calls for radiologists to be fully engaged with emergency physicians, hospitalists, and primary care physicians (PCPs) as part of a collaborative solution toward **appropriate image utilization** and improved outcomes. Radiologists have always served as strong, albeit silent, patient advocates around imaging appropriateness, but as healthcare orga-

> **KEY CONCEPT: A Seat at the Table**
>
> All business decisions result in winners and losers. Any stakeholder who does not participate in the decision-making process is assured of being on the losing end. Radiology and other non-patient-facing specialties can be overlooked when creating decision-making teams. "If we do not have a seat at the table, then we will end up being on the menu."

nizations move from fee-for-service models to fee for value, the value needs to be quantifiable and measurable. In guiding and defining the future of radiology, the ACR seeks to affirm the role of radiologists as physician consultants [21]. The ACR's "Face of Radiology" campaign conveys patients that the "radiologist is the physician expert in diagnosis, patient care, and treatment through medical imaging."

Radiology needs to have a strong voice in enterprise information technology (IT) purchasing decisions, and in policy decisions that impact how care will be provided.

OUR EXPERIENCE: Wasteful Imaging

A seat at the table is critical to expressing the logic behind the means to curtail two major policy issues that are driving increased utilization of diagnostic imaging: self-referral [22] and defensive medicine. According to a recent survey [23], the cost of defensive medicine is estimated at $650–$850 billion, or between 26 and 34% of annual healthcare costs in the USA. A massive cultural revolution, incentivizing a move away from blind defensive medicine, is needed to address a number of cascading key trigger points in support of appropriate imaging. It is not just the swell of patients' demands for more imaging, triggered by consumer-directed marketing promoting the availability and benefits of procedures such as full-body scans. Nor is it just the disturbing and proven relationship between physician self-referrals and higher imaging utilization, perhaps to feed costs associated with acquiring expensive imaging equipment. Over time, many physicians end up practicing "rule-out medicine" as opposed to actual "diagnostic medicine" in fear of liability and expensive litigations from possible missed diagnoses [20].

Radiology, along with the rest of healthcare, is facing widespread challenges in care delivery, escalating healthcare costs and healthcare reform amid louder calls for newer care models that embrace value-based care that emphasizes rewarding better outcomes, safety, and satisfaction. Imaging informatics has a tremendous opportunity to capitalize on what may be the perfect storm of needs and capabilities to lead the charge with new thinking, new technologies, and compelling innovations and not just weather the storm of value-based care, but come out winning on the other side.

15.5 External Relationships

External relationships are just as critical as internal relationships within the health system. Note that many of the challenges with existential consequences tend to have more of an outside-in influence. If the goal of leadership is to be proactive and have the ability to make informed decisions, instituting the right roles to interface with the external world then becomes critical.

15.5.1 Vendor Partners

Many success stories in the world of business can be attributed to successful partnerships. Even in the imaging industry, we have seen successful models over time of industry partnering with healthcare organizations and universities to not just capture new technical

KEY CONCEPT: Vendor Partnerships

Be wary of vendor promises of "strategic partnerships" or other proposals of teamwork. Your institution needs assurances that the vendor will make changes at your request. The vendor must supply resources such as support personnel and software at their expense, so that they have "skin in the game."

knowledge and validate assumptions but to truly innovate and connect with care settings and improve patient health outcomes:

- The more invested the university or healthcare organization is into the partnership, the more the chances of success. (The same is true for the industry partner.)
- For these endeavors to thrive, both parties must trust each other [8].
- Every sales quarter, we see an overuse of cheesy phrases such as "strategic partners." Cutting a purchase order is clearly "strategic" for the vendor as a means to an end for the sale of their products or services. And while a signed purchase order may create a vendor-customer relationship that may even end up with a positive return on investment (ROI), this should not be confused with true **strategic** partnerships.
  - Not every vendor-customer relationship is ripe for a strategic partnership since this type of partnership often calls for a framework that is the opposite of executing against a predefined contract.

> **OUR EXPERIENCE: Vendor Partnerships**
>
> A health system partnered with their exclusive CT/MR vendor to create a next-generation PACS. Millions of dollars were funneled into a research laboratory on the academic campus, where expert programmers and IIPs used agile programming architecture to test concepts and mock-ups in a simulated real-world environment. Radiologists' salaries were paid to ensure that they had the time to participate in development. The health system was responsible for creating a new user interface, while the vendor was responsible for modifying their existing PACS to fit the novel models being created in the laboratory.
>
> Here are some key reflections on the lessons learned – and these essentially constitute a list of things to consider in similar strategic vendor partnerships: 1. Understand that existing vendors often have existing install bases and may be risk averse to real change for fear of alienating existing customers. 2. Be mindful of legacy workflow that needs to be supported, even while building newer widgets and tools. Also equally important is the need to integrate with legacy code bases. Building the new while not letting go of the old can dramatically cripple progress. 3. Watch out for the vendor's need to 'feed the beast' of quarterly sales.

- The right role for the leader to liaise with the external world need not just be one person's responsibility. A **medical director of imaging**, for example, could be the point person to proactively liaise with vendor partners, and facilitate the interactions between radiologists, clinicians, and leaders in various committees tasked with taking recommendations and processing purchase or contract decisions:
  - The medical director would also partner with the right leaders in the health system charged with information technology (such as the chief information officer and their team), the procurement team (often with leaders such as the chief supply chain officer, and the chief financial officer, and their teams), and the strategy and innovation leaders (such as the chief strategy officer and the chief innovation officer).

- The medical director would have to have firsthand knowledge of the pain points on the ground, as well as the clinical workflows and relationships on the care-delivery side.
- The director would also need to be able to translate this knowledge to "vendor-speak," and vice versa.
- This translator role is also critical in getting the right messages transmitted effectively between health system executives and clinical staff. Many vendors tend to speak to their products and solutions in more broad-based descriptors that are generalized across large swaths of possible customers. Industry terms such as "cloud-based," "AI platform," and "APIs" may not mean much to clinicians who may have heard these terms, but may not have been formally trained to understand what they really mean, or their broader implications.

- Vendors want their customers to succeed – for it is in their best interest, financially and from a business development perspective. The **vendor liaison** role entails managing through the procurement process as well as in two additional critical areas: training and support:
  - When a new solution is introduced into a group, the efficacy of the training and rollout could determine the success of change management. The medical director should be tasked with working with the leaders and clinical staff in the department, including the clinical champions, as well as with the enterprise information technology team and others to ensure that there is a well thought through *pre*-training workflow analysis, and well-coordinated series of training sessions, including train-the-trainer sessions as needed, and the right *post*-training follow-ups such as spot training and refreshers (see **Chap. 26**).
  - Coordination is just as critical in the upkeep and continued use through the lifetime of the product. The goal should be to generate continued value over the course of the usage, tracking the return on investment (ROI) and ensuring that any changes in user requirements or any development in technologies or capabilities are well translated.
  - Some partnerships can be more strategic, with an eye toward having more "skin in the game" as well as "co-creation." This level of a strategic partnership is not for everyone, but under the right construct, the partners could benefit from co-investments in product development and commercialization. It is important to keep your eyes open to signs of a healthy vendor relationship while focusing on a robust problem solving orientation, value optimization, fair and reasonable flexibility and continuous building of trust. It is important to be wary of any commitments vendors may make and any product roadmaps that may be shared. Product roadmaps sometimes create a false illusion of future certainty. While transparency is important, accountability is just as critical - and key to nurturing healthy vendor relationships is to communicate effectively and collaborate meaningfully.

15.5.2 External Organizations

Maintaining meaningful relationships with external organizations should not fall under the responsibility of one individual alone. Given the wide array of organizations and the different focus areas, it makes sense to match a leader's interest with a targeted set of activities conducted with any of the external organizations:

- Member-based organizations can benefit imagers in many ways. Broader based organizations such as the Radiological Society of North America (RSNA), the European Society of Radiology (ESR), and the American College of Radiology (ACR) have a wide reach, and often have the muscle to influence industry trends, policies, and regulations [18]. As an example, radiologists can immerse themselves in engaging in and influencing policy decisions, by actively working with the ACR, who have the depth and breadth of engaging both private payers and the government.
- Imagers also have a role in public health. Increasing awareness and implementation of screening programs could have a significant impact on public health.
- Specialty-based organizations can add to the overall strategic pursuits of the health system. These organizations – such as the Society of Abdominal Radiology (SAR), the Society of Breast Imaging (SBI), and the American Society of Neuroradiology (ASNR) – are typically smaller than the broad-based organizations, but tend to have more specialized levels of focus that often result in deeper levels of dialogue and action.
- Informatics and technology-focused societies such as the Society for Imaging Informatics in Medicine (SIIM) and the European Society of Medical Imaging Informatics (EuSoMII) can involve a multidisciplinary community comprised of physicians from radiology, pathology, and other specialties, as well as PACS administrators, corporate-level administrators, engineers, IT directors and managers, as well as industry vendors. Leaders in these roles should be encouraged to become a CIIP, which entails getting certified from the American Board of Imaging Informatics (ABII), and demonstrating that an individual has mastered the necessary:
- Technical, clinical, and business skill sets to invest in quality improvement, be at the forefront of the profession, and innovate within the field of imaging informatics.
- Organizations such as the Healthcare Information and Management Systems Society (HIMSS) offer a broad array of opportunities for leaders in all information technology-related roles from analysts and managers to directors and CIOs. Of note are cross-functional groups such as the HIMSS-SIIM Enterprise Imaging Community that offer greater cross-disciplinary opportunities.

INTERNATIONAL CONSIDERATIONS

The European Society of Medical Imaging Informatics (EuSoMII) is the European counterpart to SIIM. The two organizations have a memorandum of understanding that enables them to share resources, content, and lecturers.

15.6 Conclusion

There is no magic bullet for the right types of partnerships, but there is also no doubt that meaningful and well-aligned partnerships can transform the face of radiology. With a positive, persuasive, and collaborative approach, synergistic partnerships based on mutual respect can be incentivized for success. Crafted correctly with the right roles and a more balanced portfolio of engagements aligned to the health system's strategic priorities, these partnerships allow organizations to be nimble, action-oriented, and strategic.

> **PEARLS**
>
> - There are well-defined departmental and enterprise roles that are similar between all institutions. Know the people in your neighborhood and what roles they play.
> - Understand how your department fits into the coordinated care of the overall enterprise.
> - Medicine is a business; understand how the medical providers and the corporate entity interact.
> - Be wary of the relationship between the enterprise and vendors. Some relationships have tremendous synergy, but others can be parasitic.

References

1. Shrestha R. Imaging: embracing the enterprise. Appl Radiol. 2015;44:26.
2. Shrestha R. The myths and realities of true enterprise imaging. Appl Radiol. 2012;41(11):26.
3. Delivery, Project Value. How Changing Mindset is the Prerequisite of Any Organizational Change. www.ProjectValueDelivery.com, 2012.
4. Shrestha R. The illusion of communication. Appl Radiol. 2016;45(7):20–2.
5. Person- and Family-Centered Care. National Quality Forum. [Online] [Cited: June 9, 2016.] http://www.qualityforum.org/Topics/Person-_and_Family-Centered_Care.aspx.
6. Singhal S, Kayyali B, Levin R, Greenberg Z. The next wave of healthcare innovation: the evolution of ecosystems. McKinsey & Company; 2020.
7. Wolff JL, Darer JD, Berger A, Clarke D, Green JA, Stametz RA, Delbanco T, Walker J. Inviting patients and care partners to read doctors' notes: OpenNotes and shared access to electronic medical records. J Am Med Inform Assoc. 2016;24(e1):e166.
8. Shrestha R, Kalafut J. Transforming radiology with the power of partnership. Appl Radiol. 2013;42:30.
9. Iglehart JK. Health insurers and medical-imaging policy—a work in progress. N Engl J Med. 2009;360:1030–7.
10. Shrestha RB. Accountable care and value-based imaging: challenges and opportunities. Appl Radiol. April 2013;42:19.
11. Mahesh M. Essential role of a medical physicist in the radiology department. Radiographics. 2018;38:1665–71.
12. Radiation dose monitoring solutions 2014. Provo: KLAS Research, 2014.
13. Porter ME, Teisberg EO. Redefining health care: creating value-based competition on results. Harvard Business School Press; 2006.

14. Shrestha R. Enterprise imaging: the imaging value chain. Appl Radiol. 2014;
15. Hillman BJ, Goldsmith JC. The uncritical use of high-tech medical imaging. N Engl J Med. 2010;363:4.
16. Paz D. The radiologist as a physician consultant. J Am Coll Radiol. 2010;7:664–6.
17. Shrestha R. Transformation through interoperability: are we there yet? Appl Radiol. 2015;
18. Knechtges PM, Carlos RC. The evolving role of the radiologist within the health care system. J Am Coll Radiol. 2007;4(9):626–35.
19. Muroff LR. Implementing an effective organization and governance structure for a radiology practice. J Am Coll Radiol. 2004;1:26–32.
20. Shrestha RB. Influencing wisely — the path forward for value-based imaging. Appl Radiol. 2015;44:30.
21. Paz D. The radiologist as a physician consultant. J Am Coll Radiol. 2010;7:664–6.
22. Kirby A. Current issues: self referral. The American College of Radiology Resident and Fellow Section. [Online] February 2, 2006. [Cited: June 10, 2015.] http://rfs.acr.org/current/referral.htm.
23. A costly defense: physicians sound off on the high price of defensive medicine in the US. Jackson Healthcare. [Online] May 27, 2011. [Cited: December 14, 2020.] https://true-costofhealthcare.org/wp-content/uploads/2015/02/defensivemedicine_ebook_final.pdf.

Self-Assessment Questions

1. Each department in the enterprise represents:

    A. A separate silo that must coordinate with other silos
    B. An independent purchasing entity
    C. An island, because a rock feels no pain and an island never cries
    D. Part of a coordinated care system designed for efficiencies of scale

2. Which of the following is a physician?

    A. PA
    B. CRNP
    C. Intern
    D. Medical student

3. Commoditization is:

    A. Removing unique elements from a product or service so that it is interchangeable between providers
    B. Reducing the cost of rendered medical services
    C. Purchasing in discrete batches to better monitor costs
    D. Not relevant to healthcare enterprises

4. Which of these people might appear in an academic practice, but not a private practice?

    A. Fellow
    B. Medical physicist
    C. Department chair
    D. Physician assistant

5. Image utilization should be scrutinized because:

   A. More imaging means less profit for the hospital.
   B. Unnecessary imaging is driving up overall healthcare costs.
   C. All imaging is harmful to patients at some level.
   D. There are too many radiologists in the world.

6. List the ten people you work with most frequently. Figure out where they belong in Table 15.1 and Fig. 15.2.

7. If you need to buy new equipment or software, who will sign off on that decision? (The answer may differ depending on what type of equipment or software.)

Chapter 16
Workflow Steps in Radiology

R. L. "Skip" Kennedy

Contents

16.1 Introduction

Workflow in medical imaging is, properly, part of the larger domains of business process analysis (BPA) and business process modeling (BPM), for which extensive literature exists in business administration outside of imaging informatics. However, some special and particular aspects of digital image management, such as the specific technical mechanisms of DICOM and HL7, as well as the interactions of these and other standards, are needed to understand how data and processes interact in the context of a fully digital imaging environment. Further, it is critical for us to expand our understanding of imaging workflow to include the overall healthcare enterprise, including the EMR (electronic medical record) and other enterprise systems, and to extend into all of the medical imaging domains including cardiology, dermatology, pathology, surgery, and ophthalmology.

Film-based medical imaging workflow revolved around the fundamental nature and limitations of film itself. Because film was a physical entity, the actual transport of film constituted much of radiology "workflow."

R. L. "Skip" Kennedy (✉)
Imaging Informatics, The Permanente Medical Group, Kaiser Permanente,
Sacramento, CA, USA
e-mail: Skip.L.Kennedy@kp.org

© The Author(s), under exclusive license to Springer Science+Business Media, LLC, part of Springer Nature 2021
B. F. Branstetter IV (ed.), *Practical Imaging Informatics*,
https://doi.org/10.1007/978-1-0716-1756-4_16

PACS has fundamentally altered these assumptions. Ubiquitous electronic imaging and reporting has changed imaging workflow from basic document management and the physical transport of film to integration with the information flow of the larger healthcare enterprise:

- In 1999 it was estimated that 14% of all imaging sites had PACS and less than 1% of these were more than 80% filmless.
- In 2021, PACS is essentially universal in developed countries.
- PACS has evolved to represent the core technology for healthcare image management and now represents the accepted standard of care. With this, and with the adoption of EMRs, standardization and formalization of digital imaging workflow becomes increasingly important for interoperability, and standardized digital imaging workflow will become essential to achieve national interoperability in healthcare.

> **FURTHER READING: Technology Adoption and Maturity Models**
>
> https://www.himssanalytics.org/emram
> United States. https://www.himssanalytics.org/north-america/digital-imaging-adoption-model
> Europe. https://europe.himssanalytics.org/

Two models of technology adoption are relevant (both are from HIMSS):

- The EMRAM (Electronic Medical Record Adoption Model) has PACS as a requirement for stage 1 of 7 defined stages. It is estimated that less than 1% of US hospitals had not reached stage 1 by 2019.
- The DIAM (Digital Imaging Adoption Model) is specific to digital imaging and also has seven stages. Both address essential elements of radiology workflow.

16.2 Understanding Basic Concepts

The formal analysis of business processes within an enterprise is a well-established domain of academic business administration programs. Much of this is directly applicable to digital imaging workflow, but there are some specific aspects of medical imaging that are unique:

- Where the DICOM and HL7 protocols interact to provide triggers for the flow of business processes, special attention must be paid to the internals of these standards to best model electronic medical image workflow.
- The capabilities and implementations of these two standards will define our options for workflow design. Fortunately, the IHE (Integrating the Healthcare Enterprise) frameworks offer particularly useful models that specifically address and leverage both HL7 and DICOM capabilities in regard to workflow design.
- While much can be gained from the standard literature for business process analysis, workflow in medical imaging can only be fully understood in the context of those two standards that provide the foundation for essentially all modern PACS, RIS, and, increasingly, the EMR.
- PACS and RIS are each an integral part of the "fully image enabled EMR."

16.3 Documentation and Process Flow

Although we must still apply the specifics of HL7 and DICOM to traditional business process analysis and modeling to be fully useful for our purposes, the tools available from the general disciplines of business administration remain extremely valuable. **Process flow diagramming** offers us great value for documentation information flow and the various event triggers that drive imaging workflow. Hit is an essential exercise for any PACS and RIS deployment to document intended workflow using standard business process documentation tools. Figure 16.1 is an example of a typical process flow diagram, incorporating RIS, PACS, report management, and EMR workflow steps. The key to this process is to **redesign workflow** to achieve desired clinical results, to the degree possible with the new systems, rather than to simply re-implement electronically those same workflows that defined film-based radiology imaging. We need to build for the present rather than rebuild workflows and processes we have utilized in the past.

FURTHER READING: Business Process Analysis

Darnton G, Darnton M. Business process analysis. International Thomson Business Press; 1997.

Harrington HJ, Esseling C, van Nimwegen H. Business process improvement workbook: documentation, analysis, design, and management of business process improvement. McGraw-Hill Professional; 1997.

Nelson M. Fundamentals of business process analysis: the capture, documentation, analysis and knowledge transfer of business requirements. Annenberg Communications Institute; 1999.

16.4 Key Steps of Workflow

One of the essential points of understanding the HL7 and DICOM aspects of digital image workflow is the concept of event triggers.

- For example, the action of a technologist clicking on a button on the CT scanner and initiating a DICOM transmission to the PACS of the completed study may trigger yet other automated actions further in the workflow, such as potentially the PACS forwarding a HL7 message to the EMR signaling new image availability.

KEY CONCEPT: Event Triggers

A single workflow event may produce a cascade of other workflow events, some of which are automated, and some of which rely on manual input.

FURTHER READING: Workflow Steps in Radiology

Siegel E, Reiner B. Workflow redesign: the key to success when using PACS. AJR Am J Roentgenol. 2002;178(3):563–6. https://pubmed.ncbi.nlm.nih.gov/11856674/

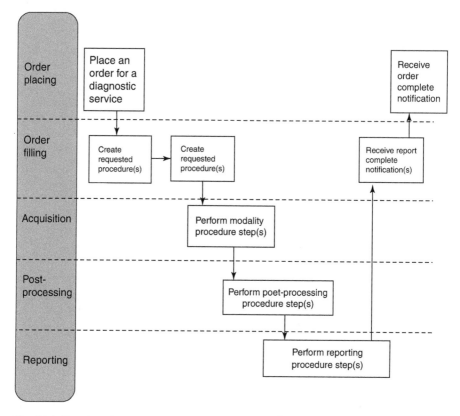

Fig. 16.1 Sample radiology workflow flowchart. (Reprinted from the IHE Radiology Technical Framework White Paper 2004–2005 with permission from IHE International)

- Understanding these workflow triggers, in most cases, involves understanding the state conditions of the underlying protocols—typically DICOM and HL7, but increasingly also web services such as SOAP—as well as the actual events that these represent in the actual business logic.
- The translation of the business logic to the appropriate protocol messaging state is the key to the implementation of functional workflow in digital imaging.

CHECKLIST: Workflow Steps

Sample workflow steps for members of the imaging team are provided below. These will vary from institution to institution and are provided only as a sample.

A. Radiologist workflow steps
  - Log in to PACS.
  - Set worklist filters/choose cases.

- Launch case.
- Collect clinical data/prior exams.
- Review and interpret images.
- Dictate report.
- Personally convey urgent or unexpected findings.
- Review and sign report (may be performed individually or as a batch).
- Protocol and check ongoing cases.

B. Technologist workflow steps
- Determine next patient/claim patient in RIS.
- Retrieve patient.
- Determine protocol.
- Obtain images.
- Check images for quality.
- Post-process to create additional images.
- Send images to PACS.
- Complete study in RIS.

C. Referring clinician workflow steps
- Order study:
  - Computerized physician order entry
  - Paper order in patient's chart
  - Verbal order to nurse or clerk
- Provide clinical information for radiologist.
- Review radiologist report:
  - Online
  - In the EMR
  - Paper report in the patient's chart
- Contact radiologist for clarification/discussion.

D. Other personnel with critical workflow
- Transcriptionist—workflow strongly determined by speech recognition and dictation software
- Nurses
  - Radiology nurses
  - Ward nurses
- PACS support personnel—need dashboards to stay ahead of hardware failures
- File room clerks—even after the transition to PACS, still needed to find comparison films and create CDs
- Ward clerks—often responsible for actually ordering the study, upon a physician's order
- Transportation personnel—take inpatients from their rooms to radiology and back

OUR EXPERIENCE: The Transition to Paperless Workflow

Today's IIPs might have difficulty imagining workflow that was driven by paper tokens handed from person to person, following the flow of the patients and their images through the departments. Changing from a paper-based to a paperless workflow was an obvious goal for improved efficiency and decreased human errors, but it was easy to get caught up in minor issues that prevented full implementation. If properly integrated with dictation and the RIS, PACS might have the software elements needed for the radiologist to abandon paper. But other personnel relied on those same paper tokens! Taking them out of the hands of the radiologists would not have been adequate until communication software between nurses, techs, and physicians was robust. For example, technologists used the paper requisitions to write notes to the radiologist, explaining why an exam was of suboptimal quality or providing new clinical information. Until the communication tools caught up with the other digital elements, it was impossible to go completely paperless.

16.5 IHE Workflow Steps

- An **order** represents a formal request, typically from a referring provider, for a specific or general service, representing certain actions or work products. Since reimbursement is closely linked to order status and processing, orders most typically originate

    DEFINITION: IHE

    Integrating the Healthcare Enterprise is an initiative that has created a framework for medical workflow in which different electronic systems can exchange information.

  from external systems, such as HIS or EMRs supporting electronic order entry. These are typically transmitted to a RIS and to PACS to support integration and automated modality worklist processing.
- A **requested procedure** represents a fundamental work unit, typically performed together within an encounter that is comprised of one or more procedure steps typically performed together during this patient encounter. Multiple procedure steps may be required to satisfy the procedure and the corresponding order. An example of this might be for a "CT head scan" within the EMR order entry system.
- A **procedure step** represents the discrete and indivisible steps that comprise the requested procedure as an entity. Since these are interrelated, they need to be performed within the encounter itself, or in a designated sequence. These are represented within a worklist, and are typically associated with specific CPT (Common Procedural Terminology) coding. In other cases, procedure steps may also represent the required steps that may or may not be performed within an encounter, such as treadmill or radionuclide injection.
- A **worklist** represents procedures and procedure steps that are to be performed. Typically, now, this is made available and transmitted to the performing modality via the DICOM Modality Worklist service, to avoid repeated manual data entry

and resulting data entry error. Design of worklist management is one of the most essential PACS design criteria, as it heavily contributes to both efficiency and data integrity of the imaging products of reports and the images themselves.

- **Reports** are most typically the result of radiologist interpretation, although there is now an increasing focus on structured reporting resulting from technologist workflow processes as well as automated content (such as protocol details and tabular data) directly from the modalities themselves.
- Defining and combining these steps and components allows us to design digital imaging workflow. The formalization and rigor of the IHE workflow model and technical framework provides us with a more exact semantic context for the steps of digital image workflow and allows us to merge different workflow models with shared context.

16.6 Structured Content

A key development in the evolution of radiology workflow has become the increased adoption of structured content both in terms of report structure (use of templates for reporting, leading to enhanced content standardization, and the adoption of standard lexicons such as RadLex) and modality-origin content such as biometrics from ultrasound or dose information from CT or IR. These enhancements bear directly to workflow design and engineering, and contribute to radiologist, and, overall, radiology efficiency.

- The radiology report is evolving from an unstructured narrative to a construct of various sources:
  - Dictation template
  - Modality SR
  - Technologist content
  - EMR content
  - Post-processing software
  - Artificial intelligence analysis
  - And, of course, the imager's own dictation
- Associated with this change has been the evolution from historical transcription workflow to real-time report delivery.
- These changes have allowed radiology reporting workflow to become a "matter of minutes" rather than hours, greatly enhancing its clinical value.

16.7 Web Services

Another development in radiology workflow has been the evolution of web-based protocol extensions to both HL7 (FHIR and FHIRCast) and DICOM (DICOMWeb) (see **Chap. 12**). These now allow the traditional protocol standards that comprise the foundation of radiology workflow to be instantiated within modern IT web infrastructure.

16.8 IHE Workflow Models

The Integrating the Healthcare Enterprise (IHE) initiative has provided us with invaluable templates for key aspects of medical imaging workflow, in the form of several key integration profiles for radiology. While the scope of IHE is now much larger than imaging itself, the reader is urged to refer to the following list as a foundation for approaching the various IHE profiles for workflow in digital imaging. These profiles address workflow, content, and pre-

FURTHER READINGS: IHE

HIMSS/RSNA. IHE Radiology Technical Framework White Paper 2004–2005. IHE-Radiology Technical Committee.

Channin D. Integrating the Healthcare Enterprise: a primer. Part 2. Seven brides for seven brothers: the IHE integration profiles. Radiographics. 2001;21:1343–1350.

IHE website http://www.ihe.net.

sentation—the former being most relevant here, but understanding the other profiles is important imaging workflow.

Workflow

- Scheduled workflow (**SWF**) integrates ordering, scheduling, imaging acquisition, storage, and viewing for radiology exams.
- Patient Information Reconciliation (**PIR**) coordinates reconciliation of the patient record when images are acquired for unidentified (e.g., trauma), or misidentified patients.
- Post-Processing Workflow (**PWF**) provides worklists, status, and result tracking for post-acquisition tasks, such as computer-aided detection or image processing.
- Reporting workflow (**RWF**) provides worklists, status, and result tracking for reporting tasks, such as dictation, transcription, and verification.
- Import Reconciliation Workflow (**IRWF**) manages importing images from CDs, hardcopy, etc. and reconciling identifiers to match local values.
- Portable Data for Imaging (**PDI**) provides reliable interchange of image data and diagnostic reports on CDs for importing, printing, or, optionally, displaying in a browser.

Content

- Nuclear medicine (**NM**) image specifies how nuclear medicine images and result screens are created, exchanged, used, and displayed.
- Mammography Image (**MAMMO**) specifies how mammography images and evidence objects are created, exchanged, used, and displayed.
- Evidence Documents (**ED**) specify how data objects such as digital measurements are created, exchanged, and used.
- Simple Image and Numeric Report (**SINR**) specifies how diagnostic radiology reports (including images and numeric data) are created, exchanged, and used.

Presentation

- Key Image Note (**KIN**) lets users flag images as significant (e.g., for referring, for surgery, etc.) and add notes.
- Consistent Presentation of Images (**CPI**) maintains consistent intensity and image transformations between different hardcopy and softcopy devices.
- Presentation of Grouped Procedures (**PGP**) facilitates viewing and reporting on images for individual requested procedures (e.g., head, chest, abdomen) that an operator has grouped into a single scan.
- Image fusion (**FUS**) specifies how systems creating and registering image sets and systems displaying fused images create, exchange, and use the image, registration, and blended presentation objects.

As these integration profiles expand and refine further, they serve as templates for vendor interoperability, fully supported by the technical specifics of DICOM and HL7 in the IHE Framework documents. Figure 16.2 details the first, and probably most fundamental, of the IHE integration profiles—the **scheduled workflow profile**. Dozens of other profiles now exist, and more are in development. Essentially all aspects of digital imaging workflow are now represented within the various IHE integration profiles currently available.

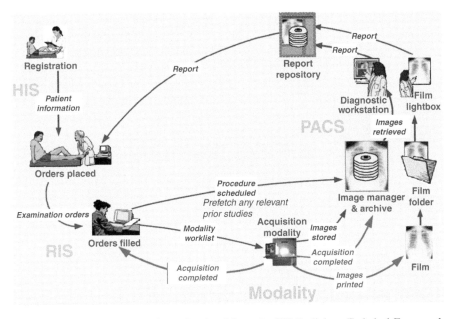

Fig. 16.2 IHE scheduled workflow. (Reprinted from the IHE Radiology Technical Framework White Paper 2004–2005 with permission from IHE International)

16.9 Goals

- The goal for any workflow analysis and workflow engineering process is, ultimately, to improve and enhance the workflows for **efficiency, reliability, fault tolerance, and transparency** to the clinical users.
- Workflow that represents many discrete steps that the clinical users must remember individually is to be avoided.
- Where possible, the concept of user interface **navigators** is particularly valuable when applied to sequential repetitive workflow.
- Where feasible, any given step that requires a **predecessor step** to be meaningful should not be available until the requisite predecessor has been completed (such as a radiologist reporting on a study for which a technologist has not yet completed or performed QA).
- **Exception workflows** for which these steps must, necessarily, be performed out of normal sequence should be available, but still allow process state recovery (as an example, the IHE profile for Patient Information Reconciliation (PIR) for reconciliation of unidentified or misidentified patient/study information.)
- A further goal for digital imaging workflow design is to facilitate **interoperability**. This is key deliverable of the IHE initiative:
  - Vendor-specific workflow is seldom capable of addressing enterprise requirements—while a "single-vendor solution" may be feasible with the confines of radiology, few, if any, vendors would be capable of addressing the needs of multiple departments and the enterprise EMR.
  - One of the fundamental goals of IHE is to facilitate vendor interoperability by the abstraction of the various system roles and the definition of standard protocol framework to the construction of workflows.

16.10 Summary

The design and testing of digital imaging workflow will be addressed more fully in **Chap. 25**, but the basics of approaching an understanding of these workflows lie in three areas:

- Leveraging existing business tools outside of informatics for workflow documentation and analysis methodologies
- Understanding the technical specifics of DICOM and HL7 as they apply to and drive digital imaging workflow
- Understanding and leveraging the IHE workflow models as templates for local workflow

A great deal of particularly valuable work has been done in developing the IHE integration profiles and frameworks, and the study of these will prove valuable to any effort regarding workflow engineering. While it is likely that not every aspect of the IHE integration profiles may apply precisely to all specific local clinical require-ments, it is equally unlikely that any institution developing and deploying PACS at this time would not find the majority of the IHE workflow models directly applica-ble and valuable. The use of the IHE technical frameworks for achieving vendor interoperability and regional institutional interoperability in the future are key developments and resources in these efforts.

Digital imaging has now moved well beyond the confines of radiol-ogy, both in terms of multiple imag-ing departments and servicing the entire enterprise as its customer base. Early implementations of PACS and RIS were, by necessity, limited in scope, but modern digital imaging workflow has as its expanded scope multiple departments and enterprise access. The culmination of these changes will almost certainly be enterprise, regional, and finally national EMRs that encompass digital imaging. We must build workflows today to support and embrace these futures.

> **FURTHER READING: RIS and PACS**
>
> Healthcare Informatics. Diagnostic imaging: PACS and radiology infor-mation systems. Nov 2007. http://www.healthcare-informatics.com/Media/DocumentLibrary/Diagnostic%20imaging.pdf.

PEARLS

- Workflows for different personnel are inextricably linked.
- IHE provides a useful framework for radiology workflow.
- Workflow improvements should address the efficiency, reliability, fault toler-ance, and transparency of workflow.
- Improved communication between different software programs allows for more efficient workflow.

Self-Assessment Questions

1. Which of these is *not* a usual element of radiologist workflow?

    (a) Obtain images.
    (b) Convey unexpected findings.
    (c) Protocol ongoing cases.
    (d) Collect clinical data.

2. Which of these is *not* a usual element of technologist workflow?

    (a) Send images to PACS.
    (b) Check images for quality.
    (c) Post-process the study to create new images.
    (d) Bring the patient to the radiology department.

3. Which of these is *not* a usual element of clinician workflow?

   (a) Order study
   (b) Dictate radiology reports.
   (c) Review radiologist report.
   (d) Provide clinical data.

4. Which of these is *not* an IHE integration profile?

   (a) Reporting workflow
   (b) Evidence documents
   (c) Consistent presentation of images
   (d) Procedure step

5. Which of these is *not* a hierarchical IHE component?

   (a) Post-processing
   (b) Order
   (c) Requested procedure
   (d) Worklist

6. If you could magically create a single piece of software, how would you address workflow inefficiencies in your own department?

7. Think of questions you would ask a vendor to make sure that their product has the IHE profiles you need.

Chapter 17
Viewing Images

Elizabeth A. Krupinski and Erik S. Storm

Contents

17.1 Introduction

Viewing images is at the core of numerous medical diagnostic tasks, and one can consider it from two perspectives (at least). On the one hand is the technology used to display the images and how factors such as luminance and display noise affect the quality of the image and hence the perception and interpretation of features in that image [1]. On the other hand, there is the human observer relying on their perceptual and cognitive systems to process the information presented to them. This aspect of viewing images is less well understood. From a purely visual perspective, we understand the physiology and basic functioning of the human visual system. What we understand to a lesser degree is how that information gets processed by the

E. A. Krupinski (✉)
Department of Radiology & Imaging Sciences, Emory University, Atlanta, GA, USA
e-mail: ekrupin@emory.edu

E. S. Storm
Departments of Radiology and Medical Education, Salem VA Medical Center,
Salem, VA, USA
e-mail: Erik.Storm@va.gov

© The Author(s), under exclusive license to Springer Science+Business Media,
LLC, part of Springer Nature 2021
B. F. Branstetter IV (ed.), *Practical Imaging Informatics*,
https://doi.org/10.1007/978-1-0716-1756-4_17

higher functioning parts of the brain. How does the radiologist process a set of features in an X-ray image and interpret that as a lung nodule versus pneumonia? These are issues that are currently under investigation by many investigators interested in medical image perception and their quest to improve reader performance. Traditionally radiology has been the clinical specialty that utilizes image data the most, but with the advent of telemedicine, other clinical specialties within the Integrating the Healthcare Enterprise (IHE) are also relying on the interpretation of digital image data for routine patient care [2, 3]. Thus, it becomes important for imaging informatics professionals (IIPs) to understand some of the key issues involved in the image interpretation process and how to optimize the digital reading environment for effective and efficient image reading.

The purpose of this chapter is to discuss some of the key issues involved in image viewing from the perspective of how to best accommodate the perceptual [4] and cognitive processes of the radiologist (or other clinician) rendering a diagnostic decision. It is important to remember two things when choosing a workstation for daily use in the viewing and interpretation of digital images. The first is that it can be a very daunting task because there are numerous products available on the market and more are continually being added and touted as the "best." The second is that there is no "one-size-fits-all" workstation that will please every user. In many situations, however, there are established practice guidelines and technology review papers that can provide at least the minimal technical requirements required for digital diagnostic viewing [1–3, 5–7].

FURTHER READINGS

Bevins NB, et al. Practical application of AAPM Report 270 in display quality assurance: a report of Task Group 270. Med Phys. 2020; https://doi.org/10.1002/mp.14227. [1]

McKoy K, et al. Practice guidelines for teledermatology. Telemed J E Health. 2016;12:981–90. [2]

Pantonowitz L, et al. American Telemedicine Association clinical guidelines for telepathology. J Pathol Inform. 2014;5:39. [3]

The Royal College of Radiologists. Picture archiving and communication systems (PACS) and guidelines on diagnostic display devices. 3rd ed. The Royal College of Radiologists, BFCR(19)2; 2019. https://bit.ly/3opnkaW.

Entz K, et al. Evaluation of the new DIN standard for quality assurance of diagnostic displays – technical review DIN 6868-157. Rofo. 2018;190(1):51–60.

17.2 Basics of Human Perception

- There are three main aspects of vision that are important for interpreting medical images – **spatial resolution, contrast resolution**, and **color vision**.

FURTHER READING

Snowden R, Thompson P, Troscianko T. Basic vision: an introduction to visual perception. Oxford: Oxford University Press; 2012. [4]

- The eye is a complex organ, but there are certain parts of this highly specialized organ that deserve a brief description here. The eyes' main function is photoreception or the process by which light from the environment changes the specialized photoreceptors (nerve cells) in the retina called rods and cones. The retina is actually located at the back of the eye, so light travels through the pupil, the lens, and the watery vitreous center before it reaches the retina itself. Within the retina are about 115 million rods and 6.5 million cones. Rods are responsible for sensing contrast, brightness, and motion and are located mostly in the periphery of the retina. The **cones are responsible for fine spatial resolution**, spatial resolution, and color vision and are **located in the fovea and parafoveal regions**. The pigments in the rods and cones undergo chemical transformations as light hits them, converting light energy into electrical energy that acts upon the various nerve cells connecting the eye to the optic nerve and subsequent visual pathways that extend to the visual cortices in the brain itself. The fact that we have two eyes accounts for our ability to see depth or for the radiologist to generate the perception of depth from two-dimensional images. The transformation of electrical nerve signals generated in the early stages of vision to the perception of the outside world takes place in a number of brain regions that are equally specialized for visual perception.
- **Spatial resolution**, or the ability to see fine details, is highest at the fovea, but declines quite sharply toward the peripheral regions of the retina. This means that clinicians must search or move their eyes around the image in order to detect lesion features with high-resolution vision. Deficiencies in spatial resolution can easily be corrected by prescription glasses. With age, spatial resolution naturally degrades and most people require corrective lenses. **Glasses specifically designed for computer viewing** can be prescribed and should be considered if a clinician is having trouble viewing softcopy images on digital displays.

KEY CONCEPTS: Foveal Vision

The human eye sees details best with the central foveal vision (the thing you are looking at directly), so clinicians need to scan or search images to detect fine or subtle features indicative of abnormalities.

- Visual acuity also depends on **contrast** – differences in color and brightness that allows one to distinguish between objects and background in an image. To determine the contrast levels that are perceptible by the human eye, tests were developed that use a sinusoidal grating pattern (alternating black and white lines where the average luminance remains the same but the contrast between the light and dark areas differ). Discrimination of the grating is described in terms of cycles per degree or the grating frequency. Contrast sensitivity peaks in the mid-spatial frequency range around 3–5 cycles/degree. This means that low-contrast lesions can often go undetected, especially when viewing conditions are not optimal.
- The cones in the retina are what make **color vision** possible. There are three types of cones, each with a different photopic spectral sensitivity – short, medium, and long wavelengths corresponding to blue, green, and red, respectively. Color vision is

KEY CONCEPT: Spatial Resolution Versus Contrast Resolution

Spatial resolution measures how small an object can be and still be detected. Contrast resolution measures how similar in color an object can be to its surroundings and still be detected. Radiology techniques are often a balancing act between spatial and contrast resolution; improving either of them can make a lesion more easily detectable.

TROUBLESHOOTING: Poor Display Quality

There are no requirements for radiologists or other clinicians to have their vision checked on a regular basis; however, an annual eye exam can detect and correct vision problems that you might not even be aware of. The solution to some complaints about image and/or display quality could be an eye exam and prescription for corrective lenses.

less important in radiology than in other medical image-based clinical specialties such as pathology, dermatology, and ophthalmology [6]. Deficiencies in color vision affect about 10% of the population (males more often than females), potentially affecting the interpretation of color and pseudo-color medical images.

17.3 Display Hardware Basics

- **Technology**: **Liquid-crystal displays** (LCDs) are the dominant technology used in the majority of medical-grade and off-the-shelf monitors. **Cathode-ray tube** (CRT) displays were prevalent until the start of the twenty-first century, but are now increasingly rare:
  - There are two categories of displays typically used in radiology. First are those typically used for image interpretation, and for the most part, these are **medical-grade (MG)** displays. **Commercial/consumer-off-the-shelf (COTS)** displays can be used for some image interpretation but are more common for technologist viewing of images during acquisition and processing as well as during interpretation for accessing additional data (e.g., accessing the electronic health record) and for report generation. MG displays tend to be more expensive, built for multi-year use, have built in calibration tools specific to medical imaging, have automated image quality assessment tools and sensors, and are more standardized in terms of features. COTS displays, especially professional-grade (PG; used for animation, graphic design, photography, video production, and related tasks), often rival MG displays in terms of spatial resolution, but many of the other features are less advanced. The advantage is they cost far less, although they do need to be replaced on a more frequent basis.
  - Very briefly, LCDs are made of a panel of liquid-crystal cells between two electrodes and polarizing filters. Light is shone through the cells, and, by adjusting the voltage between the electrodes, the conformation of the crystals within the cells is changed, affecting the amount of light that can pass through to create an image for the viewer. Color is created by adding filters that allow transmission of select wavelengths. There are three basic panel types used in LCDs: **twisted nematic (TN)**, **in-plane switching (IPS)**, and **vertical alignment (VA)**. TNs have been around the longest and so are the least expensive. They are limited by narrow viewing angles (i.e., when viewing from off-center, contrast is lost) and poor color rendition. IPS improves these two features but can suffer from backlight bleeding (light leakage around display edges). VA is the newest technology and has better viewing angles than TNs and less backlight bleeding than IPS displays.
  - The light source for LCDs was initially a cold-cathode fluorescent lamp (CCFL), but now is mostly light-emitting diodes (LEDs) that are far more energy efficient, provide better light uniformity, are brighter, and are thinner than CCFLs allowing for thinner and lighter displays. Emissive displays using organic LEDs (OLEDs) are commonly used in laptops, tablets, smartphones, and televisions. microLEDs are a new technology that use very small (<1 mm) LEDs that require fewer layers and thus even thinner displays. These are still a few years away from wide adoption.
  - Most displays in medical imaging are two-dimensional displays in which depth information is only poorly rendered. There are dedicated displays avail-

able for 3D viewing, but their use in medical image interpretation is quite limited.

- **Stereoscopic displays** allow for better perception of depth but generally require the use of special glasses to see the depth information. These displays often rely on basic stereoscopic "tricks" to display depth. Two images are acquired of the same objet but from slightly (about 15°) different angles. In its most familiar form, one image is coded in red and the other in green. A simple pair of glasses with red and green filters then sends one image to one eye and the other image to the other eye. The brain then fuses the images and there is the perception of depth. More sophisticated technologies exist for viewing stereoscopic displays, but they are all based on this basic premise. True 3D displays are available and may be useful for viewing certain types of images, especially 3D and tomographic reconstructions of radiologic images. The technology used in these displays varies depending on the manufacturer. One common technique is to layer the display so that some pixels are in one plane and others in another, weaved together in a sense so every other pixel or so is in either the back or forward plane. Once again, the system relies on the ability of the human brain to fuse the information into a perception of depth although this time without the need for special glasses.

  It is interesting to note that stereoscopic displays have never really caught on in radiology even though data are acquired from two angles on a regular basis. Aside from the issues involved in creating and viewing stereoscopic images and the increased time it takes to view them, another reason that stereoscopic displays may not be useful is that there is not much information gained. As noted, in order to create stereoscopic images, the most common technique is to acquire images of the same scene from two different angles. This does not double the information, however, since in order to perceive stereoscopic depth the images need to be highly correlated.

- **Virtual and augmented reality (VR & AR) displays** are increasingly being touted as possible tools for many clinical applications including radiology. Although there may be some utility for interpretation of diagnostic images, more likely uses so far are for interventional and other procedural-based specialties and for simulation-based teaching and training applications [8, 9]. In VR the user is in a completely immersive environment, typically using a headset that literally blocks out all other sources of visual input, so only the images created within the virtual environment are perceived. Most of these headsets are tethered and provide manual devices to allow the user to navigate through and manipulate "objects" in the virtual world. AR does not replace the "real" visual input but rather enhances or augments it with images or other data projected on top of the "real" world. For this, transparent "smart" glasses with miniature projectors are typically used, although smartphone apps and games also incorporate AR.

  Perceptually there are some aspects with both VR and AR that can be challenging. Some VR users cannot properly focus on or fuse the images in VR resulting in double or distorted images. The lag between navigation/manipulation actions and system display response, as well as vection (the illusion of self-movement in the display when the body is not moving causing conflict between visual and vestibular systems), can cause cybersickness (a type of motion sickness). AR users do not suffer from these issues as much, but some find it difficult to focus when faced with the overlying transparent image, and some do experience a bit of lag and thus nausea when moving the head too fast and the overlying image does not fit with the real scene any longer.

- **Matrix size or resolution**: Display resolution is the total number of pixels in a panel. It is usually reported as either the total number of pixels or how many are present in the x- and y-dimensions (e.g., 4096 × 1260 or 4K). Current displays range from 1 to 12 megapixels:

  - **Small matrix** (1 or 2 MP) displays are typically used for small matrix radiographic images such as CT, MRI, and ultrasound; clinical (i.e., non-diagnostic or those used by non-radiologists, technologists, clinical staff) review; and non-radiology specialties (e.g., dermatology, ophthalmology).
  - **Large matrix** (3 MP and higher) displays are typically used for digital radiography (e.g., chest, bone); digital mammography; and digital (a.k.a. virtual) pathology. Large displays are really only warranted when the resolution of the displayed images needs the increased resolution. Since these displays are generally more expensive than small matrix displays, their use should be reserved for cases where they are needed (mammography, etc.). The goal when choosing which format to use is to allow for the greatest amount of inherent resolution to be displayed without the use of zoom and pan to access higher-resolution data, since zooming and panning result in more time being spent per image and there is the chance that the user may forget to use it or not use it systematically over the entire image.
  - **Orientation**: Most radiology images are more appropriately viewed using displays in portrait mode (although CT, MRI, and US can use landscape), while most other medical images can be viewed using landscape.

- **Display pixel size**: Display pixel size is a more accurate measure of display resolution. Visual acuity and contrast sensitivity indicate that 2.5 cycles/mm or **200-micron pixel size is best**. Pixel pitch refers to the distance between neighbor-

> **DEFINITION: Megapixels**
>
> MP is the number of pixels contained in the display, measured in millions of pixels.

> **KEY CONCEPT: Image Size**
>
> A typical CT or MRI image is 256 or 512 pixels per side. A conventional radiograph is 1000–2000 pixels per side. A mammogram may be up to 5000 pixels per side!

> **KEY CONCEPTS: Choosing Display Matrix Size**
>
> Matrix size should be as close as possible to the original acquired image data sent to the display (known in radiology as "for processing"), or the full-resolution data should be attainable with magnification.

ing pixels. It is inversely related to resolution – the lower the pixel pitch, the higher the resolution. This is important because two displays with the same resolution but different pixel pitch will look different – the one with the higher pixel pitch will look fuzzy or granular at closer viewing distances (which is common in radiology).

- **Monochrome vs. color**: Nearly all displays, both off-the-shelf and medical-grade, come in both monochrome and color versions. **Monochrome displays** are sometimes still recommended for large matrix images (CR, DR, and digital mammography) as monochrome displays tend to have lower intrinsic noise than color displays. Color displays are often used in radiology for small matrix images such as CT, MRI, and ultrasound. Radiology images that utilize pseudo-color (e.g., 3D reconstructions) should use color displays. Non-radiology medical images such as those from dermatology, pathology, and ophthalmology should all use color displays of the appropriate matrix size.

- **Moving images**: Medical images for the most part are not actual moving images in the traditional sense (i.e., movies). However, radiologists do view stacks of images that simulate moving images, and zooming/panning large images (e.g., mammograms and pathology whole-slide images) requires some of the same hardware features as for movies (which are really a series of single-image frames). There are two features that are important to consider. **Refresh rate** is the number of times the screen is updated per second and is measured in hertz (Hz). Perceptually it is reflected in how smooth the motion appears to be as opposed to flickering or tearing with low refresh rates. Refresh rates of 60 Hz or higher are better but are more expensive. **Response time** refers to how long it takes for a pixel to switch from one color to another or from black to white or vice versa. It is measured in milliseconds (msec or ms), and the lower it is, the better it is, although with today's technology most people do not notice.

- **Calibration**: Display monitors and corresponding video graphics cards must be calibrated to and conform to the current DICOM grayscale standard display function (GSDF) perceptual linearization methods [1, 10–12]. Color displays can also be calibrated to the DICOM GSDF to display monochrome images properly. Methods for color calibration also exist [2, 6], although there is little consensus on exactly which color gamut

> **DEFINITION: GSDF**
>
> The grayscale display function is a DICOM method that defines the relationship between the pixel value of an image and the luminance of the display. It is designed to optimize human perception and is a necessary part of display calibration in radiology.

(amount of a specific color space or range of colors, such as the mix of the three basic colors red, blue, and green) or standard (e.g., standard red, green, blue (sRGB); cyan, magenta, yellow, black (CMYK)) is the most appropriate or useful in terms of optimizing displays for accurate and efficient color medical image interpretation.

- **Display luminance**: Luminance is the amount of light generated by the display technology and can be measured objectively (commonly using candelas or cd/m²). Brightness is often used incorrectly to describe displays but is actually the subjective perception of light intensity. Both are affected by ambient light settings or illuminance that is typically measured in lux (20–40 lux recommended for image interpretation). The ratio of maximum to minimum luminance (contrast) should be at least 50. Maximum luminance of grayscale monitors used for viewing digital conventional radiographs should be at least **250 cd/m²**. Mammography has separate requirements, discussed later in this chapter. Most manufacturers of medical-grade displays meet this specification. A significant number of off-the-shelf displays meet it as well, but the specifications should be checked before purchasing if the displays are to be used for primary interpretation.

> **KEY CONCEPT: Display Calibration**
>
> Most medical-grade displays come with the hardware and software for calibration. Basic hardware can also be purchased for less than $250, and DICOM GSDF test patterns such as the SMPTE monitor test pattern can be downloaded for free from various sources [1, 10–12]. Some vendors also offer remote performance monitoring, calibration, and quality control.

> **KEY CONCEPT: Ambient Lighting**
>
> The light level in the room can dramatically affect the visibility of objects on an image. Radiologist may prefer to work in a brightly lit room, but that reduces their effectiveness.

- **Contrast response**: Should comply with AAPM guidelines [1, 10], DICOM grayscale standard display function (GSDF) recommendations, and not deviate by more than 10%. Most manufacturers of medical-grade displays meet this specification. Most off-the-shelf displays do not come with the software (or luminance meters) to carry out the DICOM calibration. These items can be purchased separately and used to calibrate any monitor. The specifications should be checked before purchasing if the displays are to be used for primary interpretation.
- **Bit depth**: A minimum of 8-bit depth (luminance resolution) is required. Higher is recommended if original or "for presentation" image data is greater than 8 bits in depth. In general, the higher the luminance ratio of the display, the larger the bit-depth resolution that is advised. Most manufacturers of medical-grade and off-the-shelf displays meet this specification. The specifications should be checked before purchasing if the displays are to be used for primary interpretation.
- **Protective shields**: Many shields add to reflections, so **shields should be avoided**. Many displays come with antireflective coatings that are quite effective at reducing glare and reflections. One of the best ways to avoid glare and reflections is to use diffuse lighting sources and avoid having displays face light sources (such as windows or other workstations) and **avoid wearing white coats**.

- **Warm-up time**: To maximize performance, most displays require about 30 minutes of warm-up time. This actually fits well with a property of the human visual system – dark adaptation. **Dark adaptation** is a process whereby the pupil dilates and the rods in the retina (via regeneration of rhodopsin) increase sensitivity as a reaction to decreased illumination (think about what happens when walking into a dark theater after being outside in the bright sunlight). The process starts almost immediately, but to become fully dark-adapted takes 20–30 minutes. Full dark adaptation is required since without it, the detection of low-contrast targets is especially compromised.

HYPOTHETICAL SCENARIO: Minimum Display Requirements

A radiologist asks whether a commercial off-the-shelf (nonmedical grade) display can be used for diagnostic reading and whether there are existing guidelines to be followed. The answer is yes – the American College of Radiology (ACR) in association with the American Association of Physicists in Medicine (AAPM) and the Society for Medical Imaging Informatics (SIIM) has published guidelines [1, 5, 10, 12] for digital radiology that include display requirements.

INTERNATIONAL CONSIDERATIONS: Display Requirements

In Europe, the Royal College of Radiologists (RCR) has published guidelines on diagnostic display devices, mentioning COTS as a sensible economical alternative to MG displays, although due attention is required regarding their application for primary diagnostics.

https://www.rcr.ac.uk/system/files/publication/field_publication_files/bfcr192_pacs-diagnostic-display.pdf.

17.4 Display Software Considerations

- **Window and level**: Adjustment tools must be available in order to display the full dynamic range of most images. Presets for window/level can make it easier for users to manipulate images. Most displays have 4096 shades of gray displayable. However, there are usually only a small range of intensities useful for most studies. Window defines this intensity range and defines the upper and lower shades to be included in the "window." The rest of the pixels that the user is not interested in for that particular view of the image are mapped to either black or white. Level is a

KEY CONCEPT: Window and Level

A CT scanner produces 12-bit data (4096 potential values), but the human eye (and most displays) can only differentiate 256 different shades of gray. Window and level is a way of mapping 12-bit scanner data to 8-bit display data, and also to focus on particular anatomic features.

related technique. It is a mathematical definition of how to map pixel values in the window to display luminances. For example, suppose someone wants to see a detail in a very dense tissue area. They could select a level that transforms an intensity difference of 1 to a luminance difference of 5 when displayed. In other words, if two dots in an image have pixel intensities of 125 and 126, the human eye cannot discern them from each other. By leveling or stretching them and increasing the luminance difference to 5, the difference is easily seen, and a subtle feature becomes obvious.

> **OUR EXPERIENCE**
>
> When deciding what vendor to use for purchasing diagnostic workstations, it is ideal to have multiple vendors come to your site on the same day for a "shoot-out" during which you can compare and use products side by side. An alternative strategy is to attend a conference with an exhibition area where multiple vendors are present.

- **Zoom and pan**: Magnification and roaming should be used to display the originally acquired image spatial resolutions. Users should not move closer to the display.
- **Image processing**: Five generic processing tools fulfill most image processing needs:
  - Grayscale rendition
  - Exposure recognition
  - Edge restoration
  - Noise reduction
  - Contrast enhancement
- **Computer-aided detection/decision (CADe/CADx), deep learning (DL), and artificial intelligence (AI) tools** have been experiencing a rapid rise not only in research but also in implementation in clinical practice (see **Chap. 14**). There are literally thousands of publications on the development and stand-alone testing of these tools with fewer on the impact on radiologists' decisions or time spent reviewing images. In general, those studies that do investigate impact have mixed results. Some studies find a positive impact on performance (increased accuracy) and reading time, while others do not. Differences as a function of level of training, years since being board certified, types of images, types of findings, subtlety/size/location of lesions, number of computer prompts, number of false positives (per image and per case), how the prompts are displayed, whether the prompt is simply an indication or contains an estimate of probability of malignancy, and a host of other factors all seem to affect whether or not an individual radiologist benefits from a given computer-based decision aid. Many of these factors are perceptually and/or cognitively based, and research is being conducted to improve our understanding of how these tools should be best integrated into clinical workflow [13–15].
- **Image rotation**: Tools for image rotation and flipping are essential.
- **Hanging protocols**: Automated tools for image sequencing and preferred display format should be available, flexible, and tailored to user preferences.

- **Response time**: The time needed to display an image stored locally (as opposed to a long-term archive) should be 3 seconds or less.
- **Data tagging**: Automated tools that accurately associate patient and study demographic information with the images are essential.
- **Measurement tools**: Tools that calculate and display linear measurements with appropriate units, regions of interest, and pixel values (mean and standard deviation) are useful.

> **DEFINITION: Compression**
>
> Compression reduces the volume of data to reduce image processing, transmission times, bandwidth requirements, and storage needs.
>
> *Lossless compression* allows for reconstruction of exact original data before compression without loss of information.
>
> *Lossy compression* uses methods that lose data once the image has been compressed and uncompressed, but provides a greater degree of compression.

- **Image compression**: If compression is applied to an image or set of images, the type (encoding method such as JPEG, and lossy vs. lossless) and amount (e.g., 10:1) should be known.
- **Total image set**: All images acquired in a study need to be accessible for interpretation. It is not necessary to display them simultaneously, but the use of dual monitors to display multiple images at full resolution is useful.
- **Acquisition parameters**: Clinically useful technical parameters of the acquired image should be accessible (e.g., mAs, kV, exposure value).

17.5 Human-Computer Interface

Workstation technologies (hardware and software) impact diagnostic accuracy, visual search, and interpretation efficiency. Hardware and software optimization techniques are often derived in part by considering the capabilities of the human visual system, especially with respect to spatial and contrast sensitivity. There are also factors related to the environment in which the workstation will be placed and how the clinician interacts with the technology that are important. Poor interface and environment can reduce diagnostic accuracy, reduce reader efficiency, increase reader fatigue, and risk injury. Ergonomics [16, 17] and good room design (see **Chap. 21**) are mandatory in the digital reading room:

- **Ambient room lights**: Ambient light sources should be kept at a minimum to reduce reflections and glare. Indirect and backlight incandescent lights with dimmer switches rather than fluorescent are optimal. Clinicians should **avoid wearing light-colored clothing** and lab coats since they add to reflections and glare. About 20–40 lux (or 0.03–0.06 Watts using yellow wavelength which the eyes are most sensitive to, since conversion varies as a function of wavelength) will avoid reflections and still provide sufficient light for the human visual system to adapt to the surrounding environment and the displays. Room lights should not be turned off completely.

- **Viewing direction**: Users should be seated as close to **on-axis viewing** as possible since some displays suffer from poor viewing angles and image contrast degrades as the viewer moves off-axis. When multiple displays are

> **DEFINITION: On-Axis Viewing**
>
> The viewer should be directly in front of the display, with line of sight perpendicular to the surface of the display.

used, they should be placed side by side and angled slightly toward each other. Large screens that are curved are on the market now, but for the most part, these are COTS, not MG displays.
- **Ambient air**: Computers, especially with dual monitors and in rooms with multiple workstations, require adequate airflow and optimal temperature and humidity controls. Direct ventilation for each workstation may be needed, and water-cooled computers should be considered if extra cooling is required.
- **Ambient noise**: Noise can distract the clinician from the diagnostic task so it should be minimized. Movable walls, sound-absorbing tiles/walls, and carpeting can be used to minimize noise between workstation areas. If dictation systems are used, it is especially important to isolate users from each other.
- **Seating**: Chairs with good lumbar support and **adjustable height controls** can help avoid injuries and fatigue.
- **Desk/tabletops**: It should be possible to adjust the height of tables and/or desks for each user.
- **Peripheral input devices**: Keyboards and mice should be comfortable for each user and placed for ease and comfort during use to avoid hand and wrist injuries. Users should consider personal mice to maximize hand comfort, so long as the mice are adequately programmable to support the PACS. Onboard programming in the mouse is helpful. Dictation tools, Internet access, and other reference tools should be readily accessible and easy to use during image interpretation. Although keyboards and the mouse are still the prevailing modes of interaction for most users, there are other that may provide some ergonomic advantages such as joysticks, graphic tablets, and speech recognition [18, 19]. To some extent, however, everyone is different and has different preferences, so all options should be considered on an individual basis rather than trying to find a one-size-fits-all solution.

17.6 Fatigue in the Reading Room

There is an increasing amount of literature and research on the topic of fatigue in the reading room, how it impacts interpretation performance and efficiency, and how we can avoid fatigue [20–26]. From a perceptual perspective, research has demonstrated that radiologists' ability to focus (accommodate) is significantly reduced after about 8 hours of clinical reading [26, 27]; and from a cognitive perspective, an fNIRS (functional near-infrared spectroscopy) study showed that after 4–5 hours of clinical reading, radiologists were subjectively fatigued and there was an apparent decrease in brain activity [25]. Additional studies with a range of image types and degree of complexity have consistently shown that after about 8 hours of clinical reading, diagnostic performance drops significantly by about 5%, as reflected by a decrease in false negatives and an increase in false positives [21, 26–30]. Interestingly, the decrease in performance is more pronounced in residents than faculty, suggesting that the overall experience of being a resident is already fatigue-inducing and stressful and that long hours exacerbate the problem. It has also been shown that fatigue actually changes the scanning patterns and the efficiency with which radiologists search images [23]. Total viewing time is often longer when fatigued, more fixations (point of gaze or where someone is looking in a scene) are generated, it takes longer to initially fixate on a lesion, and the times associated with positive decisions (both true and false) are longer.

OUR EXPERIENCE: Computer Vision Syndrome

With the switch from hardcopy film to softcopy digital reading in radiology, radiologists are spending long hours in front of computers doing "near reading." Long hours of near reading from computer displays can lead to computer vision syndrome characterized by blurred vision, double vision, dry eyes, the inability to focus properly, and headaches. We measured radiologists' ability to focus properly (or accommodate) on a target at the beginning of the day before reading images and after a long day of continual softcopy image reading. We found that there was more error in accommodation after a day of reading than before, especially for targets closer to the eyes. As radiologists are having difficulty focusing on discrete targets, this leads to increased errors as a function of reader fatigue [26, 27].

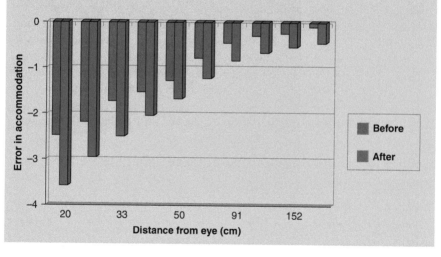

17.7 Special Considerations for Mammography, Tomosynthesis, and Breast Imaging

Breast imaging and its component modalities mammography and tomosynthesis have unique display requirements. Mammography is one of the only radiology specialties to have specifically codified federal regulations for medical imaging. Mammography IT needs to balance recommendations from professional organizations (e.g., ACR, SIIM, AAPM, RCR) versus legal requirements (e.g., MQSA regulations [31]). The areas most germane to the discussion of mammography display monitors include resolution, luminance, and response rate. Related factors include display configuration (i.e., dual portrait vs. large format/widescreen), monochrome vs. color, and the availability of appropriate onboard image processing and quality assurance (QA) tools [32, 33].

> INTERNATIONAL CONSIDERATIONS: Mammography QA
>
> European guidelines for quality assurance in breast cancer screening and diagnosis.
> https://www.euref.org/downloads?download=24:european-guidelines-for-quality-assurance-in-breast-cancer-screening-and-diagnosis-pdf.

> FURTHER READING
>
> Krupinski EA, Morgan MB, Siegel EL. ACR–AAPM–SIIM practice parameter for determinants of image quality in digital mammography [34]

- **Widescreen vs. portrait display**: Widescreen large-format dual displays capable of matching the technical performance of individual stand-alone displays have become recently available. Current widescreen monitors offer equivalent resolution to their portrait-oriented counterparts, with superior performance characteristics. Widescreen units typically contain two identical displays within a single external housing, without the need for a separating bezel. Whether these displays significantly impact reader efficiency is controversial [35–37].
- **Monochrome vs. color**: Color displays were until recently not considered appropriate for mammography, as they could not typically offer sufficient performance with respect to resolution and luminance. Modern color displays have overcome this limitation and are now considered a preferred option because breast imaging interpretation frequently includes color modalities such as ultrasound and MRI.
- **Resolution**: According to Shannon's theorem for the information capacity of a communication channel, as long as the pixel size of an image display is equal to

or lesser in size than the smallest image element (i.e., detector pixel size), then there will be no loss of information. Therefore, the spatial resolution of the display should match the spatial resolution of the image source.

The 200-μm pixel pitch of a 3-MP display translates a resolution of 2.5 line pairs per mm (lp/mm); the 165-μm pixel pitch of a 5-MP display translates to 3 lp/mm. But the native resolution of screen-film mammography is up to **20 lp/ mm**! This corresponds to a native resolution varying from 2400 × 3070 (7.4 MP) on the low end (GE) up to 4800 × 5200 (25 MP) on the high end (Sectra). As of the time of this writing, the maximum resolution of commercially available display units is 6 MP per display (12 MP widescreen). Even this resolution translates to a pixel pitch of only 169 μm, far less than the native resolution of film, and less than the ~100-μm resolution of the digital mammogram detector. It is therefore technically impossible at present to meet the desired goal of matched detector/display resolution.

Is it acceptable to interpret mammography on a digital display? The DMIST trial concluded that not only was digital mammography equivalent to traditional screen-film mammography, but that it was **more accurate** for younger women who are more likely to have dense breast tissue. The latter finding is attributable to the large dynamic range of the digital mammogram, providing increased contrast resolution [38].

– **Why is 5 MP recommended in mammography?**

The historic preference for 5 MP over standard 3 MP displays derives from the limitations of CRT technology. CRT displays exhibited lower than expected net observable resolution due to subtle blurring from anisotropy [39]. A 5-MP CRT monitor with its smaller pixel pitch was felt to help compensate for this theoretical discrepancy. Modern LCD displays do not suffer this same limitation, and the observable resolution remains true to the technical specification.

The time it takes to review a study depends on how much the radiologist needs to pan and zoom. The larger the difference between native image resolution and display resolution, the more manipulation will be required to view the entire image. Compared to 3-MP displays, 5-MP displays require less zoom, reduce the amount of work required to read the exam, and thus potentially increase radiologist efficiency. An additional concern is whether all users will take the time to fully zoom/pan the entire study, especially when reading high volumes. This could lead to diagnostic error.

• **Recommendations versus requirements**: The recommendation for individual displays to have a minimum resolution of 5 MP is **not** a legal requirement under MQSA. Although it is mandatory for a **facility** to be accredited, including its mam-

> **DEFINITION: MQSA**
>
> The Mammography Quality Standards Act and Program of the US Food and Drug Administration define numerous standards by which institutions become accredited to perform mammography [31].

mography imaging units, MQSA only **recommends** that displays be FDA-approved.

- The performance of mammography interpretation as a function of display resolution has been extensively studied in the literature for displays ranging from 3 to 5+ MP, and the consensus among these authors is that there is overall no significant difference in accuracy.

FURTHER READING

Bevins N, Flynn M, Silosky M, Marsh R, Walz-Flannigan A, Badano A. AAPM report 270: display quality assurance. American Association of Physicists in Medicine; 2019 [40].

- **Luminance**: Despite the intense scrutiny placed on display resolution, the more important factor in determining quality and appropriateness for diagnostic interpretation is luminance. The range of luminance available on a display is the ratio of light reaching the eye between a fully lit display pixel and a completely off pixel. This is a theoretical value, as the luminance we actually observe from a given pixel is affected by additional factors such as ambient light (Lamb), and the luminance of adjacent pixels. For mammography displays Lmax is recommended to be at least 450 cd/m^2. Most diagnostic displays offer much higher values, even greater than 2000 cd/m^2. The higher Lmax recommended for breast imaging in practice may help to compensate for the decreased native resolution of digital mammography relative to that of screen-film mammography [40].

- **Response rate**: Digital breast tomosynthesis is an advanced form of mammography in which each of the four usual projections (bilateral CC/MLO) is displayed as a cine of 25–100 tomosynthetic slices. The rate at which the display can turn an individual pixel on or off defines the rate-limiting step with respect to how fast each image in the stack can be replaced with the next. LCD displays designed and/or FDA-approved for tomosynthesis must have a high response rate (e.g., 17 ms) in order to perform at optimum efficiency.

PEARLS

- The solution to some complaints about image and/or display quality could be an eye exam and prescription for corrective lenses.
- Most medical-grade displays come with the hardware and software for calibration. Basic hardware can also be purchased for less than $250, and DICOM GSDF test patterns such as the SMPTE monitor test pattern can be downloaded for free.
- When deciding what vendor to use for purchasing diagnostic workstations, it is ideal to have multiple vendors come to your site to compare products side by side.
- Mammography requires higher-resolution imaging than any other area in medicine. This results in special IT requirements for mammography.

References

1. Bevins NB, Silosky MS, Badano A, Marsh RM, Flynn MJ, Walz-Flannigan AI. Practical application of AAPM Report 270 in display quality assurance: a report of Task Group 270. Med Phys. 2020; https://doi.org/10.1002/mp.14227.
2. McKoy K, Antoniotti NM, Armstrong A, Basjshur R, Bernard J, Bernstein D, Burdick A, Edison K, Goldyne M, Kovarik C, Krupinski EA, Kvedar J, Larkey J, Lee-Keltner I, Lipoff JB, Oh DH, Pak H, Seraly MP, Siegel D, Tejasvi T, Whited J. Practice guidelines for teledermatology. Telemed J E Health. 2016;12:981–90.
3. Pantanowitz L, Dickinson K, Evans AJ, Hassell LA, Henricks WH, Lennerz JK, Lowe A, Parwani AV, Riben M, Smith D, Tuthill JM, Weinstein RS, Wilbur DC, Krupinski EA, Bernard J. American Telemedicine Association clinical guidelines for telepathology. J Pathol Inform. 2014;5:39.
4. Snowden R, Thompson P, Troscianko T. Basic vision: an introduction to visual perception. Oxford: Oxford University Press; 2012.
5. Ruckdeschel TG, Keener CR, Kofler JM, Nagy P, Samei E, Andriole KP, Krupinski E, Seibert JA, Towbin AJ, Bevins NB, Lewis DA. ACR-AAPM-SIIM technical standard for electronic practice of medical imaging. 2017. https://www.google.com/url?sa=t&rct=j&q=&esrc=s&source=web&cd=&ved=2ahUKEwi1kpfS0qzrAhWHnOAKHZ-lAOIQFjAAegQIBxAB&url=https%3A%2F%2Fwww.acr.org%2F-%2Fmedia%2FACR%2FFiles%2FPractice-Parameters%2Felec-practice-medimag.pdf&usg=AOvVaw2lDxY5useu0iV_lclhBK9Z.
6. Badano A, Revie C, Casertano A, Cheng WC, Green P, Kimpe T, Krupinski E, Sisson C, Skrovseth S, Treanor D, Boynton P, Clunie D, Flynn MJ, Heki T, Hewitt S, Homma H, Masia A, Matsui T, Nagy B, Nishibori M, Penczek J, Schopf T, Yagi Y, Yokoi H, Summit on Color in Medical Imaging. Consistency and standardization of color in medical imaging: a consensus report. J Digit Imaging. 2015;28:41–52.
7. Abel JT, Ouillette P, Williams CL, Blau J, Cheng J, Yao K, Lee WY, Cornish TC, Balis UGJ, McClintock DS. Display characteristics and their impact on digital pathology: a current review of pathologists' future "microscope". J Pathol Inform. 2020;11:23.
8. Elsayed M, Kadom N, Ghobadi C, Strauss B, Al Dandan O, Aggarwal A, Anzai Y, Griffith B, Lazarow F, Straus CM, Safdar NM. Virtual and augmented reality: potential applications in radiology. Acta Radiol. 2020;61(9):1258–65. https://doi.org/10.1177/0284185119897362.
9. Uppot RN, Laguna B, McCarthy CJ, De Novi G, Phelps A, Siegel E, Courtier J. Implementing virtual and augmented reality tools for radiology education and training, communication and clinical care. Radiology. 2019;291:570–80.
10. American Association of Physicists in Medicine. Task Group 18: assessment of display performance for medical imaging systems. https://www.aapm.org/pubs/reports/detail.asp. Last accessed 25 Aug 2020.
11. Monitor Calibration Methods. http://www.drycreekphoto.com/Learn/monitor_calibration.htm. Last accessed 7 May 2008.
12. American College of Radiology Practice Guideline for Digital Radiography. https://www.google.com/url?sa=t&rct=j&q=&esrc=s&source=web&cd=&ved=2ahUKEwjQi9jUnbfrAhXodN8KHY2gCdQQFjAAegQIARAB&url=https%3A%2F%2Fwww.acr.org%2F-%2Fmedia%2FACR%2FFiles%2FPractice-Parameters%2FRad-Digital.pdf&usg=AOvVaw0_I3Pp50hchLkpWHicxLMr. Last accessed 25 Aug 2020.
13. Dikici E, Bigelow M, Prevedello LM, White RD, Erdal BS. Integrating AI into radiology workflow: levels of research, production, and feedback maturity. J Med Imaging. 2020;7:016502.
14. Kotter E, Ranschaert E. Challenges and solutions for introducing artificial intelligence (AI) into daily clinical workflow. Eur Radiol. 2021;31:5–7. https://doi.org/10.1007/s00330-020-07148-2.
15. Jacobson FL. Medical image perception research in the emerging age of artificial intelligence. Radiology. 2020;294:210–1.

16. Seidel RL, Krupinski EA. Optimizing ergonomics in breast imaging. J Breast Imaging. 2019;1:234–8.
17. Degnan AJ, Ghobadi EH, Hardy P, Krupinski E, Scali EP, Stratchko L, Ulano A, Walker E, Wasnik AP, Auffermann WF. Perceptual and interpretative error in diagnostic radiology – causes and potential solutions. Acad Radiol. 2019;26:833–45.
18. Texeira PAG, Leplat C, Lombard C, Rauch A, Germain E, Waled AA, Jendoubi S, Bonarelli C, Padoin P, Simon L, Gillet R, Blum A, Nancy Radiology Ergonomics Group. Alternative PACS interface devices are well-accepted and may reduce radiologist's musculoskeletal discomfort as compared to keyboard-mouse-recording device. Eur Radiol. 2020;30:5200–8.
19. Grigorian A, Fang P, Kirk T, Efendizade A, Jadidi J, Sighary M, Cohen-Addad DI. Learning from gamers: integrating alternative input devices and AutoHotkey scripts to simplify repetitive tasks and improve workflow. Radiographics. 2020;40:141–50.
20. Taylor-Phillips S, Stinton C. Fatigue in radiology: a fertile area for future research. Br J Radiol. 2019;92:20190043.
21. Zhan H, Schartz K, Zygmont ME, Johnson JO, Krupinski EA. The impact of fatigue on complex CT case interpretation by radiology references. Acad Radiol. 2021;28(3):424–32. https://doi.org/10.1016/j.acra.2020.06.005.
22. Stec N, Arje D, Moody AR, Krupinski EA, Tyrell PN. A systematic review of fatigue in radiology: is it a problem? Am J Roentgenol. 2018;210:799–806.
23. Hanna TN, Zygmont ME, Peterson R, Theriot D, Shekhani H, Johnson JO, Krupinski EA. The effects of fatigue from overnight shifts on radiology search patterns and diagnostic performance. J Am Coll Radiol. 2018;15:1709–16.
24. Waite S, Kolla S, Jeudy J, Legasto A, Macknik SL, Martinez-Conde S, Krupinski EA, Reede DL. Tired in the reading room: the influence of fatigue in radiology. J Am Coll Radiol. 2017;14:191–7.
25. Nihashi T, Ishigaki T, Satake H, Ito S, Kaii O, Mori Y, Shimamoto K, Fukushima H, Suzuki K, Umakoshi H, Ohashi M, Kawaguchi F, Naganawa S. Monitoring of fatigue in radiologists during prolonged image interpretation using fNIRS. Jpn J Radiol. 2019;37:437–48.
26. Krupinski EA, Berbaum KS, Caldwell RT, Schartz KM, Kim J. Long radiology workdays reduce detection and accommodation accuracy. J Am Coll Radiol. 2010;7:698–704.
27. Krupinski EA, Berbaum KS. Measurement of visual strain in radiologists. Acad Radiol. 2009;16:947–50.
28. Krupinski EA, Berbaum KS, Schartz KM, Caldwell RT, Madsen MT. The impact of fatigue on satisfaction of search in chest radiography. Acad Radiol. 2017;24:1058–63.
29. Krupinski EA, Berbaum KS, Caldwell RT, Schartz KM, Madsen MT, Kramer DJ. Do long radiology workdays affect nodule detection in dunamic CT interpretation? J Am Coll Radiol. 2012;9:191–8.
30. Krupinski EA, Schartz KM, van Tassell MS, Madsen MT, Caldwell RT, Berbaum KS. Effect of fatigue on reading computed tomography examination of the multiply injured patient. J Med Imaging. 2017;4:035504.
31. US Food and Drug Administration. Radiation-emitting products: frequently asked questions about MQSA. https://www.fda.gov/radiation-emitting-products/consumer-information-mqsa/frequently-asked-questions-about-mqsa.
32. US Food and Drug Administration. Mammography facility surveys, mammography equipment evaluations, and medical physicist qualification requirements under MQSA. Guidance document. Docket FDA-2009-D-0448. 13 Sept 2005.
33. US Food and Drug Administration. Display devices for diagnostic radiology – guidance for industry and Food and Drug Administration staff. 2 Oct 2017. https://www.fda.gov/media/95527/download.
34. Krupinski EA, Morgan MB, Siegel EL. ACR–AAPM–SIIM practice parameter for determinants of image quality in digital mammography.
35. Strudley CJ, Young KC, Warren LM. The role of imaging in screening special feature: full paper. Mammography cancer detection: comparison of single 8MP and pair of 5MP reporting monitors. Br J Radiol. 2018;91:20170246.

36. Krupinski EA. Diagnostic accuracy and visual search efficiency: single 8 MP vs. dual 5 MP displays. J Digit Imaging. 2017;30(2):144–7.
37. Yabuuchi H, Kawanami S, Kamitani T, Matsumura T, Yamasaki Y, Morishita J, Honda H. Detectability of BI-RADS category 3 or higher breast lesions and reading time on mammography: comparison between 5-MP and 8-MP LCD monitors. Acta Radiol. 2017;58(4):403–7.
38. Pisano ED, Gatsonis C, Hendrick E, Yaffe M, Baum JK, Acharyya S, Conant EF, Fajardo LL, Bassett L, D'Orsi C, Jong R. Diagnostic performance of digital versus film mammography for breast-cancer screening. N Engl J Med. 2005;353(17):1773–83.
39. Blume H. CRT-based display systems in radiology. In: SID symposium digest of technical papers, vol. 30, No. 1. Oxford: Blackwell Publishing Ltd; 1999. p. 968–71.
40. Bevins N, Flynn M, Silosky M, Marsh R, Walz-Flannigan A, Badano A. AAPM report 270: display quality assurance. American Association of Physicists in Medicine; 2019.

Self-Assessment Questions

1. Lossy data compression does all but which of the following?

   (a) Allows for storage of more data compared to no compression
   (b) Loses data once the images have been compressed and uncompressed
   (c) Slows down transmission of image data over networks
   (d) Allows for reconstruction of exact original data as before compression without loss of information

2. Three of the key visual properties important for the interpretation of medical images are:

   (a) Contrast resolution, spatial resolution, and the color of the eyes
   (b) Night vision, contrast resolution, and spatial resolution
   (c) Color vision, spatial resolution, and blink rate
   (d) Spatial resolution, contrast resolution, and color vision

3. Display pixel size is a more accurate measure of display resolution and should be what size?

   (a) 50 microns
   (b) 100 microns
   (c) 200 microns
   (d) 300 microns

4. Monochrome displays for diagnostic viewing and interpretation of images should be calibrated to what standard?

   (a) DICOM grayscale standard display function
   (b) HDTV display standards
   (c) SMPTE display standard

5. Ambient room lights should be indirect or backlight and set to what level?

   (a) Turned off completely
   (b) 40–60 lux
   (c) 20–40 lux
   (d) 0–20 lux

6. Small matrix (1 or 2 MP) is appropriate for all of the following types of images except what kind?

    (a) CT
    (b) Digital mammography
    (c) MRI
    (d) Ultrasound

7. Contrast sensitivity peaks in the mid-spatial frequency range around 3–5 cycles/degree and is important for what aspect of image viewing?

    (a) Distinguishing between objects and background in an image
    (b) Measuring the size of an abnormality
    (c) Distinguishing blue-stained cells in a pathology slide from red-stained cells
    (d) Detecting fine features in an image

8. The ratio of maximum to minimum luminance of a display should be at least:

    (a) 25
    (b) 50
    (c) 75

9. Full dark adaptation takes about how long?

    (a) 0–10 minutes
    (b) 10–20 minutes
    (c) 20–30 minutes
    (d) 30–40 minutes

10. What types of displays are most appropriate for diagnostic interpretation?

    (a) VR
    (b) AR
    (c) COTS
    (d) MG

11. For mammography displays, maximum luminance (Lmax) should be at least what value?

    (a) 300 cd/m²
    (b) 450 cd/m²
    (c) 1000 cd/m²
    (d) 2500 cd/m²

12. Which of the following is *required* of displays used for primary interpretation of mammography, according to the Mammography Quality Standards Act (MQSA)?

    (a) Have a minimum pixel pitch of 200 μm (3-MP spatial resolution).
    (b) Display must be FDA-approved for digital mammography and tomosynthesis.
    (c) Only monochrome displays are permissible.
    (d) All of the above are correct.
    (e) None of the above are correct.

13. The display technical factor relating to digital breast tomosynthesis image scrolling on an LCD monitor which of the following?

    (a) Response rate
    (b) Refresh rate
    (c) Restore rate
    (d) Replace rate

14. Which of the following is true with respect to mammography displays?

    (a) The resolution of modern digital detectors now approaches that of traditional screen-film.
    (b) Reading on a 5+ MP versus a 3-MP display enables full-screen image viewing at native 1:1 resolution without the need for zoom/pan.
    (c) Digital mammography has been shown to be more accurate than traditional screen-film mammography for detection of breast cancer in women with dense breast tissue.
    (d) A color display is required for interpretation of digital tomosynthesis.

Chapter 18
Reporting and Dictation

Woojin Kim

Contents

18.1 Introduction

- The radiology report is the radiologist's primary work product that communicates imaging findings, interpretations, and recommendations. Therefore, abnormalities in the radiology reports need to be conveyed in both interpretable and actionable manners.

W. Kim (✉)
VA Palo Alto, Palo Alto, CA, USA

© The Author(s), under exclusive license to Springer Science+Business Media, LLC, part of Springer Nature 2021
B. F. Branstetter IV (ed.), *Practical Imaging Informatics*,
https://doi.org/10.1007/978-1-0716-1756-4_18

- While radiology reports have traditionally been in prose format, there have been increasing efforts toward using **structured reporting**. The structured reporting is a part of a more considerable effort to promote greater standardization within radiology, including standard **lexicons**, such as RadLex.
- In addition to interpretations, radiology reports often communicate urgent findings and recommendations.
- Radiology has been one of the early adopters of **speech recognition** technology in medicine, and many radiologists use speech recognition to generate their reports today.

DEFINITION: Structured Reporting

While there is no set definition for this term, there are three attributes structured reporting can have: uniform **format**, consistent **organization**, and standard **terminology** [10].

DEFINITION: Lexicon

A lexicon is a common vocabulary to standardize and enhance communication and potentially reduce healthcare-related communication errors.

DEFINITION: Speech Recognition

Machine or software's ability to identify and convert spoken language into text.

SYNONYMS: Speech Recognition

Automatic speech recognition
Computer speech recognition
Speech-to-text

18.2 Structured Reporting

- Although the term structured reporting is commonly used in radiology, there is no set, agreed-upon definition of the term. Instead, it is used to describe various reporting techniques.
- Many have promoted structured reporting over free-text, prose-style reporting, but it is not without issues. Implementation of structured reporting is complex, with potentially a significant impact on

FURTHER READING: Radiology Reports

Langlotz CP. The radiology report: a guide to thoughtful communication for radiologists and other medical professionals. San Bernardino: CreateSpace Independent Publishing Platform; 2015.

radiologists' workflow. Hence, its implementation and use should be carefully planned and should involve all affected parties. Wider adoption of structured reporting depends on both the radiologists and vendors.

- As there is no uniformly accepted definition of the term "structure reporting," we will use the three distinct attributes described by Langlotz, format, organization, and terminology:

  - **Format** refers to the visual layout of the radiology report. A consistent format is necessary for ease of consumption by people and computers. For example, are the section headers in all capital letters so that they stand out? (Remember that you cannot use bold or font size in most electronic medical record systems.)

    > **DEFINITION: Template**
    >
    > A formatted report outline in which blanks can be filled in with pertinent information. Templates are helpful to maintain strict organization in reports. Templates may be pre-populated or may have blanks where the content is added.

  - Standard ordering of information enhances the comprehension of what you want to convey. The report's consistent **organization** includes dividing the report text into sections with headings (e.g., "IMPRESSION:"), which most radiolo-

    > **FURTHER READING: Terminology**
    >
    > The Radiological Society of North America has created an ontology called RadLex for use in radiology reports (http://www.radlex.org).

    gists already do. But organization also refers to a consistent organization of the imaging observations within the text (e.g., the liver is always discussed first, then the gallbladder, then...). Some have described this as itemized reporting, which can be created using conventional dictation, speech recognition, or point-and-click interfaces. Standard reporting templates can aid in this process and ensure each report is consistently organized. However, this level of organizing reports has created controversy among radiologists and is not universally accepted.

  - The third attribute of structured reporting is the use of **standard terminology**:

    > Two radiologists can report the same findings and interpretations using very different wording (e.g., a focal area within the lung filled with fluid may be called an "opacity", "infiltrate", or "consolidation" – although they **sound** like precise terms,

    > **DEFINITION: Structured Data Elements**
    >
    > In the context of structured reporting, SDE are tags or labels applied to the words in a report that cannot be seen when you read the report but are helpful for data mining or other computer applications.

    these words mean different things to different people).

Likewise, two referring providers can interpret the same report differently.

Standard terminology appears most reliably in mammography reporting.

- Some people view a report with section headings as a structured report, while many will not use that term until formal itemized reporting is used. Some will go further, using the terms **itemized** or **template reporting**, and reserve the term structured reporting for reports with structured data elements stored in the backend that also utilize standard terminology.

18.2.1 Advantages of Structured Reporting

- Referring physicians prefer a structured reporting format over the free-text format.
- Improved readability, especially when making comparisons to prior reports.
- Improved visibility of critical/urgent findings.
- Improved tumor localization and staging assessment.
- Improved surgical planning.
- Reduced omission of pertinent information to allow for higher completeness of reports.
- The American College of Radiology (ACR) provides guidelines on a radiology report's components, such as relevant clinical information, procedures and materials, findings, potential limitations, clinical issues, comparison studies and reports, and impression including follow-up recommendations, which can be satisfied through the usage of a structured report template.
- The templates utilized in structured reporting can serve as a checklist for the radiology trainees.
- Guideline-based decision trees used in some structured reporting solutions can aid in greater completeness, particularly complex pathology descriptions.
- Potential for standardization in report formats and increased use of standard lexicons.
- Potential benefits not commonly utilized:
  1. Automate functions (e.g., tumor, node, metastasis (TNM) staging).
  2. Integrate with other data sources (e.g., radiomics, laboratory results).
  3. Share data with external entities (e.g., registries).
  4. Perform data mining for research, education, quality improvement, and operational enhancements.
  5. Generate quality metrics, including those needed for meeting requirements like the Merit-based Incentive Payment System (MIPS), which can have financial consequences.
  6. Train artificial intelligence algorithms. The reports generated by radiologists can be used as the reference standard for AI training.

DEFINITION: Turnaround Time

In radiology, TAT often refers to the time between completing a study and when the final report is signed. However, the start time and end time can vary depending on the person and situation. Hence, it is essential to clarify both the start time and end time when TAT is used.

- Reduced grammatical and nongrammatical errors.
- Potential for improved **turnaround times**.

18.2.2 Disadvantages of Structured Reporting

- Elevated risk of distraction from increased time looking at the reporting solution screen instead of the images. This may decrease interpreting accuracy.
- Increased reporting times from cumbersome decision trees, especially in point-and-click solutions.
- Saying normal phrases can help the radiologist to ensure that all elements of the scan are interpreted.
- Templates may lead to constrained thinking, in which diagnoses not listed in the template are ignored.
- Obscure findings that require more in-depth action may be overlooked to avoid the added burden of documentation.
- Uniformity of reports leading to commoditization of radiology.
- Oversimplification of reports by using report templates that can limit consolidating associated findings to synthesize an overall impression due to predefined formats within the report templates.

18.2.3 Recommendations

- When it comes to defining the structured reports' content and organization, they should match the clinical requests and circumstances and be concise while containing all the required elements. For example, when describing pancreatic cancer, the radiology report needs to document findings relevant to surgical planning, such as a detailed extent of the lesion's vascular involvement.

INTERNATIONAL CONSIDERATIONS

The European Society of Radiology (ESR) has outlined additional challenges in designing structured reporting, such as categorizing medical procedures and clinical situations, deciding which authority body to define structured reports, considering intellectual properties, and incorporating appropriate imaging biomarkers.

- When available, standardized reporting criteria, such as the TNM staging systems, should be used.
- Data formats
  - Management of Radiology Report Templates (MRRT) is the IHE integration profile dedicated to reporting templates.
  - Common Data Elements (CDEs) specify a data entity's name, data type, and allowed values.
  - DICOM introduced structured reporting with its Supplement 23 Structured Reporting Object.
- Protocols
  - MRRT uses Hypertext Transfer Protocol (HTTP).
  - DICOM Structured Reporting uses traditional DICOM messaging as well as DICOMweb.
- The RSNA, in conjunction with the ESR, has developed a free online library of reporting templates with CDEs at radreport.org. Each template has been designed utilizing appropriate terminology (e.g., RadLex) and is based on best practices and established technical standards:
  - Many of the **RadReport** templates are currently based on the IHE MRRT profile and were converted from the Extensible Markup Language (XML) format, encoded using the Regular Language for XML Next Generation (RELAX NG):
      The format of the templates used an extension of HTML5.
      MRRT profile defines the transportation mechanism to query, retrieve, and store templates [9].
  - The Template Library Advisory Panel is a joint committee of the ESR and RSNA to provide expertise in developing these templates and to review submitted templates.
- Integration into the existing workflow is essential:
  - Structured reporting solutions should be incorporated in a speech-driven workflow as many radiologists use speech recognition to generate their reports.
  - Templates should be linked to the study codes so that the appropriate template can automatically appear at the start of dictation.
  - Reporting solutions should integrate with external data sources so that specific fields within the report template can be automatically populated, which can reduce errors, improve efficiency, and ensure complete documentation:
      Clinical indication can be automatically inserted from the computerized physician order entry (CPOE) data, EMR, or RIS.

> **FURTHER READING: TNM**
>
> TNM is a classification system used for staging the extent of cancer. https://www.cancer.gov/about-cancer/diagnosis-staging/staging.

> **DEFINITION: RadElement Common Data Elements**
>
> RadElement CDEs are standardized sets of questions and allowable answers in radiology [19]. For example, for a lung nodule, a query may be "nodule diameter," which has an ID of RDE607, with the answer being a numerical value in mm unit with a step value of 0.1. CDEs can enhance radiology reporting, data analysis, research, and decision support and improve data exchange [25].

The imaging technique field can be automatically populated based on the imaging study performed and contrast type and dose.

Medication information can be automatically imported from the EMR.

Measurements from ultrasound scans, dual-energy X-ray absorptiometry (DXA) scans, or AI applications can be populated within the appropriate fields.

Radiation dose estimates (which is a reporting requirement in certain states in the United States) can be incorporated to save time and enhance compliance.

OUR EXPERIENCE

Reporting automation can dramatically affect radiologists' efficiency. At the University of Pennsylvania, we automated reporting of DXA studies, which significantly reduced the reporting time and error rates. By automatically incorporating ultrasound measurements, Dr. Steven Horii reduced the time to generate first-trimester US reports by 40% and second-trimester reports by 30%.

18.2.4 Implementation Strategies

- Respect current radiologists' workflow, including speech-driven reporting.
- Radiologists need to understand the benefits and added value of structured reporting so that they have buy-in.
- Incorporate radiologists and referring providers' input when designing the report templates, as often the main challenge is not technical but sociologic.
- Take baby steps – start with standard report headings and then move on to standard report templates (ideally utilizing RadLex and based on RadReport templates).
- Consider a pilot introduction of the above steps to gain experience and adoption before broader implementation. Training will be an essential component as modern reporting solutions offer shortcuts, workarounds, and several advanced options.
- Find superusers and early adopters who can assist with change management and encourage their colleagues (see **Chap. 26**). Trainees are often best at this.
- Provide flexibility with the template elements for individual users.
- Consider templates with areas for free-text input.
- Make compliance with structured reporting a part of internal quality audits.
- A point-and-click option may be beneficial in certain situations. However, extra considerations and efforts are needed to ensure it fits the radiologist workflow.
- The structured report format can be garbled after the reports are transmitted through various interfaces. Hence, it is important to review the reports' format from the referring providers' view and make necessary adjustments and modifications.
- Certain types of reports (e.g., renal ultrasound, mammography) are more amenable to structured reporting. Implement in these areas first.

INTERNATIONAL CONSIDERATIONS

Adoption of ontologies outside of the United States is even more challenging, as regional linguistic differences in the use of English can complicate agreement on how terms are used. Extending these principles to other languages requires substantial additional work.

18.3 Lexicons, Coding Systems, and Ontologies

Examples of current lexicons, coding systems, and ontologies in medicine:

- Current Procedural Terminology (CPT, American Medical Association) – code set that describes medical, surgical, and diagnostic services [2].

DEFINITION: Ontology

In computer science and information science, an ontology is a set of concepts and the relationships between those concepts for a particular subject. For example, RadLex is an ontology focused on the subject of radiology.

- Foundational Model of Anatomy Ontology (FMA; Structural Informatics Group, University of Washington) – an ontology for human anatomy [27].
- International Classification of Diseases (ICD; World Health Organization (WHO)) – diagnostic classification standard for clinical and research purposes. It is currently in its tenth revision, hence ICD-10 [31].
- Logical Observation Identifiers Names and Codes (LOINC) standard for identifying medical laboratory observations [12].
- SNOMED CT (SNOMED International) – covers diagnosis, clinical findings, diagnostic procedures, observables, body structures, organisms, substances, pharmaceutical products, physical objects, physical forces, and specimens [26].

KEY CONCEPT: Lexicon Versus Ontology

A lexicon is vocabulary, but an ontology is something more – it is a set of concepts and the relationships between those concepts.

- Unified Medical Language System (UMLS; National Library of Medicine) is a set of files and software that provides mapping and enhanced interoperability among various health and biomedical vocabularies that can be used by the developers in the medical informatics space [28].

18.3.1 ACR Reporting and Data Systems

- The **Breast Imaging Reporting and Data System (BI-RADS)** has become the standard way of reporting breast imaging findings:
  - Provides a set of clearly defined terms for breast imaging with accompanying atlas, and its final assessment categories provide actionable conclusions.

- BI-RADS was the first successful approach to standardize the process of radiology communication.
- Modeled after BI-RADS, the ACR Reporting and Data Systems (RADS) have created additional standardized frameworks for reporting imaging findings in other areas of radiology:
  - C-RADS (CT colonography)
  - CAD-RADS (coronary artery disease)
  - HI-RADS (head injury)
  - LI-RADS (liver)
  - Lung-RADS
  - NI-RADS (head and neck)
  - O-RADS (ovarian-adnexal)
  - PI-RADS (prostate)
  - TI-RADS (thyroid) [4]

18.3.2 RadLex [21]

- A **controlled terminology** for radiology designed to meet the need for standard terminology to:
  - Improve the clarity of radiology reports.
  - Standardize key elements of the radiology reports.
  - Reduce radiologist variation.
  - Enable access to imaging information.
  - Link report information to the EMR.
  - Provide data collection and analysis in imaging research.
  - Retrieve data from teaching files and research repositories.
  - Improve the quality of practice.
- Often it has two concept or term types, called *preferred name and synonyms*. There are additional attributes, such as *RadLex ID, definition*, and ontological relationships.
- Provides the foundation for the LOINC/RSNA Radiology Playbook, RadElement Common Data Elements, and RadReport radiology report templates.
- RadLex Term Browser is available online with also information on additional access methods [22].
- Designed for use in software applications, such as structured reporting, coded radiology teaching files, data registries, and decision support [10, 24].
- Available for free for commercial and noncommercial uses.

18.3.3 LOINC/RSNA Radiology Playbook

LOINC/RSNA Radiology Playbook provides a standard system for naming radiology procedures, using elements like modality and body part [20].

18.3.4 RadElement Common Data Elements

RadElement CDEs are standardized sets of questions and allowable answers in radiology [19].

18.4 Communications

- Radiology reports communicate findings and recommendations to referring providers and patients. Therefore, effective and timely communication is essential. In addition to preliminary and final reports, there may be needs for **nonroutine communications**.
- Failure to communicate results of a radiologic study is a commonly cited cause of medical malpractice.

18.4.1 Radiology Reports and Patients

- The radiology reports have been traditionally designed to communicate with the referring physicians. However, with increasing access by the patients to their radiology reports through online patient portals, patient interactions have become an essential consideration with increasing attention placed on the interpretability of the reports by the patients.
- Various deficiencies in the patient portal's radiology section have been documented, including the need for patient-friendly radiology reports that are often not met due to insufficient time and staffing [1].
- Embedding radiologist contact information with the radiology reports can enhance radiologist visibility to the patients but may be opposed by radiologists who fear being overwhelmed by patient discussions.
- Several patient-centered methods have been proposed to enhance the interpretation of radiology reports [10, 14, 16]:
  - Use standardized language.
  - Avoid abbreviations.
  - Quantify the level of diagnostic certainty using percentages.
  - Provide the radiologists with feedback about their reports.
  - Incorporate hypertext linking text elements to supplemental information.
- Despite the possibility of miscommunication through the text reports, direct communication to the patients from the radiologists is a controversial topic. Many referring physicians do not favor direct contact by the radiologists. They are concerned that it may lead to patient confusion, increased patient anxiety, and a loss of the referring physician-patient relationship. However, other studies have shown that patients desire improved turnaround time and expertise through direct communication with the radiologists [7].

- When dealing with self-referred patients, the responsibility for communicating results, including appropriate follow-ups, falls on the radiologists. Similar duties may also apply when dealing with third-party referred patients.

18.4.2 Critical Results and Actionable Findings

- According to the ACR Practice Parameter for Communication of Diagnostic Imaging Findings, three situations warrant nonroutine communication to the referring provider or the provider's designee with the option of conveying the results directly to the patients if the referring provider cannot be contacted:
  1. Findings that require immediate or urgent intervention.
  2. Findings that have clinically significant discrepancies with a prior interpretation of the same imaging study.
  3. Nonurgent findings that can have serious adverse effects if not addressed [3].
- According to the ACR, these nonroutine communications should be documented, ideally in the radiology report or the patient's medical record. When documenting, the following should be included, along with the finding:
  - Time
  - Method of communication
  - Name of the person to whom the communication was delivered to [3]
- Communication by telephone or in-person is preferred. Other forms of communication that provide documentation of receipt may also suffice. Regardless of the methods used, one must comply with appropriate privacy requirements, such as HIPAA [3].
- Every medical imaging department should establish a policy on communication following best-practice guidelines [3].
- The ACR formed the Actionable Reporting Work Group to address IT's role in the communication of imaging findings. They classified all findings that require nonroutine communication as **actionable findings (AF)**. Different authors and institutions have used various approaches to categorize the level of urgency. The Actionable Reporting Work Group used categories 1, 2, and 3 for findings that require communication within minutes, hours, and days, respectively. Category 3 findings are often referred to as "incidental" or "unexpected."

> **DEFINITION: Actionable Finding**
>
> Any imaging finding that requires nonroutine communication to the ordering physician or patient. This includes urgent findings that might immediately affect patient care and also nonurgent findings that might slip through the cracks. Personal phone conversation is the preferred mode of communication. This task must be documented in the report.

- IT has a different role for each category of urgency.
  - Category 1:
    Identify and locate the referring provider.

Remind the radiologist when AF is present within the report text to ensure the site's communication policy is followed.

Facilitate documentation of communication within the radiology report.

Keep a record of the documentation.

Assist with the auditing needs.

- Category 2:

In addition to all of the above, acknowledge receipt of the report (as these findings may not be directly verbally communicated).

- Category 3:

In addition to all of the above, flag reports with AF

Assist with follow-up management

Facilitate the scheduling of follow-up studies and procedures with reminders.

- Additional requirements:

The system should be customizable based on local preferences and needs.

Fit into the radiologists' workflow [11].

- A software solution designed to handle critical result reporting and management is called **Critical Test Results Management** (CTRM), also known as Critical Test Results Reporting and Closed-Loop Reporting [30]. For example, when a radiologist encounters a finding that is considered an AF, the communication can be triggered, which will send information about the AF to the referring provider via text messaging, secure email, pager, or voice mail with a predetermined escalation process. Upon opening the message, the software will record the confirmation of receipt. The software also manages the audit trails and record-keeping. One of the main challenges with CTRM to keep in mind is maintaining the referring contact information up to date.

- There are **natural language processing** applications that detect AF within the report text and determine whether communication has been documented.

> **DEFINITION: Critical Test Results Management**
>
> Software and processes to ensure that important radiologic results are properly communicated and do not slip through the cracks.

> **SYNONYMS: CTRM**
>
> - Critical Test Results Management
> - Critical Test Results Reporting
> - Closed-Loop Reporting

> **INTERNATIONAL CONSIDERATIONS**
>
> The ESR states that timely communication of urgent incidental findings is the shared responsibility of the institution and the radiologist, and that institutions should support all initiatives that improve the timely communication of imaging findings and prompt action on the part of referrers. Radiologists must ensure that they have robust protocols to transmit reports in a timely, reliable, and consistent way.
>
> https://www.ncbi.nlm.nih.gov/pmc/articles/PMC3292650/
>
> https://www.researchgate.net/publication/319400728_Report_Communication_Standards

18.5 Speech Recognition

18.5.1 How Does Speech Recognition Work?

- Early speech recognition systems have been replaced by probabilistic methods like the hidden Markov model (HMM), including hybrid models that use HMM with deep neural network (DNN) [15].
- Speech recognition is a very complex area in computer science. The following is a significantly simplified explanation of how speech recognition works:
  1. An analog-to-digital converter (ADC) converts analog sound waves to digital data.
  2. An ADC signal is divided into tiny parts, and the speech recognition engine matches them to **phonemes**.
  3. Two mathematical models analyze the sound information. The **acoustic model** deals with the probability of a word given the sounds (e.g., phonemes). The **language model** uses previous words to estimate the probability of a word (e.g., a trigram language model uses the previous two words to estimate the probability of the third word) [10].

KEY CONCEPT: VR Versus SR

Some people use the term voice recognition interchangeably with speech recognition. However, it should be noted that voice recognition refers to identifying a speaker based on idiosyncrasies in voice patterns, whereas speech recognition refers to identifying words and phrases. Voice recognition can be used as a security biometric (e.g., saying "my voice is my password" to access your bank account over the phone).

DEFINITION: Phoneme

A phoneme is a basic block of sound that makes up words. English has about 42 phonemes (different opinions exist on the exact number). For example, the word, "speech," has four phonemes: /s/p/E/ch/ [8].

18.5.2 Advantages of Speech Recognition

- Decreased turnaround times, often by more than 90% [5].
- Speech recognition can be used to navigate within different fields of a structured report template. Also, verbal commands can operate other functionalities within the reporting software (e.g., "sign off report").
- Shorter reports.
- Cost-effectiveness (possibly). Costs are lower if transcriptionists are replaced. However, there may be increased costs from increased editing time by physicians who are paid higher than transcriptionists.

18.5.3 Disadvantages of Speech Recognition

- Decreased productivity with increased time spent on document creation, dictation, and especially correction [5]
- Increased error rates:
  - Three types of errors often cited are substitution, deletion, and insertion.
  - Error rates range from 4.8% to 38% for self-edited speech recognition-generated reports. These errors can be reduced with secondary review by a transcriptionist (correctionist model) or with self-correction [32].
  - Native language and accent can affect error rates.

18.5.4 Speech Recognition Errors and Possible Remedies

- Many radiologists underestimate their own error rates [18].
- Although radiologists are familiar with speech recognition errors, they must be reminded to emphasize manual revision and editing.
- Train the speech engine so that it is tailored to the individual user's voice and speech pattern.
- Initiate and maintain quality control with regular report audits.
- Use **macros and templates**.
- Incorporate automation, such as filling of specific structured report fields from external data sources, whenever possible.
- Apply automatic mandatory spellchecks.
- Incorporate advanced technology like NLP-based tools to detect and correct errors, including wrong laterality and gender-related discrepancies.
- Test efficacy regularly, especially after any substantial changes.

> **DEFINITION: Macro**
>
> In the setting of speech recognition, a macro is a short phrase that represents a more complex set of keystrokes, text, or actions. The dictator speaks the macro and the report automatically populates with a large amount of text. This text may have blanks built in that need to be filled.

> **KEY CONCEPT: Macros Versus Templates**
>
> Macros and templates are essential features of both structured reporting and speech recognition that can shorten reporting time. While many people use the terms interchangeably, a macro is a shortcut or a command that performs a preset sequence of tasks. A macro can output predefined words, phrases, paragraphs, and reports. A reporting template is a sample report that has formatting but with blanks filled either by the radiologists or data from external sources. There is overlap; for example, a macro can be used to output a report template.

- Keep up with hardware and software upgrades, but check functionality afterward! [13, 17, 23, 29]

> **VIEW TO THE FUTURE**
>
> Small words like "no" or "none" are frequently misconstrued by speech recognition software. They are also easy to overlook when manually correcting reports. Unfortunately, these words can make a sentence mean the opposite of the intended meaning. Artificial intelligence vendors are attempting to combine image analysis with natural language processing to detect subtle omissions or inaccuracies in radiologists' reports.

18.5.5 Implementation

- Choose the best speech recognition model for your institution:
  - **Self-edit mode** will achieve better TAT and cost savings.
  - **Transcriptionist mode** is more acceptable to radiologists who struggle with accuracy. It is more expensive.
  - Some sites use a hybrid model, allowing radiologists to choose between the two modes.
- Assess speech engine accuracy, keeping in mind the limitations of short-term evaluation
- Ensure the language model used is specific to radiology
- Observe multiple levels of users (trainees, junior staff, senior staff) at a site visit
- Evaluate the level of integration with PACS and RIS *specifically* as it pertains to your software and setup
- Assess radiologist workflow specifically on the navigation through text while eyes are on the PACS viewer images

> **DEFINITION: Self-Edit Mode**
>
> Users dictate, edit, and sign reports without the aid of a human backend transcription. The reports can be completed one at a time or batched.

> **DEFINITION: Transcription Mode**
>
> Users dictate using speech recognition. After each report is completed, both the text and voice files are sent to a human transcriptionist, who then performs edits. The edited report with corrections is sent back to the radiologist, who then finalizes it.

> **DEFINITION: Batch Mode**
>
> A radiologist may sign each report as it is dictated or dictate several reports and sign them all in a batch.

- Ensure both initial and ongoing application support. Will you or the vendor be training new users and supporting current ones?
- Evaluate the upgrade path and roadmap of future enhancements
- Observe how dual reads, resident workflow, and addenda are handled
- Keep the speech recognition vendor engaged not only throughout the training process, but also afterward to monitor accuracy and error rates and detect individuals who may need additional training or a new speech profile.

> **DEFINITION: Addendum (*Plural*: Addenda)**
>
> Once the radiologist has finalized a radiology report, it cannot be modified, as it is a permanent part of the medical record. Any changes and/or clarifications must be appended to the end of the report as a separate section without modifying the original report.

- Problem-solving
  - Microphone:

    When asked to troubleshoot, first check that the microphone is connected correctly.

    A proper microphone position is essential. Some use headset microphones to maintain consistent positioning of the microphone and to keep the hands free. Similarly, some have used unidirectional microphones attached to the monitor or a stand for hands-free operations, especially when working from home or an individual office.

    If the handset is used for a microphone, programmable buttons can facilitate increased efficiency in navigation. However, be aware of repetitive injuries, especially to the thumb.

    Ergonomics. Consider using interface devices other than the mouse and keyboard (**note**: the modern mouse has side buttons that can be programmed to control various microphone-/handset-related functions).

    If the microphone is left on record mode while not speaking, the system will have more errors and may freeze as it tries to convert background noise into text.
  - Timing errors:

    There is often a split-second delay after a navigation command while the system responds. Users must be aware of this and time their dictation accordingly; otherwise, the system can freeze or create errors.

    Likewise, there is a split-second delay when the microphone is turned on before the system is ready to accept spoken dictation. Users who are used to speaking simultaneously with pushing the record button will find the first syllable of their opening word truncated, leading to errors.
  - Recognition:

    Some words, even for the best users, will be problematic. Try to add and train a word or phrase with the **vocabulary editor**, if available.

Make sure that users understand to use the vocabulary editor or correction command when making corrections:

- In addition to training, if the speech recognition engine's dictionary is not radiology-specific, you will need to delete irrelevant words to improve recognition.

A typed correction typically does not train the software, and thus accuracy will not improve.

If repeated attempts at correcting a single word fail, encourage users to train phrases (i.e., leverage the trigram language model) rather than individual words.

Users with heavy accents will often require more training and more use of the vocabulary editor.

Encourage users who are having recognition difficulty to take advantage of macros.

Encourage users to contact the vendor for help with words that are used frequently but are not well recognized by the software.

- Environment:

Soundproofing techniques, such as the use of carpeting/floor mats, acoustic ceiling tiles, and acoustical wall panels, are beneficial and should be considered in every reading room design.

Consider the use of a white noise generator for problem areas.

- Use of macros:
  - Using macros can shorten the reporting process.
  - Macros work particularly well in conjunction with structured reporting.
  - Alert the radiologist with a beep every time a macro has been inserted.
  - The reporting solutions often use different font colors to differentiate the macro text versus text that was typed or dictated, which allows the user to focus only on the non-macro text when looking for errors.
  - Users should be trained on how to generate and use macros. The macros can also be shared with other users and modified individually.
  - It is advisable to have system-wide standard report templates. Each site may want to find a balance between the personal and system-wide macros and templates. However, this may be difficult to achieve (even for standard templates) given the individuality of radiology reports.
- Navigation:
  - Radiologists need to navigate the speech recognition system and PACS simultaneously. A sound navigation system should allow the radiologists to control both the speech recognition system and PACS using a combination of voice commands and buttons while maintaining their eyes on the images.
  - Different users will have their own preferences, so flexibility is essential.

18.6 Interfaces and Integration

- Interoperability with EMR/RIS and PACS is essential. A *standalone reporting system* is virtually worthless in terms of department workflow and end-user efficiency.
- EMR/RIS integration:
  - A two-way interface. The accession number for a particular study is passed from the EMR/RIS to the reporting solution. The report text is passed back to the EMR/RIS for archiving and distribution.
  - Finalizing (radiologist signing) and creating an addendum of reports should be available in the reporting system, EMR/RIS, and often PACS.
  - The interface should accommodate multiuser (resident or dual read) workflow.
- PACS integration:
  - Most PACS now use an application programming interface (API). Be sure to include these costs in the project budget.

> **DEFINITION: API**
>
> An application programming interface allows software engineers from your institution to create customized software that uses functions from the vendor's software.

- Speech recognition embedded in PACS:
  - Some PACS vendors are embedding speech recognition software within their products.
- Speech recognition embedded in EMR/RIS:
  - EMR/RIS vendors are likewise offering an embedded speech engine within their product and some currently available mammography structured reporting products.
  - While this may seem like the ideal solution at first glance, EMR/RIS vendors need to offer similar functionality to the dedicated radiology reporting solutions for the product to be worthwhile. This is rarely the case, so be wary.

18.7 The Radiology Report of the Future

- Standard formatting with standard terminology to reduce confusion and variability.
- A pertinent summary of clinical history (e.g., from the EMR) is presented concisely to the radiologist and pre-populated in the report.
- Relevant prior report findings are summarized and presented.
- Automatic pre-population of report elements:
  - Lesion measurements
  - AI analysis

- Macros and CDEs increase reporting efficiency.
- NLP ensures accurate grammar and internal consistency.
- Autosuggestions promote standardized terminology.
- Reporting software provides decision support:
  - Related or similar cases
  - Online references
  - Peer-reviewed literature
  - Clinical guidelines
  - Differential diagnosis
- Advanced NLP:
  - Minimize errors within reports, such as laterality and sex
  - Ensure completeness of documentation to support billing and fulfill regulatory requirements
- Impressions can be auto-generated based on findings described by the radiologist in the radiologist's style.
- Overall global assessment codes like BI-RADS are suggested and inserted.
- The reporting software ensures evidence-based follow-up recommendations are made with appropriate imaging modality and time intervals.
- Free-text dictation is converted into structured reports, minimizing the need to navigate through blank fields within the reporting solution, thus allowing the radiologists to spend more time looking at the images.
- The report can be reformatted using AI to be tailored to the recipient (e.g., referring physician, surgeon, patient).
- The use of hyperlinks within reports can link to key images and additional information.
- The report content is parsed and stored in a structured data format that can be leveraged further for data mining and training of AI.
- Advanced analytics take advantage of the structured data elements to provide analysis of operational and clinical quality metrics.
- Past reports are rapidly searched for pertinent prior exams using an advanced search engine.
- Integrated peer review and peer learning workflows.
- The patient's EMR is populated with data elements from the report text, which can alert the referring providers of abnormal findings and recommendations or send out reminders.
- Automated participation in national registries.
- Compliance with AF notification and documentation.
- Follow-up recommendations are tracked to minimize follow-up failures.
- Feedback such as pathology-radiology correlation is communicated back to the radiologists.
- **Multimedia reports** include images, tables, and charts from the examination to support conclusions and direct referring physicians to the findings of interest [6].

A VIEW TO THE FUTURE

The radiology report of the future will leverage standard terminology and structured data backend with better interconnectivity with external systems. All relevant clinical information will be presented to the radiologist in a concise and easy-to-consume manner and appropriately pre-populated within the report. Artificial intelligence will create a preliminary report that the radiologist can confirm or edit. The reporting system will be designed to allow maximum interaction with the images and interpretation task while minimizing the words that need to be spoken, including auto-generation of impressions and recommendations. Intelligence within the system will reduce errors and comply with billing requirements while providing valuable feedback to the radiologists for continuous learning. Embedded multimedia such as hypertext links to literature and patient images also enhance the radiology report, with appropriate differential diagnoses, evidence-based guidelines, and recommendations while answering the clinical question tailored to the report's recipient.

PEARLS

- Remember to evaluate workflow functionality and not just report creation for both speech recognition and structured reporting
- Take steps to maximize user accuracy in speech recognition including microphone position and proper dictation techniques
- Plan on at least temporary productivity decreases when implementing speech recognition or structured reporting
- Introduce structured reporting slowly in stages
- Encourage the use of macros and templates in both speech recognition and structured reporting
- Ensure that actionable findings are communicated appropriately
- Become familiar with RadLex, CDEs, and other lexicons and ontologies

References

1. Alarifi M, Patrick T, Jabour A, Wu M, Luo J. Full radiology report through patient web portal: a literature review. Int J Environ Res Public Health. 2020;17(10):3673. https://doi.org/10.3390/ijerph17103673.
2. AMA. CPT®. American Medical Association. n.d. Retrieved September 5, 2020, from https://www.ama-assn.org/practice-management/cpt.
3. American College of Radiology. ACR practice parameter for communication of diagnostic imaging findings. n.d. p. 9. https://www.acr.org/-/media/ACR/Files/Practice-Parameters/CommunicationDiag.pdf.
4. American College of Radiology. Reporting and data systems. n.d. Retrieved September 5, 2020, from https://www.acr.org/Clinical-Resources/Reporting-and-Data-Systems.

5. Blackley SV, Huynh J, Wang L, Korach Z, Zhou L. Speech recognition for clinical documentation from 1990 to 2018: a systematic review. J Am Med Inform Assoc. 2019;26(4):324–38. https://doi.org/10.1093/jamia/ocy179.

6. Dunnick NR, Langlotz CP. The radiology report of the future: a summary of the 2007 intersociety conference. J Am Coll Radiol. 2008;5(5):626–9. https://doi.org/10.1016/j.jacr.2007.12.015.

7. Gunn AJ, Sahani DV, Bennett SE, Choy G. Recent measures to improve radiology reporting: perspectives from primary care physicians. J Am Coll Radiol. 2013;10(2):122–7. https://doi.org/10.1016/j.jacr.2012.08.013.

8. How to count phonemes in spoken words. n.d. http://wp.auburn.edu/rdggenie/home/lessons/phoncount/.

9. Kahn CE, Genereaux B, Langlotz CP. Conversion of radiology reporting templates to the MRRT standard. J Digit Imaging. 2015;28(5):528–36. https://doi.org/10.1007/s10278-015-9787-3.

10. Langlotz CP. The radiology report: a guide to thoughtful communication for radiologists and other medical professionals. 1st ed. San Bernardino: CreateSpace Independent Publishing Platform; 2015.

11. Larson PA, Berland LL, Griffith B, Kahn CE, Liebscher LA. Actionable findings and the role of IT support: report of the ACR Actionable Reporting Work Group. J Am Coll Radiol. 2014;11(6):552–8. https://doi.org/10.1016/j.jacr.2013.12.016.

12. LOINC. LOINC. n.d. Retrieved September 5, 2020, from https://loinc.org/.

13. Minn MJ, Zandieh AR, Filice RW. Improving radiology report quality by rapidly notifying radiologist of report errors. J Digit Imaging. 2015;28(4):492–8. https://doi.org/10.1007/s10278-015-9781-9.

14. Mityul MI, Gilcrease-Garcia B, Mangano MD, Demertzis JL, Gunn AJ. Radiology reporting: current practices and an introduction to patient-centered opportunities for improvement. Am J Roentgenol. 2018;210(2):376–85. https://doi.org/10.2214/AJR.17.18721.

15. Nassif AB, Shahin I, Attili I, Azzeh M, Shaalan K. Speech recognition using deep neural networks: a systematic review. IEEE Access. 2019;7:19143–65. https://doi.org/10.1109/ACCESS.2019.2896880.

16. Oh SC. PORTER: a prototype system for patient-oriented radiology reporting. J Digit Imaging. 2016;29(4):450–4.

17. Paulett JM, Langlotz CP. Improving language models for radiology speech recognition. J Biomed Inform. 2009;42(1):53–8. https://doi.org/10.1016/j.jbi.2008.08.001.

18. Quint LE, Quint DJ, Myles JD. Frequency and spectrum of errors in final radiology reports generated with automatic speech recognition technology. J Am Coll Radiol. 2008;5(12):1196–9. https://doi.org/10.1016/j.jacr.2008.07.005.

19. RadElement. n.d. Retrieved September 5, 2020, from https://www.radelement.org/.

20. RadLex Playbook. n.d. http://playbook.radlex.org/playbook/SearchRadlexAction.

21. RadLex Radiology Lexicon. n.d. Retrieved September 5, 2020, from https://www.rsna.org/en/practice-tools/data-tools-and-standards/radlex-radiology-lexicon.

22. RadLex Term Browser. n.d. Retrieved September 5, 2020, from http://radlex.org/.

23. Ringler MD, Goss BC, Bartholmai BJ. Syntactic and semantic errors in radiology reports associated with speech recognition software. Health Informatics J. 2017;23(1):3–13. https://doi.org/10.1177/1460458215613614.

24. Rubin DL. Creating and curating a terminology for radiology: ontology modeling and analysis. J Digit Imaging. 2008;21(4):355–62. https://doi.org/10.1007/s10278-007-9073-0.

25. Rubin DL, Kahn CE. Common data elements in radiology. Radiology. 2017;283(3):837–44.

26. SNOMED. 5-Step briefing. n.d. Retrieved September 5, 2020, from http://www.snomed.org/snomed-ct/five-step-briefing.

27. Structural Informatics Group. Foundational model of anatomy. n.d. Retrieved September 5, 2020, from http://www.si.washington.edu/projects/fma.

28. Unified Medical Language System (UMLS). [List of Links]. U.S. National Library of Medicine. n.d. Retrieved September 5, 2020, from https://www.nlm.nih.gov/research/umls/index.html.

29. Voll K, Atkins S, Forster B. Improving the utility of speech recognition through error detection. J Digit Imaging. 2008;21(4):371–7. https://doi.org/10.1007/s10278-007-9034-7.
30. Wikipedia. Critical test results management. 2019. https://en.wikipedia.org/w/index.php?title=Critical_Test_Results_Management&oldid=930955989.
31. Wikipedia. International classification of diseases. 2020. https://en.wikipedia.org/w/index.php?title=International_Classification_of_Diseases&oldid=973693987.
32. Zhou L, Blackley SV, Kowalski L, Doan R, Acker WW, Landman AB, Kontrient E, Mack D, Meteer M, Bates DW, Goss FR. Analysis of errors in dictated clinical documents assisted by speech recognition software and professional transcriptionists. JAMA Netw Open. 2018;1(3):e180530. https://doi.org/10.1001/jamanetworkopen.2018.0530.

Self-Assessment Questions

1. All of the following pertain to the use of macros and templates *except*:

   (a) Using macros can shorten the reporting process.
   (b) System-wide standard report templates can promote uniformity.
   (c) Individual radiologists should not be trained on how to generate their own macros.
   (d) Templates should be linked to the study codes so that the appropriate template can automatically appear at the start of dictation.

2. When troubleshooting a radiologist complaining of poor accuracy in speech recognition, you should do everything *except*:

   (a) Check that the microphone is connected correctly.
   (b) Encourage the radiologist to make typed corrections.
   (c) Discourage the user from speaking and pushing the record button simultaneously.
   (d) Encourage consistent positioning of the microphone.

3. Which of the following provides a standard system for naming radiology procedures, using elements like modality and body part?

   (a) RadElement Common Data Elements
   (b) LOINC/RSNA Radiology Playbook
   (c) ICD-10
   (d) FMA

4. All of the following is true of RadLex *except*:

   (a) Is a controlled terminology for radiology designed to meet the need for standard terminology
   (b) Often has two concept or term types, called preferred name and synonyms
   (c) There is a licensing fee for commercial uses
   (d) Is designed for use in software applications

5. RadElement Common Data Elements:
   - (a) Specify a data entity's name, data type, and allowed values
   - (b) Is a set of commonly used critical results
   - (c) Contains complete, best-practice reporting templates
   - (d) Found universally in every radiology report

6. Which of the following represents the standard way of reporting breast imaging findings?
   - (a) LI-RADS
   - (b) PI-RADS
   - (c) BI-RADS
   - (d) TI-RADS

7. Langlotz described all of the following attributes of structured reporting *except*:
   - (a) Standard terminology
   - (b) Uniform format
   - (c) Consistent organization
   - (d) Variable voice pattern

Chapter 19
User Governance

Christopher J. Roth

Contents

19.1 Introduction

Hospitals set missions and strategic plans and must invest large capital and operational sums in information technology, data management, and associated staffing to achieve those ends. Faced with hospital risk-sharing payer arrangements and a keen focus on cost-effective, high-quality care, hospitals must pressure their hospital information technology budgets to decrease expenditures. A primary intent of enterprise imaging governance is to ensure high-value investment and health returns by aligning imaging operations with the institutional mission, strategic plan, and adhering to best practices and statutory or regulatory requirements.

C. J. Roth (✉)
Department of Radiology, Duke University, Durham, NC, USA

Duke Health, Durham, NC, USA
e-mail: Christopher.roth@duke.edu

© The Author(s), under exclusive license to Springer Science+Business Media, LLC, part of Springer Nature 2021
B. F. Branstetter IV (ed.), *Practical Imaging Informatics*,
https://doi.org/10.1007/978-1-0716-1756-4_19

There are numerous definitions of "governance" as it relates to IT:

- According to CIO.com, IT governance is "…a formal way to align IT strategy with business strategy."[1]

- According to Gartner, IT governance is defined as "the processes that ensure the effective and efficient use of IT in enabling an organization to achieve its goals. IT demand governance (what IT should work on) is the process by which organizations ensure the effective evaluation, selection, prioritization, and funding of competing IT investments; oversee their implementation; and extract (measurable) business benefits. IT demand governance is a business investment decision-making and oversight process, and it is a business management responsibility. IT supply-side governance (how IT should do what it does) is concerned with ensuring that the IT organization operates in an effective, efficient and compliant fashion."[2]

> **FURTHER READINGS:**
> **Governance**
>
> Biggs E. Healthcare governance: a guide for effective boards. ACHE management. Health Administration Press; 2011.
> Weill P, Ross J. IT governance: how top performers manage IT decision rights for superior results. Harvard Business School Press; 2004.
> Roth CJ, Lannum LM, Joseph CL. Enterprise imaging governance: HIMSS-SIIM collaborative white paper. J Digit Imaging. 2016;29: 539–46.

- According to Weill and Ross, IT governance is "…systematically determining who makes each type of decision (a decision right), who has input to a decision (an input right) and how these people (or groups) are held accountable for their role." [1]

- According to the HIMSS-SIIM Enterprise Imaging Community, enterprise imaging governance is "the decision-making body, framework, and process to oversee and develop strategies for the enterprise imaging program, technology, information, clinical use, and available financial resources." [2]

19.2 Roles of Governance, Mission, and Principles

19.2.1 Mission Statement

- Your imaging informatics governance committee (IGC) should have a statement of purpose. The author's institutional imaging governance committee mission statement is: "The IGC is constituted as the body convening clinical, administra-

---

[1] CIO.com. https://www.cio.com/video/98547/what-is-it-governance. 10/7/2019.

[2] Gartner Glossary. https://www.gartner.com/en/information-technology/glossary/it-governance.

tive, and technology experts to govern imaging clinical care, technology, information, and available financial resources across (the health system). IGC will create and oversee the framework and processes for evaluating and implementing solutions to accomplish (the health system) imaging needs."

DEFINITION: Mission Statement Versus Vision Statement

A mission statement defines the purpose of a company, institution, or working group. Mission statements include current objectives and the approach to those objectives.

A vision statement, on the other hand, is aspirational – what do we want to become?

In other words, mission statements focus on today, while vision statements focus on tomorrow.

DEFINITION: IT Governance

The structure around how organizations assign roles and make IT decisions.

19.2.2 Roles of Governance

- **Strategic alignment**: Governance can align IT staff and leadership attention around the strategic initiatives for the capture, storage, indexing, management, distribution, viewing, sharing, reporting, and corresponding electronic health record (EHR) imaging workflows for all patient care and research multimedia (still image, video, audio). That is reason enough to care about governance. In addition to composing an on-paper enterprise imaging strategic roadmap, an imaging governance body can serve as a contributing body to institutional strategies that incorporate imaging, such as those for telehealth, artificial intelligence research, information security and data protection, and population health management and cost-conscious care.
- **Quality of care improvement**: Governance meetings are an opportunity for more mature imaging specialties to educate, demonstrate leadership, and share best practices learned from decades of experience. Providers embracing standard workflows, devices, software, and operational policies limit clinical variation and promote more appropriate, high-quality care. An imaging governance body can additionally serve as an informatics design resource for those looking to develop, innovate, and drive projects and ideas toward favorable cost and effectiveness.
- **Culture**: Frosty or suspicious relationships between some clinical specialties over many years may have resulted in an apathetic or resistant culture around

imaging informatics governance. Unfamiliar colleagues can quickly and easily commiserate around shared institutional technology shortcomings if they are known already. Setting an expectation that physicians **check their specialty at the door** permits governance committee members to ultimately choose what is right across specialties and all hospital patients.

- **Communication**: Governance provides a venue for transparency, collegiality, and collaboration. Governance provides an engagement point for the stakeholders as decisions are made, as well as a unified outbound voice communicating direction, strategy, and timelines out to the broader community stakeholders. Sometimes this **unified voice** can serve to cover individuals on the committee if an ultimately appropriate strategic direction or clinical care policy is unpopular with their constituents.
- **Expense reduction**: As clinical networks integrate and hospital consolidations progress, expensive and redundant imaging equipment, storage, and viewer systems must be managed with expert clinical and technical insight.
- **Financial oversight**: Requiring that imaging strategic planning and business plans come through a governing body demonstrates transparency and fairness in resource deployment. Such an expectation also sets a higher bar of planning and execution for future purchase requestors. This higher bar quickly leads to more thoughtful and comprehensively prepared requests.
- **IT talent retention**: Retaining and appreciating the talented staff assigned to support these systems is vital; employees becoming disgruntled or leaving because of mismanaged projects hurt all involved. Governance provides a singular, respected direction to staff regarding the highest priority activities.
- **Technology evolution and expansion**: Healthcare data grows daily by petabytes. Single-copy annual storage requirements for a hospital's diagnostic medical imaging and multimedia usually dwarf that hospital's single-copy electronic health record data requirements. Documentation images are increasingly commonly stored across many care settings. Mobile phone image capture is part of routine clinical care. Upcoming investments for digital pathology and widespread clinical video capture portend further large outlays for on premise and/or public cloud storage. Governance permits oversight of current trends and technology advances across several important axes and care specialties.
- **Ethical imaging data secondary use**: Health systems are sitting on valuable and high profile data available for secondary use. Governance body clinical subject matter experts are often in tune with their specialty's current thinking on appropriate and secure data reuse. Such opinions are helpful for institutional risk mitigation for researchers and quality improvement staff.
- **Thorny problems**: A multispecialty, highly functional governance body can be invaluable for answering difficult policy and procedure questions.

19.3 Necessary Components of Imaging Informatics Governance

19.3.1 Clinical Governance

- **Care oversight**: Governance should recognize high-quality patient care as its top priority. Providers have the pulse on the efficacy and user satisfaction from the deployed portfolio of workflows and applications. They also appreciate the need to maintain patient privacy, security, regulatory compliance, ethical conduct, and mitigate risk.
  - The portfolio of applications and associated workflows for clinical oversight includes diagnostic viewers, image sharing applications, virtual and augmented reality software, artificial intelligence software, clinical decision support, image capture and storage, resulting applications, and more. Clinical imaging governance should be at least familiar with the relevant supporting hardware includes those for the above capabilities, medical devices, 3D printing, mobile and handheld capture devices, and diagnostic modalities.
  - Clinicians as part of imaging governance can detail ideal workflow, train (and retrain) their colleagues, adopt culture change and standardization, develop policy, monitor data generated, and follow relevant success metrics. Clinicians also may be called to vet and perform ongoing monitoring of locally developed and commercially purchased artificial intelligence algorithms to ensure accuracy on a hospital's local patients and acquisition protocols.
- **Incoming clinical technology testing oversight**: Clinical governance leaders should vet incoming new applications, application upgrades, and prospective devices across a diverse user base and multiple workflows:
  - Clinical leaders must appreciate the **spectrum of end users** using new, integrated solutions. The university site physician may have unique preferences compared to community private practice locations. Specialties with larger budgets (typically primarily procedural oriented or subspecialized disciplines) may be willing to spend more on preferred infrastructure, while specialties less flush with cash (typically primary care) may not.
- Leaders of imaging governance will need to decide where their job ends, and other committees begin. Some medical centers classify the below example capabilities out of scope for imaging governance:
  - Clinical decision support, which may be governed at least in part by a dedicated point-of-care alerts committee
  - User training, which may be governed by a group of enterprise-wide imaging and non-imaging trainers
  - Patient imaging engagement, which may be governed by those in charge of the patient portal
  - Scanned document images, which almost always are governed by a dedicated health information management group

19.3.2 Data, Information, and Knowledge Governance

- **Image and information management policies and process oversight**: The American Health Information Management Association has developed eight principles of information governance: accountability, transparency, integrity, protection, compliance, availability, retention, and disposition.[3] These principles of information management also apply to multimedia data and metadata. Among the implications, imaging governance bodies must:

> **DEFINITION: Data Governance**
>
> Governance includes monitoring data quality to ensure that the organization successfully realizes its desired outcomes and receives business value from data management activities.

  - Ensure ethical, verifiable, and transparent information distribution within the legal and regulatory limitations, and consistent with the health system needs.

> **FURTHER READING: Data Governance**
>
> Office of the National Coordinator for Health Information Technology https://www.healthit.gov/playbook/pddq-framework/data-governance/

  - Balance adequate protection from breach, corruption, and loss while also extracting appropriate value from information for further innovation, research, and patient care process improvement. In particular, these concepts extend today to the de-identification of DICOM imaging data for institutional or commercial artificial intelligence research and development purposes.

> **KEY CONCEPT: Principles of Information Governance**
>
> - Accountability
> - Transparency
> - Integrity
> - Protection
> - Compliance
> - Availability
> - Retention
> - Disposition

  - Fully comply with applicable laws, regulations, standards, and organizational policies, notably image life-cycle management and retention.
  - Work to scale agile and sustainable platforms and data models as technology evolves.
  - Discourage parochialism and commit to data, tool, and process reusability across stakeholders. Once one group makes improvements to a report or data

---

[3] https://library.ahima.org/doc?oid=107468#.X1QT7flKgcE.

mart, like with clinical applications and processes, all users have access to those outputs and can build off of them.

– Insist on clean and standardized data collection for secondary use in population health and artificial intelligence analytics.

• **Data analytics oversight**: Imaging governance will decide what still image pixel/audio/video data and metadata are mandatory, conditional, and optional to collect, and how to associate those data

– In some cases, imaging governance will not have direct authority to create and implement complex dashboards, scorecards, business intelligence reports, or predictive analytics. Imaging governance bodies will collaborate with process engineers, dedicated report writers, data visualization analysts, data scientists, and data warehouse experts who specialize in such needs.

– Similarly, imaging governance should expect to inform and educate those analytics experts on imaging data and metadata, such as DICOM tags.

– Imaging governance may play a significant role in engaging data requestors. Often governance bodies understand the evolving analytics capabilities and current limitations in data collection and visualization. Governance offers pointed expertise between workflow and data, partnering with data requestors to curate requests to design high-yield analytics. Finally, partnering governance with requestors can elucidate if the end user has clearly and comprehensively considered what to do with the requested product.

19.3.3 Technology Governance

• **Architecture oversight**: IT members should fully understand the dataflows, interfaces, and data storage, and have standards expertise to determine if prospective applications and devices would be successful in local or cloud environments.

• **Application oversight**: Understanding current and potential future version features and functionality for both internally developed and commercial products is the responsibility of IT members of imaging governance. They should own educational documentation that a support service desk would rely on to troubleshoot issues with a user, especially after system upgrades.

• **Capture device oversight**: Clinical engineering and device support at your institution support a bewildering hardware inventory and specific secure connectivity protocols. They also must review and document findings on prospective new devices. They must consider physical plant wireless and wired connectivity in ways and locations that clinical users would use the devices. IT members of imaging governance must be familiar with these, plus the related enabling services, such as servers, networking, and information security.

OUR EXPERIENCE: Point-of-Care Ultrasound

A years-long ungoverned approach to point-of-care ultrasound (POCUS) modality procurement caused Duke Health to have more than 100 models of point-of-care ultrasound across more than 20 vendors by 2014. This spectrum of over 400 legacy devices caused technical data semantic inconsistencies, minute-to-minute support challenges, and redundant software solutions and prevented the deployment of innovative clinical workflows due to heterogeneous wireless and DICOM data export capabilities. It also led to operational clinical care confusion, contracting variation, and difficulties with privileging, infection control, and revenue capture.

A POCUS governing body underneath enterprise imaging was created, including members of all relevant clinical specialties performing POCUS, plus administrative members from credentialing, safety, risk management, compliance, revenue cycle, and information technology. Three physicians from emergency medicine, radiology, and critical care led the group. A narrow group of standard ultrasound modality vendors was determined, workflows were agreed upon, and outputs of clinical POCUS care were available for the necessary quality and safety, and revenue processes. POCUS process oversight was transitioned back to operational owners as technical optimization progressed.

KEY LESSONS LEARNED

- Identify and rectify governance issues early.
- Create a cadence of discussion and a culture of respect.
- Ensure decision-makers both respect the clinical need and technical capabilities of existing systems and available alternatives.

- **User securities oversight**: While a parallel team likely is responsible for adding staff to authentication databases and provisioning their login and password, imaging governance often is responsible for adjudicating and provisioning security authorizations. As staff onboard, the imaging IT teams for viewers, the electronic health record, and similar applications work with the authentication support team to assign users the correct permissions:
    - Many users request permissions beyond their expected scope of activity. Imaging governance should require specific documented reasons for additional permissions and thoroughly investigate such requests. In general, governance groups should adhere to the principle of least privilege (POLP). POLP minimizes the attack surface, limits malware propagation, and supports sensitive data protection in the event of a **security breach**.

> **DEFINITION: Principle of Least Privilege**
>
> The concept that any user, process, or application should be granted the bare minimum authorization privileges needed to fulfill its responsibilities.

SYNONYMS: POLP

- Principle of least privilege
- Principle of minimal privilege
- Principle of least authority

HYPOTHETICAL SCENARIO: POLP

An employee in the Image Library only responsible for CD or electronically shared image ingestion was given limited EHR permissions commensurate with POLP. A phishing attack duped this employee into giving up his login and password. If this employee had also been provisioned full access to view and edit driver's license or social security numbers, a cybercriminal's potential damage could be more severe.

CHECKLIST: Capture Devices

- Endoscopes
- Microscopes
- Point-of-care ultrasound
- Diagnostic modalities
- Clinical video
- Mobile photos
- Handheld camera
- Et cetera

19.3.4 Financial Governance

- **Cost and revenue oversight**:
  - Duplicative applications, devices, functionality, and technical services remain entrenched across many health systems. Individual physician preference is a frequently mentioned cause. Part of the responsibility of imaging governance is to identify such redundancy and then **consolidate and standardize** aggressively to reduce costs.

HYPOTHETICAL SCENARIO: Financial Governance

Radiography, venous and arterial ultrasound, and pain management injections are commonly performed and billed for by several hospital services. You are asked to lead an effort to standardize workflow for one such clinical procedure performed by many clinical departments. Revenue and turf governance discussions can be particularly sensitive. Do not be afraid to call in administrative oversight from both clinical + financial governance early to navigate the complex incentives.

– Annual imaging CPT code updates and system maintenance activities necessitate frequent revenue cycle representation.

– Health systems are increasingly experimenting with payer-specific scheduling, innovative pre-certification and peer-to-peer processes, and risk-sharing relationships as part of responding to Protecting Access to Medicare Act clinical decision support mandates. These process changes take significant electronic health record analyst

> **DEFINITION: CPT Code**
>
> Current Procedural Terminology codes indicate which procedure was done to a patient by a physician. These can be physical examinations, operations, or interpreting radiologic tests. CPT codes should not be confused with ICD codes, which are used by hospitals (and other facilities) to indicate patient diagnosis.

resources to deploy and require imaging governance resource oversight.

– In some systems with more immature imaging governance, financial governance may play a relatively small role in the monthly imaging governance committee activities. In those instances, members responsible for finance would provide process instructions for device or software procurement, and share the annual capital and operational budget cycle events and budgetary outcomes.

– In many medical centers, final approvals for purchase and budgeting are centered in a senior-level committee.

19.3.5 Program Governance

- **Strategic oversight**: Program governance performs duties of project management, current issue/troubleshooting tracking, communications, and aligning imaging activities with departmental and institutional strategic planning.
- **Procurement oversight**: Many hospitals are pursuing a consolidated, narrow set of industry partners from which to procure equipment and software. Doing so permits the best pricing power, a simplified and comprehensive relationship, easier contracting, early access to new technologies, more consistently created data, and "one throat to choke" for the institution and its governances.
- **Governance oversight**: Program governance ensures that different facets of governance function and communicate well together. Committee members and the broader community should recognize that the purpose of governance is toward long-term strategic enablement, not erecting roadblocks.

19.4 Imaging Governance Operations

19.4.1 Imaging Governance Composition

- **Specialties producing still images, video, audio, and other multimedia** should have a representative on the committee. These specialties include cardiology, dermatology, emergency medicine, endoscopy, obstetrics and gynecology, ophthalmology,

> **KEY CONCEPT: Levels of Governance**
>
> Information flow between "higher" and "lower" levels of governance is vital for governance and strategic success.

operative suite, pathology, radiology, etc. It is recommended that all levels of experience, from seasoned physicians to medical school learners and residents (if applicable), are included. Curmudgeon physicians who do not engage technology well are particularly encouraged on governance bodies, as if they can adopt workflows under consideration with minimal effort; the workflows are more likely to be broadly acceptable.
- **Medical specialties that do not typically create many images** should also be invited as **pure consumers** of the images and the processes surrounding the images, such as clinical decision support and interfacility image sharing. These may include family practice, internal medicine, and pediatrics.
- Other hospital **disciplines**, such as nursing, pharmacy, technologists, and transport, may also have standing memberships or be extended invitations to relevant conversations.
- Additional **administrative leadership**, such as compliance, risk management, revenue cycle, project management, and scheduling, are commonly offered standing committee membership.
- Critical **IT team members** such as those from the electronic health record, image storage and management services, clinical applications, workstation support, modality support and clinical engineering, interfaces, business continuity/disaster recovery, patient and external physician portals, and information security also may commonly be part of the committee.
- Having an **inclusive and diverse** imaging governance committee membership is essential because committee members may also serve in semi-related hospital roles elsewhere. Asking governance committee colleagues to be on the lookout for imaging-related initiatives while involved in other strategic and operational groups serves a valuable communication need.
- As suggested by Biggs above, convening a 60 minute physician and high-level administrative personnel meeting is expensive, and a precious opportunity; such a meeting may cost high four, low five figures depending on the group's size. Prioritizing governance with **dedicated administrative time** is necessary for well-governed, cohesive, strategic organizations.

19.4.2 Top-Down Approach

"Top-down" governance tends to centralize decision-making into a few team members in more senior administrative positions:

- A single council of chairs, chief officers, senior directors, and similar leadership may make up these decision-makers. These leaders communicate with imaging governances to share guidance on acceptable levels of risk to the institutional board, budget planning and approval updates, cost allocations to imaging, new facility planning, and health policy impacting institution governances.

> **INTERNATIONAL CONSIDERATIONS: Top-Down Governance**
>
> In some countries, national decision-makers determining strategic priorities and budgetary constraints will often strongly influence your enterprise imaging strategy and governance decisions.

- Such a governance structure may be seen in Fig. 19.1, where enterprise imaging governance functions as a broad, crosscutting horizontal group similar to the way the electronic health record and research applications apply to many medical specialties and hospital administrative areas.
- One downside of a narrow top-down governance committee of decision-makers is that these leaders may be heavily administrative rather than familiar with existing systems' **frontline pain points**.

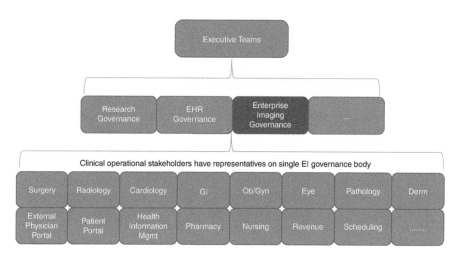

Fig. 19.1 Schematic governance hierarchy for imaging. Information flow up and down the governance chain is crucial in such a model. (Adapted from Roth CJ, Lannum LM, Joseph CL. Enterprise imaging governance: HIMSS-SIIM collaborative white paper. J Digit Imaging. 2016;29:539–46)

- In many cases, governances in other areas of the health system, for example, HIM, compliance, and risk management, will make policies and standard operating procedures imaging governance will need to account for. While not necessarily above imaging governance on a hospital organizational chart, their position and expertise within the organization dictate strategy in other areas.

> **KEY CONCEPT: Top-Down Versus Bottom-Up Governance**
>
> Top-down governance is the traditional method in which leaders make decisions that filter down to the workers. Bottom-up governance enables the workers to be the decision-makers. Many institutions use mixed models.

- Some healthcare enterprise governance activities are mandated by state and federal law, such as the 21st Century Cures Act of 2016, the Protecting Access to Medicare Act of 2014 (PAMA), or the Health Insurance Portability and Accountability Act of 1996 (HIPAA).

19.4.3 Bottom-Up Approach

Bottom-up or **inside out** governance is a mindset of ownership, positive culture change, and a bias toward improvement within imaging governance and the broader imaging institutional community. While this mindset is encouraged by senior leadership, it is owned and self-perpetuated on the ground level by effective frontline subject matter leadership who understand the current systems. Practically, a blend of top-down and bottom-up governance for imaging is favorable:

- Bottom-up distributed governance must be incentivized and cultivated so that workflow changes are consistently adopted, and more effective ways of working sought.
- Productive, cordial, and lively discussion is the norm in high-performing organizations with a culture of bottom-up governance.
- Your imaging governance committee must not just be a group of **rubber-stamping gatekeepers**.
- Grassroots leaders and culture may manage gripes and reeducate before the gripes get out of hand.

19.4.4 Systems for Prioritizing

- Loud voices, authoritative physicians, and a regular influx of "top priority" projects face imaging governance committees. Some systems have created and utilized transparent scoring systems to manage difficult prioritization decisions (see checklist used at the author's institution). These scoring systems have several benefits:

(i) **Scoring rubrics** quickly and transparently illustrate that the governance body is being systematic, not playing favorites, and that there are many institutional projects in the pipeline. An unpopular but thought-out governance body decision is more acceptable for all. When there is a monthslong backlog of projects that score highly, governance bodies can leverage the systematic approach toward contract or full-time hire justification.

(ii) Scoring rubrics attempt to reconcile many important axes, such as health outcomes, project complexity, the number of users impacted, cost reduction, potential revenue generation, research, and innovation. Such rubrics can keep governance committees out from being stuck in the middle.

CHECKLIST: Prioritizing Activities

Scoring system used by author's institution to prioritize activities specifically for the team responsible for image and video capture into the enterprise archive and electronic health record. Scores are summed, and higher total scores are prioritized.

Security risk resulting from current practices

No risk (0) = Following best practices (e.g., secure, encrypted storage) or no current storage
Small (1) = Overall secure, possible exposure of PHI (e.g., mobile phone images showing PHI)
Medium (2) = Large storage secure, but not encrypted or otherwise hardened
High (3) = PHI exposed and transported frequently or left unattended/unlocked, or with no backup

Potential annual billing/revenue increase if images stored in VNA and linked to patient chart

None (0) = Net neutral/no additional billing opportunities by moving image management to VNA
Small (1) = Potential to support/recoup/net gain of 0–$25,000 per year
Medium (2) = Potential to support/recoup/net gain of $25,000–$100,000 per year
Large (3) = Potential to support/recoup/net gain of >$100,000 per year

Annual cost reduction/savings (not considering archive costs)

None (0) = No cost reduction
Small (1) = Potential to save 0–$25,000 per year (e.g., eliminate cost of scanner printer paper or CDs)
Medium (2) = Potential to save $25,000–$100,000 per year
Large (3) = Save >$100,000 per year (e.g., could retire a dedicated PACS)

Value of image review by other users

None (0) = Images essentially will never be reviewed again (e.g., a historical migration of images from long ago)
Low (1) = Images only reviewed locally (e.g., in same clinic), at predictable points in time (e.g., clinic appointment), or uncommonly (medicolegal, QA, or rare case finding)
Medium (2) = Highly desirable to access images via EHR because of clinical care impact outside of the originating service line/clinic
High (3) = Urgent/emergency image accessibility required at unpredictable times and across service lines and multiple physical locations

Workflow improvement and time savings

None (0) = Current image storage already fully automated, or were saving no images prior

Low (1) = Small amount of non-MD time saved (<1 h/day)

Medium (2) = Large amount of non-MD time (>1 h/day), plus small amount of MD time saved (<1 h/day)

High (3) = Large amount of MD time expended in managing and distributing images (>1 h/day); anticipate large morale win among physicians and staff

Research/publication value

None (0) = No current research potential

Low (1) = Defined unfunded research project with need for image storage; occasional mining by users to locate images to be used in case series papers

Medium (2) = Grant funding submission requiring centralized image storage; IRB submission in place

High (3) = Grant funding approved requiring a centralized image storage solution

Teaching value

None (0) = No teaching potential

Low (1) = Rare to occasional review of images as an unusual/teaching case

Medium (2) = Occasional to frequent review of image files, with storage of image metadata for search and referencing outside of clinical care setting anticipated

High (3) = Images obtained recently are remotely reviewed frequently across multiple clinical teams and during rounds, with extensive use of imaging metadata

Value of images to patients

None (0) = No significant interest outside of internal staff

Low (1) = Providers would routinely show patients these images during follow-up

Medium (2) = Many patients would be interested and would download images from patient portal

High (3) = Healthcare news media worthy

Culture/readiness of clinical specialty to adopt new workflows and responsibilities/roles

Not ready (0) = High user satisfaction with current approach, no physician champion, no chair sign-off, little interest in storing

Low readiness (1) = Interest in storage, physician champion, and chair sign-off in place, but no real impetus to change

Medium readiness (2) = Physician champion and chair sign-off in place, staff and physicians can envision the potential for improved services

Full readiness (3) = Strong culture for solution, with enterprise wide sign-on by all staff roles

Readiness of technical infrastructure

Unknown (0) = Clinical engineering has not vetted the modalities

Not ready (1) = >$5000 unpaid/unbudgeted upgrades are required before imaging device can send to VNA (e.g., DICOM licenses)

Nearly ready (2) = <$5000 upgrade cost for configuration of software and hardware necessary to send to VNA (e.g., wireless dongle)

Completely ready (3) = Imaging device is DICOM-licensed and network-connected

Expected ease of implementation

Uncertain (0) = Uncertain or >500 FTE hours to deploy; system not yet fully evaluated
Difficult (1) = 100–500 FTE hours to deploy (complex clinic workflows, multiple device types, non-DICOM images, suitability of general purpose viewer needs to be evaluated)
Medium (2) = 25–100 FTE hours to deploy (new orders required, workflows similar across health system but need to be standardized, one or two standard imaging devices in use, industry-standard (e.g., DICOM) image file formats, files viewable by general purpose viewer)
Easy (3) = <25 FTE hours to deploy (EHR imaging orders already used, workflows already established, industry-standard (e.g., DICOM) image file formats, files viewable by general purpose viewer)

19.5 When You Present to Imaging Governance

- You must know your institutional strategic priorities, and, if possible, any balanced scorecard metrics for the department or the governing body decision-makers. Your presentation should speak to the different roles and interests on the governance committee:
  - Clinical governance members will want to see you have considered patient satisfaction, physician/employee satisfaction outcomes, patient access, efficiency and automation, quality improvement and best practice adoption, associated research opportunities, expected training, and communication plan, and have specifically accountable, identified operational owners/champions.
  - Administrative members, by contrast, may care more about capital and operational budgeting impact, revenue increases, per year total cost of ownership, federal and state law compliance, contracting, strategic vision, data and analytics, risk management, and any potential for publicizable awards and recognitions.

> **DEFINITION: Total Cost of Ownership**
>
> TCO includes the initial cost of a system, plus the costs of installation and maintenance, as well as upgrade costs.

> **KEY CONCEPT: Total Cost of Ownership**
>
> When you purchase a car, the dealer quotes you dollars out the door for the car. The dealer typically does not include your insurance, fuel, tolls, repairs, or expected maintenance costs.
>
> Similarly, when purchasing a commercial software product, you must include both costs for the software, plus additional costs to install (such as analyst time and enabling services like interfaces, virtual servers, and storage), maintain, and upgrade over a period of years, often five or seven. Thus, even "free trials" have noteworthy costs to consider!

- Central IT groups are always highly valued in an organization, although they are an expense nonetheless. IT members will be listening for opportunities to impact cost, IT talent retention, cybersecurity, data protection, maintenance, and support, and will be keen on learning the implementation project plan and teams involved.

HYPOTHETICAL SCENARIO: Presenting to Imaging Governance

You are advocating for a new clinical software package and an incremental support FTE for that application. When presenting the application for approval, you need to provide a simple, quantified, confident, concise pitch that speaks to decision-maker expected job results and institutional strategic priorities. Your pitch should include specific dollar and time requests, and reasonable, projected gains if the project and FTE are approved, such as:

- "Top line revenue increase of the project requiring the new hire is estimated by Finance to be 825K, enough to fund the position for 6 years."
- "Hiring an analyst with these skills will help us build integrations so we can turn off Systems A, B, and C on January 1st, saving us 350K annually."
- "This project would support the institution's Innovation strategic goal, as we would be first to deploy a method like this in our local catchment according to _____."
- "85% of peer comparison AMCs have already _____. None of our current systems can deploy this capability."
- "Because of 2 patient deaths, the hospital is committing funds for 2/3 of the new FTE to support building this EHR component. Joint Commission asked for this build when they were here 2 years ago."
- "With no action, we expect to have to choose between meeting deadlines for Strategic Project A or Strategic Project B, risking at least 575K."

- Some quantifications will be straightforward to quantify, such as costs in sunsetting a system or any highly likely revenue generations. Some must be informed prognostications, such as patient and employee satisfaction improvements.
- Demonstrate you have considered contingencies.
- Be nice!

FURTHER READINGS:
Being Nice

Carnegie D. How to win friends and influence people. 1936.
See **Chap. 23**: Customer Relations.

References

1. Weill P, Ross J. IT governance: how top performers manage IT decision rights for superior results. Harvard Business School Press; 2004.
2. Roth CJ, Lannum LM, Joseph CL. Enterprise imaging governance: HIMSS-SIIM collaborative white paper. J Digit Imaging. 2016;29:539–46.

Self-Assessment Questions

1. A physician at your hospital approaches your boss, the chief medical information officer (CMIO), interested to purchase a new imaging software application. The application seems redundant with software you already have, and has significant associated security risks associated. Your CMIO asks you to investigate. Of the options below, what is your best next course of action?

    (a) Ask the physician for a ticket to be placed to purchase the new application.
    (b) Decline the referring physician request outright given the perceived redundancy.
    (c) Do not discuss the new software until your upcoming imaging governance meeting.
    (d) Meet with the commercial vendor to understand their platform.
    (e) **Meet with the requesting physician to understand the clinical need, share your concerns, and open up dialogue.**

2. Which of the following is most representative of "top-down" governance?

   (a) **Decision-making tends to centralize with senior leadership.**
   (b) Grassroots culture change drives users to solve their own problems.
   (c) Through enthusiastic discussion, distributed and empowered frontline subject matter experts may engage and reeducate colleagues.
   (d) All of the above are representative of "top-down" governance.
   (e) None of the above are representative of "top-down" governance.

3. Which of the following is an outcome of weak imaging governance?

   (a) An agreed-upon strategic roadmap for clinical imaging technology adoption reflecting current and near future capabilities
   (b) Effective and consolidated software applications with broad user acceptance
   (c) Consistent imaging best practice end user adoption
   (d) **High IT talent turnover due to ineffective decision-making and project mismanagement**
   (e) Productive and easily flowing communication regarding project management and strategic initiatives

4. Which of the following is a way that EHR governance and imaging governance committees are alike?

   (a) Both EHR and imaging governances have broad subject matter familiarity across the user base.
   (b) **Both EHR and imaging governances require transparent and collegial dialogue for success.**
   (c) Both EHR and imaging governances use generally single-vendor technology.
   (d) Both EHR and imaging governances use identical data transmission standards.
   (e) None of the above.

5. You are presenting at the imaging governance committee for approval to purchase a new point-of-care ultrasound transducer, image storage, and reporting system. What information do you want as part of your presentation?

   (a) Five-year total cost of ownership.
   (b) Operational owners and project champions.
   (c) Project timelines.
   (d) Projected revenue increases from outpatient fee for service charges.
   (e) **All of the above are valuable in your presentation.**

6. Name five barriers to successful enterprise imaging user governance.

7. Name five axes your imaging governance committee could use to prioritize projects.

8. Pretend you must convince your CMIO to purchase a new artificial intelligence application to quickly diagnose strokes, quantify stroke size, and exclude the presence of bleeding in the brain. What metrics and outcomes would you consider evaluating to determine return on investment and return on health for this application? How would you calculate or estimate these outcomes?

9. State or write the imaging governance committee mission statement and objectives at your institution. If your institution does not have one, write one you may use later.

10. If your site does not have an imaging governance committee, compose a mock committee with the names of members or departments/areas who would send members.

Chapter 20
External Data

Safwan S. Halabi

Contents

20.1 Introduction

There are several reasons why data sharing is critical to imaging:

- As patients obtain care in different healthcare settings and from different providers, the portability and accessibility of their medical data, especially medical imaging, become critical to providing consistent and appropriate care across disparate environments.
- Digitization of diagnostic imaging and medical records is essential for population health and for research initiatives.
- Machine and deep learning applications require large amounts of collated data for supervised and unsupervised training to create artificial intelligence models.
- Standardization of image storage, portability, and curated data are paramount for guiding public health initiatives, patient and healthcare provider access, and the creation of artificial/augmented intelligence tools.

S. S. Halabi (✉)
Ann & Robert H. Lurie Children's Hospital of Chicago, Chicago, IL, USA

KEY CONCEPT: Ditch the Disk

The Ditch the Disk Initiative (#ditchthedisk) is a group of imaging societies, industry partners, and medical providers that is urging the healthcare industry to support a new application programming interface that makes it easier for patients to authorize clinicians to transfer their images.

KEY CONCEPT: Image Share Validation Testing

The RSNA Image Share Validation Testing Program tests the compliance of healthcare IT vendor systems with standards for the exchange of medical images used in the Image Share Network. Vendor products that successfully pass a set of rigorous tests receive the RSNA Image Share Validation seal. This stamp of approval communicates to current and future customers the vendor's image-sharing capabilities.

20.2 Image Transfer

- Image transfer has become a critical component of modern healthcare practice.
- There has been a slow and steady transition from the use of physical media storage like CD/DVD to digital and cloud platforms to transfer images.

20.2.1 Image Transfer Protocols

- IHE (Integrating the Healthcare Enterprise) is an initiative to improve how computer systems exchange medical information, including images and reports.
- IHE is not a standard but uses established standards, like DICOM and HL7, to accomplish specific medical workflows called **integration profiles**.
- A medical image workflow, like sharing images with reports, involves multiple systems, standards, and interfaces that work together to accomplish that workflow or integration profile.
- IHE (Integrating the Healthcare Enterprise), **XDS** (Cross-Enterprise Document Sharing), and XDS-I (Cross-Enterprise Document Sharing for Imaging) integration profiles leverage DICOM, HL7, and other standards to define a consistent methodology to exchange images and medical information between institutions.

DEFINITION: XDS

One of the integration profiles for IHE. The Cross-Document Sharing profile defines how institutions exchange medical information, including images.

- Two IHE integration profiles are of particular interest for exchanging images with reports:
  - **XDS (Cross-Enterprise Document Sharing)** is an IHE integration profile for sharing medical record documents with other healthcare providers. These documents could be radiology reports, lab results, clinical notes, CDAs (clinical document architectures), or a variety of other medical record documentation, including JPEG photographs.
  - **XDS-I (Cross-Enterprise Document Sharing for Imaging)** is an IHE integration profile that extends XDS to include the sharing of DICOM images, presentation states, key image notes, and other related imaging content (Fig. 20.1).

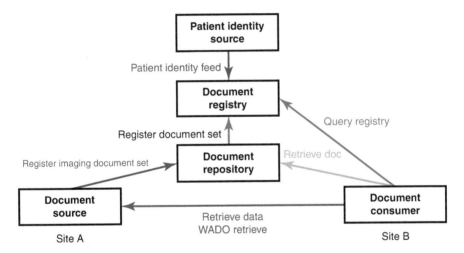

Fig. 20.1 XDS-I workflow for moving images from site A to site B. XDS-I is a variation of XDS and was developed to address images as a document type. The workflow references established standards and profiles drawn from other IHE profiles. The imaging document source sends a manifest (i.e., list of available images) to the document repository (for storage of metadata) and the document registry (for a convenient query). The images themselves are not stored in the registry or the repository. When site B (the image document consumer) wishes to learn of the existence of prior images and view them, it queries the document registry. The document registry informs the image document consumer of the existence of the images and directs it to the manifest stored in the document repository. Upon retrieving the manifest, the imaging document consumer communicates directly with the imaging document source by means of either WADO (Web Access to DICOM Objects) or C-move (a DICOM service for moving data) commands to obtain the images and display them at site B (based on IHE wiki https://wiki.ihe.net/index.php/Cross-enterprise_Document_Sharing_for_Imaging)

- The approach used by XDS and XDS-I is not a point-to-point "push" but rather a "push/pull."
- A group of hospitals and clinics that want to share images together form an IHE XDS affinity domain.

DEFINITION: XDS Affinity Domain

A group of healthcare enterprises that agree to work together using a common set of policies and share a common infrastructure.

- Medical record documents or DICOM imaging studies that are eligible to be shared in that affinity domain are registered into a central XDS registry that is shared by all the participating clinics and hospitals.
- Documents are stored in one or more XDS document repositories accessible to all participating clinics and hospitals (Fig. 20.2).
- With XDS-I, the DICOM images usually remain in each local or regional XDS imaging document source (usually a PACS or VNA).
- For each imaging study, an imaging manifest document is created that describes the image content and is then saved as a document in the XDS document repository and indexed in the XDS registry, just like any other document.

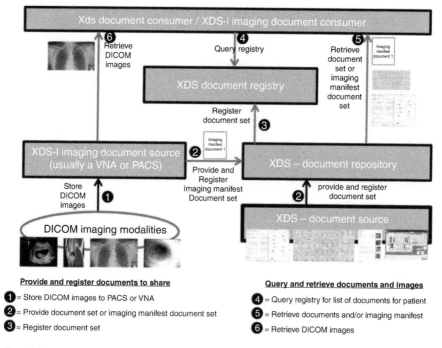

Provide and register documents to share

❶ = Store DICOM images to PACS or VNA

❷ = Provide document set or imaging manifest document set

❸ = Register document set

Query and retrieve documents and images

❹ = Query registry for list of documents for patient

❺ = Retrieve documents and/or imaging manifest

❻ = Retrieve DICOM images

Fig. 20.2 Document and image sharing in the XDS and XDS-I integration profiles. The flowchart shows how documents and images are shared between sources and consumers using actors and transactions based on IHE integration profiles. Documents are stored in an XDS document repository and registered. DICOM images are stored in an imaging document source, and an imaging manifest document is created, stored in an XDS document repository, and registered. (From Vreeland et al. [7])

- New "standards-based" DICOM **RESTful** web services are available which hold the promise to fuel the next generation of secure healthcare image and information exchange solutions in both traditional web-based and mobile environments. These include:
  - QIDO-RS (Query based on ID for DICOM Objects by RESTful Services) to query for images
  - WADO-RS (Web Access to DICOM Objects using RESTful Services) to retrieve images
  - STOW-RS (Store Over the Web by RESTful Services) to store imaging data
- **DICOMweb** is based on RESTful standards and has web service specifications for the next generation of DICOM communications.
- IHE has created new integration profiles, MHD (Mobile Access to Health Documents) and MHD-I (Mobile Access to Health Documents for Imaging) that utilize the FHIR and DICOMweb interfaces to augment the XDS and XDS-I integration profiles (see **Chap. 12**).

VIEW TO THE FUTURE: The ONC's Cures Act Final Rule

The Office of the National Coordinator for Health Information Technology has created a rule that is designed to give patients and their healthcare providers secure access to health information. It also aims to increase innovation and competition by fostering an ecosystem of new applications to provide patients with more choices in their healthcare. The rule includes a provision requiring that patients can electronically access all of their electronic health information (EHI), structured and/or unstructured, at no cost.

20.2.2 Inbound and Outbound Image Transfer

- There is variable compliance with transfer standards among the medical imaging vendors.
- Some vendors use **proprietary file formats** instead of DICOM on their CD/DVDs.
- The process of transferring a patient's images and medical documents from one institution to another can vary widely by institution.

KEY CONCEPT: Transfer of Medical Records

It is common practice to have patients that are transferred from one hospital to another to be transported with a paper or digital copy of their medical notes and images on physical media like CD/DVD. It is incumbent on the receiving hospital to view and ingest those data into their systems.

- Organizations often wrestle with how to integrate outside images into the existing local environment, tools, and workflows.

- Managing exams with physical media-based workflows is usually a manual process, triggered through paper forms and CD/DVDs.
- The real value in image exchange comes from transforming this into a proactive service that makes the outside images available to the appropriate departments in their familiar local tools (EMR, PACS, VNA, enterprise clinical image viewer, etc.) with minimal manual effort on the part of the clinicians.

> **DEFINITION: Outside Study**
>
> An imaging study that was performed at another institution but needs to be viewed, compared, or dictated locally.

- Direct digital transfer via the electronic health record and third-party systems has become the preferred mode to send and receive medical records and images but is not always available.

20.2.3 Outside Image Consultation and Interpretation

- Healthcare providers and centers receive imaging studies and other medical data generated at outside institutions for patients they are providing care for.

> **DEFINITION: St. Elsewhere**
>
> Any hospital that is not part of your own enterprise. (It's a reference to a 1980's soap opera.)

- There is no uniformity about how to handle these imaging studies performed at outside institutions, often referred to as "outside films" or "outside studies."
- Providers and institutions have to decide whether or not to:
  - Ingest outside studies into their internal PACS.
  - Officially report the studies (second read or opinion).
  - Bill third-party payers for interpretation.
  - Repeat the study locally.

> **DEFINITION: Second Read**
>
> When a patient is transferred, radiologists at the new hospital may provide an interpretation of the scans from the other institution. This second read is sometimes billable at a lower rate than the primary interpretation.

- Mini-PACS and temporary storage are alternatives for outside studies, but the studies must be easy to view and compare to local exams. The same user interfaces as the main PACS is desirable.
- Advantages to providing a second read or opinion service:
  - Reduction in cost to the patient
  - Avoiding a repeat or redundant imaging examination
  - Eliminating delays to patient care
  - Improving interpretation of concurrent examinations with access to prior imaging
  - Increasing patient and provider satisfaction

- Third-party software is available to import DICOM-based CDs and modify DICOM headers to reconcile with the preferences of the receiving institution.

> **KEY CONCEPT: Wisely and Gently**
>
> The Image Wisely (https://www.imagewisely.org/) and Image Gently (https://www.imagegently.org/) campaigns seek to inform healthcare professionals and the general public on ways to curb inappropriate and unnecessary imaging studies and thus reduce the amount of radiation exposure to patients. When patients are transferred to a new healthcare facility or receive care from a new provider, they need access to a patient's prior medical record and imaging to avoid additional costs and potential exposure to ionizing radiation to patients. The ability to securely and quickly transfer patient records between providers directly supports the Image Wisely and Image Gently campaigns.

20.3 Imaging Repositories and Research

Research and clinical trials require the sharing of patient data, including images. Solutions have been developed and continue to evolve to allow data and image sharing for research.

20.3.1 Multi-institutional Image Sharing

- Multi-institutional collaborations based on centrally shared patient data face privacy and ownership challenges.
- Depending on the intended use of the data, sharing imaging between facilities or third parties may require:
  - A data use agreement (DUA)
  - A business associate agreement (BAA)
  - Institutional research board (IRB) approval

> **DEFINITION: Data Use Agreement**
>
> A data use agreement (DUA) is a specific type of agreement that is required under the HIPAA Privacy Rule and must be entered into before there is any use or disclosure of data from the medical record to an outside institution or party usually for one of the three purposes: (1) research, (2) public health, or (3) healthcare operations.

> **DEFINITION: Business Associate Agreement (BAA)**
>
> Any individual or entity that performs functions or activities on behalf of a HIPAA-covered entity and has access to PHI is considered a business associate, according to Health and Human Services (HHS). Examples include a consultant who does hospital utilization reviews or an attorney who has PHI access while providing legal services to a healthcare provider. Business associates must have a documented BAA that ensures HIPAA Privacy Rules are followed and that PHI is protected.

- Physical media including encrypted hard drives and CD/DVD have been used to share imaging between institutions.
- Digital and cloud-based platforms have become ubiquitous and ensure increased availability of imaging studies in space and time, geographically, and among multiple healthcare providers at the point of care.

> **OUR EXPERIENCE: Image Sharing**
>
> - The ACR Transfer of Images and Data (TRIAD) system has been used extensively in multicenter trials of the ACR Imaging Network.
> - This system allows multi-institutional imaging research to occur in an anonymized, uniform environment.

- **Federated learning** is a novel paradigm for data-private multi-institutional collaborations, where model learning leverages all available data without sharing data between institutions, by distributing the model training to the data owners and aggregating their results:
  - The model itself has much lower storage requirements than the patient data and does not contain any individually identifiable patient information.
  - The distribution of deep learning models across institutions can overcome the weaknesses of distributing the patient data (see **Chap. 14**).

20.3.2 Health Information Exchanges (HIEs)

- Electronic HIEs allow doctors, nurses, pharmacists, other healthcare providers, and patients to appropriately access and securely share a patient's medical information electronically.
- **Directed exchange** is used by providers to securely send patient information—such as laboratory orders and results, patient referrals, or discharge summaries—directly to another healthcare professional.

- **Query-based exchange** is used by providers to search and discover accessible clinical sources on a patient:
  - Query-based exchange is often used when delivering unplanned care.
- **Consumer-mediated exchange** and **personal health records (PHRs)** provide patients with access to their health information, allowing them to manage their healthcare online, including:
  - Providing other providers with their health information
  - Identifying and correcting wrong or missing health information
  - Identifying and correcting incorrect billing information
  - Tracking and monitoring their own health

> **DEFINITION: RHIO**
>
> Regional Health Information Organizations are not-for-profit organizations that encourage providers to participate in health information exchanges between competing healthcare enterprises.

- There are well-established national, regional, and international HIEs. One of the best-known examples is the **Canada Health Infoway**.

> **VIEW TO THE FUTURE: HITECH**
>
> In the USA, under the 2009 Health Information Technology for Economic and Clinical Health (HITECH) Act, the plan is to adopt health information technology in order to build a nationwide information infrastructure. The aim is to start by setting policies to achieve widespread use of electronic health records (EHRs) which, as a result, will later facilitate the exchange of data. Then, under the same act, incentive programs, commonly called the Meaningful Use programs, have been initiated to encourage healthcare organizations and providers to participate in HIE. The government in this program provides financial incentives for the adoption of EHRs that conform to national standards and where providers meet certain performance thresholds. Regional Health Information Organizations (RHIOs), which are generally not-for-profit regional organizations created to bring together provider organizations and initiate health data exchange, are one of the known efforts in the USA to support HIE.

20.3.3 Research Repositories

- Multi-institutional research requires the sharing of patient data, including images.
- Solutions developed to share information between institutions and for patients have been extended into the research domain.
- Clinical trials and other prospective studies require precise terminology used and the uniformity of data elements in the research.
- Trials and studies require strict adherence to imaging protocols.

- Automatically determining if the technical aspects of the acquisition have been adhered to can be accomplished by examining the associated DICOM metadata (e.g., slice thickness, milliamperes, repetition time/echo delay time).
- Another important difference between clinical and research requirements arises from the need in a clinical trial or research study to de-identify patient information to protect the privacy and maintain the security of health-related records.
- Must be able to compare de-identified images acquired in the same patient over a period of time and often at different sites.
- Pertinent rules and regulations vary from one facility to another, and the addition of investigational review boards (IRB) and their own local requirements adds another layer of complexity.
- DICOM header de-identification and removing patient identifying information from the pixel data are other requirements to keep health-related records secure.
- More information on research databases is in **Chap. 11**.

OUR EXPERIENCE: Research Repositories

- The National Cancer Institute (NCI) has developed common data elements that are used to describe metadata (data descriptors) for NCI-sponsored research.
- Cancer Biomedical Informatics Grid (caBIG) facilitates the appropriate collection, processing, archiving, and dissemination of biospecimens to the research community, not only within an individual medical institution but also in a network across multiple institutions [16].
- The Cancer Imaging Archive (TCIA) is a service that de-identifies and hosts a large archive of medical images of cancer accessible for public download.

DEFINITION: Sync for Science (S4S)

Sync for Science (S4S) is a public-private collaboration to develop a simplified, scalable, and secure way for individuals to access and share their electronic health record (EHR) data with researchers. S4S uses and builds upon open-source standards that allow researchers to securely receive EHR data from a third-party application programming interface (API) used by a patient.

PEARLS

- Image sharing provides the following benefits:
  - Availability of a historical exam during the interpretation of a current study may improve the quality of interpretation.
  - Inappropriate utilization (duplicate exams) is decreased by making prior and complementary exams easily accessible, thus reducing health-care costs.
  - Radiation exposure is decreased, to the individual patient and the general population, by avoiding exam duplication.
  - Diagnostic information from one imaging exam, which is often needed by multiple care providers when caring for the same patient, can be made available at various sites.
  - Images and reports can be contemporaneously available at the point of care.
- IHE (Integrating the Healthcare Enterprise), XDS (Cross-Enterprise Document Sharing), and XDS-I (Cross- Enterprise Document Sharing for Imaging) integration profiles leverage DICOM, HL7, and other standards to define a consistent methodology to exchange images and medical information between institutions.
- Electronic health information exchanges (HIEs) allow doctors, nurses, pharmacists, other healthcare providers, and patients to appropriately access and securely share a patient's vital medical information electronically.
- Clinical or health consumer-based image sharing platforms can also be leveraged for research and clinical trial purposes with differences including the need to adhere to strict imaging protocols, de-identification of DICOM metadata and pixel-based identifiers, and compliance with local and federal rules.

References

1. Smith-Bindman R, Miglioretti DL, Larson EB. Rising use of diagnostic medical imaging in a large integrated health system. Health Aff (Millwood). 2008;27(6):1491–502. https://doi.org/10.1377/hlthaff.27.6.1491.
2. Smith-Bindman R, Kwan ML, Marlow EC, et al. Trends in use of medical imaging in US health care systems and in Ontario, Canada, 2000-2016. JAMA. 2019;322(9):843–56. https://doi.org/10.1001/jama.2019.11456.
3. https://ditchthedisk.com/. Accessed 1 Oct 2020.
4. https://www.radiologybusiness.com/topics/imaging-informatics/technology-company-urge-radiologists-ditch-disk#:~:text=%E2%80%9CDitch%20the%20Disk%2C%E2%80%9D%20as,16. Accessed 1 Oct 2020.

5. https://www.rsna.org/en/practice-tools/data-tools-and-standards/image-share-validation-program. Accessed 1 Oct 2020.
6. Mendelson DS, Bak PRG, Menschik E, Siegel E. Image exchange: IHE and the evolution of image sharing. Radiographics. 2008;28(7):1817–33. https://doi.org/10.1148/rg.287085174.
7. Vreeland A, Persons KR, Primo HR, et al. Considerations for exchanging and sharing medical images for improved collaboration and patient care: HIMSS-SIIM collaborative white paper. J Digit Imaging. 2016;29(5):547–58. https://doi.org/10.1007/s10278-016-9885-x.
8. Mendelson DS, Erickson BJ, Choy G. Image sharing: evolving solutions in the age of interoperability. J Am Coll Radiol. 2014;11(12, Part B):1260–9. https://doi.org/10.1016/j.jacr.2014.09.013.
9. https://wiki.ihe.net/index.php/Cross-Enterprise_Document_Sharing. Accessed 1 Oct 2020.
10. https://wiki.ihe.net/index.php/Cross-enterprise_Document_Sharing_for_Imaging. Accessed 1 Oct 2020.
11. Khoshpouri P, Khoshpouri P, Yousem KP, Yousem DM. How do American radiology institutions deal with second opinion consultations on outside studies? Am J Roentgenol. 2019;214(1):144–8. https://doi.org/10.2214/AJR.19.21805.
12. https://www.imagegently.org/. Access 1 Oct 2020.
13. Sheller MJ, Edwards B, Reina GA, et al. Federated learning in medicine: facilitating multi-institutional collaborations without sharing patient data. Sci Rep. 2020;10:12598. https://doi.org/10.1038/s41598-020-69250-1.
14. Chang K, Balachandar N, Lam C, Yi D, Brown J, Beers A, et al. Distributed deep learning networks among institutions for medical imaging. J Am Med Inform Assoc. 2018;25(8):945–54. https://doi.org/10.1093/jamia/ocy017.
15. https://www.healthit.gov/topic/health-it-and-health-information-exchange-basics/what-hie. Accessed 1 Oct 2020.
16. https://biospecimens.cancer.gov/relatedinitiatives/overview/caBig.asp. Accessed 1 Oct 2020.
17. Aryanto KY, Oudkerk M, van Ooijen PM. Free DICOM de-identification tools in clinical research: functioning and safety of patient privacy. Eur Radiol. 2015;25(12):3685–95. https://doi.org/10.1007/s00330-015-3794-0.
18. https://www.healthit.gov/topic/sync-science. Accessed 1 Oct 2020.
19. https://www.healthit.gov/curesrule/. Accessed 1 Oct 2020.

Self-Assessment Questions

1. Which of the following is an image transfer protocol "standard" defined by IHE (Integrating the Healthcare Enterprise)?

   (a) DICOM
   (b) HL7
   (c) **XDS-I**
   (d) CD/DVD

2. Which type of multi-institutional data sharing rubric allows for the evaluation of artificial intelligence models locally?

   (a) **Federated learning**
   (b) Image Wisely
   (c) Image Gently
   (d) TRIAD

3. Which of the following is typically required when sharing images for purposes of clinical trials or research compared to sharing for clinical purposes?

   (a) DICOM format
   (b) **De-identification**
   (c) Encryption
   (d) Radiology report

4. Which of the following is a benefit of clinical image sharing?

   (a) Faster image acquisition
   (b) Improved patient access to imaging services
   (c) **Decrease in repeat imaging**
   (d) Increased revenue to the imaging department

5. What health information exchange (HIE) mechanism is best used in the setting of unplanned care?

   (a) **Query-based exchange**
   (b) Consumer-mediated exchange
   (c) Directed exchange
   (d) Physician-mediated exchange

6. Sharing imaging between disparate facilities or third parties may require which of the following?

   (a) ACR certification
   (b) **Business associate agreement**
   (c) JCHAO accreditation
   (d) Image use agreement

7. Which government program incentivizes health systems and providers to participate in health information exchange (HIE)?

   (a) **Meaningful Use**
   (b) HIPAA
   (c) RHIO
   (d) TCIA

8. Personal health records (PHRs) can help patients with which of the following?

   (a) Reducing insurance deductibles
   (b) Reducing the cost of medications
   (c) Providing geolocation to ambulance services
   (d) **Tracking and monitoring their own health**

9. Which initiative is specifically geared toward reducing radiation exposure and unnecessary imaging examinations for children?

   (a) Image Wisely
   (b) **Image Gently**

    (c) Image Slowly

    (d) Image Softly

10. What are the barriers to adopting image exchange standards? How can those barriers be overcome?

11. How long do you anticipate healthcare systems will continue to use CD/DVD to transfer imaging to patients and to other facilities? What will happen when CD/DVD drives go away (which is already happening)?

12. How will government mandates (e.g., ONC's Cures Act Final Rule) that require healthcare systems and providers to share healthcare data with patients including imaging catalyze the image exchange initiatives and standards?

13. Data science research pertaining to artificial intelligence and deep learning in medicine will need access to a significant amount of data. How can external data and image exchange help with the five Vs of Big Data (e.g., volume, velocity, variety, veracity, and value)?

Part V
Work Environment and User Training

Chapter 21
Reading Room Design

Eliot L. Siegel, Steven C. Horii, and Bill Rostenberg

Contents

E. L. Siegel (✉)
Diagnostic Radiology and Nuclear Medicine, University of Maryland, School of Medicine, Baltimore, MD, USA
e-mail: esiegel@umaryland.edu

S. C. Horii
Department of Radiology, Hospital of the University of Pennsylvania, Philadelphia, PA, USA

Center for Fetal Diagnosis and Treatment, Children's Hospital of Philadelphia, Philadelphia, PA, USA
e-mail: steve.horii@pennmedicine.upenn.edu, horiisc@email.chop.edu

B. Rostenberg
Architecture for Advanced Medicine, Greenbrae, CA, USA

© The Author(s), under exclusive license to Springer Science+Business Media, LLC, part of Springer Nature 2021
B. F. Branstetter IV (ed.), *Practical Imaging Informatics*, https://doi.org/10.1007/978-1-0716-1756-4_21

21.1 Introduction

One consequence of the transition from film-based to digital image capture, review, and transmission is the legitimate concern about improperly designed reading rooms and related spaces where digital images are displayed. This chapter will focus on the optimization of radiology room design to maximize productivity while reducing radiologist fatigue and discomfort as well as discuss airflow design and recycling.

21.2 History and Evolving Impact of Reading Room Design

The term "ergonomics" originates from the Greek words **ergon** (work) and **nomos** (natural laws). The International Ergonomics Association has divided the field into three domains: physical, cognitive, and organizational. Practitioners of ergonomics study room design, environmental factors, and the specific job-related tasks of people in an effort to improve performance and promote safe work environments.

> **DEFINITION: Ergonomics**
>
> The study of human efficiency in the work environment. It encompasses physical (human responses to physical and physiological loads), cognitive (mental processes such as perception, attention, and cognition), and organizational (organizational structures, policies, and processes) elements.

21.2.1 The Impact of Reading Room Design

- Quality in the imaging chain includes image acquisition, then image processing, storage and transmission, and ultimately display quality on computer monitors.
- Radiologists require optimal environmental conditions that promote an appropriate degree of comfort while mitigating factors that lead to visual and physical fatigue. Radiologists must maintain focus and visual acuity while diminishing distractions throughout their work shift. These parameters impact radiologist stress levels, endurance, and accuracy of interpretation.
- Image interpretation has become a highly active process because imaging modalities now acquire such large and complex studies. Radiologists are presented with imaging studies that require multiple tools to review numerous image sequences in multiple planes within a single study. The process often occurs with the fusion of multiple modalities such as PET and CT, as well as during the comparison of prior and current studies using multiple window/level (contrast/brightness) settings.

- Quality interpretation requires an optimal reading environment (often called the cockpit). Poor workspace design can lead to loss of radiologist confidence and accuracy in interpretation due to:
  - Reduced interpretation speed
  - Fatigue
  - Stress
  - Repetitive motion injuries
  - Headaches
  - Eyestrain
  - Neck and back pain

CHECKLIST: What Makes an Uncomfortable Read for Radiologists?

Symptom	Frequency
Physical discomfort	87%
Eye fatigue	66%
Neck strain	56%
Neck pain	52%

https://www.barco.com/en/news/2014-09-30-what-makes-a-good-read-for-radiologists

21.2.2 Reading Room Locations

Diagnostic images are interpreted in various locations throughout the hospital enterprise and also remotely; each site poses unique challenges. Where image viewing takes place outside of the standard radiology reading room, such as PACS review stations in emergency departments, ICUs, or general acuity nursing units, special care must be taken to protect private patient information. Additionally, it is ideal to seek locations with minimal physical and mental distractions and where it is easy to control lighting and sound:

- The emergency department and intensive care units may have a significant amount of background noise and security challenges due to workstation locations being in high foot-traffic areas.
- Physician offices may be challenged with network bandwidth requirements.
- Team rooms may lack height-adjustable ergonomic desks.
- Operating rooms will have sterility requirements
- Home offices often have personal distractions

In mammography, for example, 60% of breast imagers report repetitive stress injuries with only 17% using an "ergonomic" mouse and only 13% reporting having any ergonomic training. There are numerous articles in the imaging literature regarding carpal and cubital tunnel syndromes associated with repetitive motion of the wrist in radiologists.

FURTHER READING: Chronic Injuries

Sze, Gordon, et al. Work-related injuries for radiologists and possible ergonomic solutions: recommendations from the ACR Commission on Human Resources. JACR. 2017;14(10):1353–1358

21.3 Challenges of Reading Room Design

Architects use the term "charrette" for interactive brainstorming sessions with their clients to address challenges associated with the creation or redesign of a radiology reading room. This includes the process of listening, envisioning, drawing, and then iterating on this process multiple times.

21.3.1 Educating the Design Team

Many existing reading rooms were designed for film interpretation. The lighting, ergonomic, and acoustic solutions for those environments were very different from (and less demanding than) current requirements. Also, radiologists may be performing image interpretation in spaces that were originally designed as generic offices or are reading from home. Without revision, these environments are rarely optimal for image interpretation. The design team should include **environmental engineers**, information technology personnel, imaging informatics professionals (IIPs), radiology administrators, radiologists, and clinicians.

21.3.2 Optimal Reading Space

- Reading rooms should make space allowances for radiologist collaboration as well as clinician collaboration. Optimal reading spaces allow spatial separation to achieve an environment that fosters less distractions while allowing collaboration with other radiologists and, to a lesser but essential degree, clinical colleagues. The design team should take into consideration that these types of in-person collaborations are more the exception than the rule.
- It is preferred to have radiologists reading rooms located near technologists and image acquisition devices such as CT and MR scanners.
- Some departments have **embedded reading rooms** in clinical areas. For example, embedding

DEFINITION: Work Area

Zone including PACS monitors and computer system; one or several people seated or standing reviewing the same set of images and data (note: architects often refer to a workstation as being the same as a work area; radiologists often refer to a workstation specifically as the PACS equipment)

FURTHER READING: The Embedded Radiologist

Tillack AA, Borgstede JP. An evaluation of the impact of clinically embedded reading rooms on radiologist-referring clinician communication. J Am Coll Radiol. 2013; 10(5): 368–372

breast radiologists in a breast center and musculoskeletal radiologists in an orthopedic clinic result in a substantial increase in frequency of radiologist-clinician interaction.

21.4 Room Configuration

Reading room *configuration and orientation of workspaces* will affect the ability of the occupants to interact with each other as well as the ability to control lighting and acoustics.

21.4.1 Subdivision of Moderately Sized Spaces

- Unless private offices are desired, consider *subdividing a moderately sized space into smaller work areas* using modular furniture.
- Each work area can accommodate several individuals collaborating at one workspace.
- Typically, a workspace designed for 1–3 people seated with adequate space for occasional groups of 4–6 individuals standing is desirable in an academic environment for teaching purposes. This arrangement can be accommodated with a minimum of 60–90 net square feet (NSF) of floor space. More space may be allocated for more generous accommodations.
- In contrast, a private modestly sized single occupancy office is usually 90–110 NSF.
- Avoid built-in casework. Ergonomically designed **fully adjustable furniture** is preferable.
- Placement of workstations along the room's perimeter requires the least amount of space, but also provides the least amount of acoustic and lighting control. Conversely, arranging the workspaces in the room's center requires additional space, but provides better opportunities to control lighting and acoustics.

> **KEY CONCEPT: NSF vs. DGSF**
>
> Net square feet = space allocation excluding fixed walls, corridors, or permanent building structure
> Departmental gross square feet = sum total of all the NSF allocations within a department plus the area accommodating wall thicknesses, permanent building structures, and departmental corridors. NSF multiplied by a "net-to-gross" multiplier (typically ranging from 1.40 to 1.65 for a radiology department) yields DGSF.

FURTHER READINGS: Reading Room Design

Rostenberg. The architecture of medical imaging. John Wiley and Sons; 2006 253–263.

Siegel E, Reiner B. Reading room design: the next generation. Appl Radiol. 2002;31(4):11–16S

Nagy P, Siegel E, Hanson T, Kreiner L, Johnson, K, Reiner B. PACS reading room design. Semin Roentgenol. 2003;38(5): 24–55B.

Rostenberg. Desperately seeking solutions to digital reading room design. Adv Imaging Oncol Administrators 2004;14(5): 31–33

Xthona. Designing the perfect reading room for digital mammography. Internal white paper of Barco n.v. Kortrijk, Belgium; 2003. www.barco.com

21.4.2 Conference Space

- It is convenient to include space for small conferences between radiologists and groups of clinicians, or for trainees in a teaching environment.
- A large display high-resolution monitor can be placed on a wall and should reflect a particular workstation or dedicated conference computer.
- A small area for seated or standing conversation should be available in front of the display.
- When floor space is at a premium, this option may not be feasible.

21.5 Reading Room Environment and Design Optimization

Most radiologists typically prefer to balance their complex image interpretation tasks with relative privacy along with controlled lighting, acoustic control, and a thermally comfortable environment. Generic "clerical" furniture may not be conducive to lighting, acoustic, or ventilation control, which is necessary for diagnostic imaging reading activities.

21.5.1 Lighting

- Provide individual lighting, and select furniture that facilitates optimal lighting when dictating in the seated or standing position.

KEY CONCEPT: Lighting

Lighting control is the reading room's single most important design consideration.

- Improper lighting can lead to overall stress, eye fatigue, headaches, and other occupational injuries, subsequently leading to suboptimal reading speed and performance.

- Contrast discrimination is best when levels of ambient light in the room and computer monitor luminance are similar. Increasing brightness of both medical grade and off-the-shelf monitors (at least 350 cd/m^2) has resulted in the ability to work under brighter background room lighting conditions.
- Each work area within a reading room should have individual controls. All lighting should be dimmable.

> **KEY CONCEPT: Monitor Luminance**
>
> The ACR's Technical Standard for Electronic Practice of Medical Imaging, Revised 2017, suggests that the standard for monitor luminance for primary image interpretation is 350 cd/m^2, which is easily achievable in both diagnostic and off-the-shelf monitors. A luminance of 420 cd/m^2 is stipulated for monitors used in mammography.

- Fluorescent lights may cause flickering. Consider LED, or less preferably, incandescent or halogen bulbs. The cost of LED lighting has dropped dramatically to less than $3 per bulb, and a variety of color temperatures are available:
  - Yellowish (warm) light in the range of 3500-degree Kelvin is similar to incandescent light and has been found to be most relaxing, while higher color temperatures such as 5000-degree Kelvin, with a bluish hue, are associated with higher levels of alertness.

> **FURTHER READING: Lighting Color**
>
> Mills PR, Tomkins SC, Schlangen LJ The effect of high correlated colour temperature office lighting on employee wellbeing and work performance. Circadian Rhythms. 2007;5(2).

  - Both parasympathetic and sympathetic nervous systems are thought to be enhanced at higher color temperatures.
  - Increased drowsiness has been observed at 3000-degree Kelvin compared with 5000 K.
- Two distinct types of lighting are needed in the reading room: ambient and supplemental.
- Dimmable ambient lighting:
  - Provides low levels of evenly distributed background illumination for image interpretation.
  - The same light sources can be adjusted for higher illumination during maintenance and housekeeping activities.

> **CHECKLIST: Ambient Lighting**
>
> - General illumination levels for computer tasks
> - Illumination for reading tasks using localized light sources such as a desk lamp
> - Balance of brightness levels in the user's field of vision
> - Control of monitor reflection

  - Should have broad beam coverage, meaning that the angle of light that spreads across the floor should be high and that narrow beams of focused light should be avoided.

- Indirect ambient lighting that bounces off a surface, such as the ceiling, is generally preferred over direct lighting where the source of illumination can be seen. A ceiling height of 9′6″ or higher may be required for proper installation of indirect lighting.

> **OUR EXPERIENCE: Building Codes**
>
> Many building codes require that all occupied rooms have some lights remain on at all times the space is occupied to aid in emergency egress.

- Supplemental task lighting:
  - Unlike ambient lighting, supplemental lighting should be narrowly focused.
  - Intended for reading paper or seeing a keyboard.
  - May be mounted to workstations or be stand-alone portable fixtures.
  - Often used intermittently.
- **Veiling glare** can degrade the quality of diagnostic images on primary display devices and should be minimized:
  - Other workstations are the biggest source of veiling glare.
  - Workstations that face each other across the room will each interfere with the other.

> **DEFINITION: Veiling Glare**
>
> Reflection of light sources on a monitor's surface. Items in a room that contrast with room color and tonal values (lightness or darkness) and particularly light sources and other monitors are the major causes of veiling glare.

  - Facing all workstations in the same direction may not be maximally space efficient but is often the best solution.
- Room illumination levels should be nearly equal to the illumination level of the primary reading monitor:
  - Thus, as brighter monitors become available with higher illumination output levels, the room's ambient illumination level can and should increase.
  - The reading room should not be completely dark.
  - Ambient lighting should be provided in such a way that the contrast between the monitor(s) and surrounding wall surfaces is not so great that it causes eyestrain. The room must be dark enough and free of glare such that images and text on a

> **KEY CONCEPT: Reading in the Dark**
>
> It is a misconception that the reading room should be excessively dark. Wall and ceiling surfaces, as well as surfaces of computers and other equipment, should be neutral in color and nonreflective in finish.

workstation monitor can be easily discerned.

– Working with one or more computer monitors for many hours causes "myopization," which is a temporary near-sightedness that can accentuate visual fatigue and eyestrain. Long hours of working with a monitor also result in a

DEFINITION: Computer Vision Syndrome

Long periods in front of a computer can cause "myopization," which is temporary nearsightedness that results in eyestrain and irritation.

decreased blink rate from an average of 22 blinks per minute to around 7 blinks resulting in "computer vision syndrome" which includes:

- Eyestrain
- Eye fatigue
- Blurred vision
- Double vision
- Tearing
- Itching
- Burning and dry eyes

– Most radiologists work closer to the screen than their resting point of vergence (RPV); educating radiologists about optimal viewing distance is a key role for the IIP. The RPV is typically 45 inches when looking straight forward and 35 inches when looking slightly downward.

DEFINITION: RPV

Resting point of vergence is the distance that the eyes naturally converge when relaxed in total darkness. This is the ideal ergonomic distance between the viewer and the display, typically 35–45 inches.

– In general, the greater the distance from the monitor, the lower the expected level of eyestrain.

– The 20/20/20 technique can reduce the eyestrain associated

KEY CONCEPT: 20/20/20

To minimize visual fatigue, the computer user should look 20 feet away for 20 seconds every 20 min.

with being too close to the monitor. This involves looking at something 20 feet away for 20 seconds every 20 minutes.

– Blue indirect lighting (e.g., suffusing the walls behind the monitor) has been shown to decrease emotional stress and increase visual acuity under low lighting conditions.

21.5.2 Acoustics

- Acoustic control within the reading room has always been an important issue. With the advent of speech recognition, it has further grown in importance.

- Two sources of acoustic noise should be addressed: computers and conversations.
  - Noise from computers and other sounds originating from within the reading room can be annoying and can detrimentally affect speech recognition systems:

    Noise travels either through the air or through walls and other surfaces.

    Noise can be controlled by utilizing sound-absorbing materials for wall, floor, and ceiling finishes as well as by utilizing **sound-absorbing partitions**, either fixed or movable.
  - Discernable **conversations** that originate from within the reading room are the most distracting kind of sounds. Overheard conversations make it difficult for radiologists to concentrate on activities of reading and image interpretation and thus detrimentally affect reading accuracy and speed:

    Where image viewing takes place outside of the reading room – such as at a PACS review station in the emergency department, ICU, or a general acuity nursing unit, special care must be taken to prevent clinical conversations from being overheard by others, in violation of HIPAA privacy regulations.
- It is difficult to provide complete acoustic control unless the reading room is a single-occupancy private office, but some degree of controlling sound can be achieved in rooms housing several work areas.
- Sound transmission is also influenced by the shape of the room. Convex surfaces tend to diffuse sound which is good, while concave surfaces can cause sound to converge in "hot spots" within the space and sound that carries long distances. Rooms with nonparallel surfaces (irregularly shaped rooms) can minimize what is known as **flutter echo** which can be distracting.
- **Sound masking systems** are engineered to match the sound frequencies of human speech and thus "mask" out distracting human conversations. These can be surprisingly effective in reducing the perception of noise in a room and are quite cost-effective. Sound masking is different from white noise which itself can sound like "static" and be quite distracting:
  - Sometimes the sound of air passing through heating, ventilation, and air conditioning (HVAC) ductwork is adequate to scramble discernable conversation.
  - Active sound cancellation as from noise reduction headphones is very difficult to achieve in an open space.
  - Some radiologists prefer to listen to music when they dictate which can reduce stress and improve concentration.

> **OUR EXPERIENCE: Sound Transmission**
>
> The ceiling is typically the one surface that will have the greatest influence on sound transmission in a room. Thus, its configuration, construction, and material composition are critical!

21.5.3 Thermal Comfort

- Thermal comfort can significantly influence one's ability to work efficiently and comfortably.
- Temperature ranges for thermal comfort vary considerably among individuals with the most frequently reported comfortable temperature of 78-degree Fahrenheit compared with the optimal temperature for productivity which is 75 degrees to as low as 63 degrees.
- If possible, provide *individual controls* for each workstation's control of temperature and airflow volume.
- Some furniture manufacturers provide options for temperature and airflow controls built into their workstation furniture.

21.6 Ergonomics

- Image interpretation is an intense **repetitive process**. As such, radiologists may be subject to work-related repetitive stress injuries, especially if the reading room and its furnishings are not ergonomically designed.
- Reading workstations may be **shared by several individuals** of varying size, shape, and age. Thus, each physical element (work surface, chair, monitor, input device, etc.) comprising the workstation should be capable of adjustment to multiple positions.
- Even if only one individual uses a given workstation, it should be capable of a range of adjustments to prevent fatigue during a work session.
- Consider reading in a variety of positions including seated, standing, and reclining.
- Three **points of contact** should be considered when designing an ergonomic work environment:
  - (i) Where the eyes meet the monitor. In general, it is less stressful on the neck to look slightly down at the center of the monitor. A simple method is to have the top of the monitor aligned with the viewer's eyebrows.
  - (ii) Where the hands and fingers contact the input device. This is if the input device is hand operated.
  - (iii) Where the body rests against the chair. Wrist rests may be useful for some people, but they can also result in pressure on the carpal tunnel. **Do** not use them ubiquitously.
- Instead of constantly relying on workstation input devices such as the standard keyboard and/or mouse, radiologists may use **alternative input mechanisms**, such as speech, foot control, or a variety of input devices derived from the electronic gaming industry.
- Proper dimensions, such as seat and work surface height, and range of adjustments should conform to guidelines established by the **Human Factors Society** (HFS) and the **American National Standards Institute** (ANSI).

- Chairs should have adjustable height armrests with lumbar support.
- Keyboards should be adjustable in height, position, and tilt. Consider using keyboard trays.
- Given that the keyboard is generally placed in front of a monitor, the **center of the space bar, not** the physical center of the keyboard, should be aligned with the center of the monitor. This avoids having a person's arms shifted to one side or the other when typing.
- Avoid built-in work counters and other types of work fixtures that do not provide an extensive range of adjustments.
- The reading room configuration and its furniture should be **scalable** in order to *accommodate future developments* in reading processes and technology. Future reading technologies may include projecting images on wall surfaces or other non-monitor surfaces or the potential use of visual or holographic headsets. Virtual, augmented reality and visual immersion studios are emerging technologies that are in limited use today and are likely to become more commonly used in the future.

FURTHER READINGS: Ergonomics

Rostenberg, Ergonomics straightens its posture at SCAR 2004. Diagnostic Imaging, September (2004) 25–31

Harisinghani M, Blake A, Saksena M, Hahn, P, Gervais D, Zalis M, Fernande L, Mueller P. Importance and effects of altered workplace ergonomics in modern radiology suites. RadioGraphics. 2004;24: 615–27

Herman Miller, Inc. A few simple facts on the risky business of office ergonomics. Zeeland: Herman Miller; 1992, 13

Rosch WN. Does your computer – or how you use it – cause health problems? PCMagazine; 1991, 491

21.7 Connectivity

- Disorganized wires and cables connecting various components of the reading station can be distracting and can even pose tripping hazards.
- Many modular furniture systems include integrated cable management systems.
- **Wireless components** may reduce cable clutter, but they may also pose **security** and transmission interference challenges and may reduce bandwidth.
- **Power and device connections** *should be located on the workstation surface to mitigate power cords and USB or audio cabling being routed on the floor.*
- Avoid placing surge protectors where they can be accidentally kicked, turning off the workstation.

- *Consider placing frequently used devices*, such as telephones, dictation handsets, etc. within close reach of the operator so that the devices can be used intuitively without having to remove focus from the data screen.

FURTHER READINGS: Radiologist Workspace

Siddiqui KM, Chia S, Knight N, Siegel EL. Design and ergonomic considerations for the filmless environment. J Am Coll Radiol. 2006

van Ooijen PMA, Koesoema AP, Oudkerk M. User questionnaire to evaluate the radiological workspace. J Digital Imaging. 2006: 52–59

Krupinski EA. Technology and perception in the 21st-century reading room. J Am Coll Radiol. 2006: 433–440

Buerger TM. Looking to a filmless future – designing a PACS reading room for tomorrow and beyond. Radiol Today. 2005;6(19):22

Chawla, AS, Samei E. Ambient illumination revisited: a new adaptation-based approach for optimizing medical imaging reading environments. Med Phys. 2007; 34(1):81–90

Uffmann M, Prokop M, Kupper W, Mang T, Fiedler V, Schaefer-Prokop C. Soft-copy reading of digital chest radiographs: effect of ambient light and automatic optimization of monitor luminance. Invest Radiol. 2005;40(3):180–5

21.8 Fatigue

- Fatigue is common among radiologists and plays a large part in interpretation accuracy:
  - Nearly 50% of participants in a multicenter survey of radiologists admitted to falling asleep while reading a study on call.
  - Respondents attributed more than 17% of missed findings to lack of sleep.
  - Nearly 30% of radiologists in one survey reported they had fallen asleep while driving after call.
  - More than 47% admitted to "microsleeps" while interpreting a study on call.

DEFINITION: Microsleep

A brief period of sleep in which the person is not even aware of dozing off.

21.9 Airflow in the Pandemic and Post-Pandemic Era

Indoor ventilation considerations have become a topic of interest since the COVID-19 global pandemic of 2020. Indoor air quality studies have increased significantly in an effort to evaluate airflow design and improve upon the ventilation in indoor public spaces. Heating, ventilation, and air conditioning (HVAC) systems are being closely evaluated to ensure airflow design is optimal for the mitigation of aerosol spread in all areas of imaging departments including radiologist reading rooms.

21.9.1 Airflow Design

- Airflow for radiologist reading rooms can be designed similarly to operating rooms in which filtered air flows in a downward direction and the return of air is near the floor. Common reasons for this design include:
  - Preventing exhaled warmer air from rising and then potentially being blown horizontally by airflow from the HVAC system.
  - Allowing for an effective "bubble" of down-flowing air around each person, even without dividers between workstations.
  - Free flow in the return/exhaust or the air flowing in a downward direction may simply turn up again as it hits the floor.
- Downward flow from ceiling source vents and back to ceiling return vents should be avoided as it can draw aerosols down, but then back up past one or more people.
- Cross airflow (horizontal) should also be avoided. There are known cases of disease spread resulting from this type of airflow.
- For the design of new reading rooms, consider a raised floor like those used for computer rooms, especially for large reading rooms:
  - This would allow for return air to be drawn down through vents in the floor.
  - As an added benefit, this configuration augments cable management and facilitates simple cable runs.
- Existing rooms can be retrofitted if the ceiling is high enough.
- The floor height does not have to be tremendously deep – likely less than a foot to accommodate a large open plenum or ducting.
- If air filtration is introduced or increased, carefully deploy to a level that will not impede airflow.

21.9.2 Air Recycling

- To conserve energy, return air in an HVAC system is often "recycled" to save the warm or cool temperature.
- Most HVAC systems filter return air, but the filtration system needs to be able to capture airborne pathogens or sanitize the air.

DEFINITION: Ventilation

According to the World Health Organization, ventilation is the intentional introduction of fresh air into a space while the stale air is removed. It is done to maintain the quality of air in that space.

- Air sanitization can be performed using short-wave ultraviolet lamps; however, using this technology can raise the return air temperature. This may be considered favorable if you are in a heating cycle and generating ozone:
  - Return air has to be mixed with sufficient fresh air to keep the ozone concentration below accepted maximum levels.
  - Catalytic converters reduce ozone by catalyzing it to normal oxygen.
  - The number of air changes per hour in a reading room should conform to those for healthcare facilities. These recommendations have changed since the COVID-19 global pandemic.
- For the incorporation of more outside air and to save energy, a **heat exchanger** could be used. The air-to-air heat exchanger could warm (or cool) the incoming air resulting in a reduction in work for the HVAC system as well as aid in the removal of excess humidity and flush out pollutants.
- Cubicles should have full-height dividers or be true separate rooms which would allow for individual airflow with a ceiling supply vent and returns on or near the floor.

FURTHER READING: Mitigating Airborne Infectious Diseases in HVAC Design

This infographic on the American Society of Heating, Refrigerating and Air-Conditioning Engineers (ASHRAE) website is a useful reference for both architects and radiologists: https://www.ashrae.org/file%20library/technical%20resources/covid-19/ashrae-covid19-infographic-.pdf

CHECKLIST: Reading Room Design

1. Room enclosure
2. Lighting
3. Acoustics
4. Ergonomics
5. Connectivity
6. Thermal comfort
7. Airflow

Self-Assessment Test

1. Sound masking in a radiologist reading room is best accomplished using:

   (a) White noise
   (b) Sounds that simulate "static"
   (c) A frequency which is close to that of human speech
   (d) Active noise cancellation
   (e) Passive noise cancellation

2. Which of these is *not* an ergonomic design consideration?

   (a) Where eyes meet the monitor
   (b) Where hands and fingers meet the input device
   (c) Where the body rests against chair
   (d) Where ears meet the speakers
   (e) The ability to change positions during the workday

3. What type of light is the *least* optimal for reading rooms?

   (a) Fluorescent.
   (b) Incandescent.
   (c) Halogen.
   (d) LED.
   (e) These are all equally effective.

4. What surface in the reading room has the greatest influence on sound transmission?

   (a) The door
   (b) The window
   (c) The wall
   (d) The ceiling
   (e) The floor

5. What amount of light is ideal for a reading room?

   (a) Almost complete darkness for image viewing which maximizes the perception that the monitors are bright
   (b) What the ambient light is approximately equal to the brightness of the monitors
   (c) Daylight only
   (d) When the ambient light is significantly lower than the brightness of the monitors to make them appear brighter
   (e) When the ambient light is significantly higher than the brightness of the monitor because even today's monitors cannot match the brightness of LED overhead lights

6. Which of the following is true about the **resting point of vergence**?

   (a) It typically is at a distance closer to the monitor than most people sit.
   (b) The resting point of vergence occurs at 20 feet in total darkness which is the reason for the 20/20/20 rule.
   (c) It represents a time point that occurs approximately every 20 minutes during which a user should rest her/his eyes.
   (d) It represents the distance that the eyes naturally converge (relax) in total darkness.
   (e) It does not vary significantly when you shift your gaze.

7. Which of these are effective ways of providing acoustic control within a shared reading room?

   (a) Sound-absorbing materials for wall, floor, and ceiling finishes
   (b) Sound masking systems
   (c) Ceiling design
   (d) All of the above
   (e) None of the above

8. What are some of the ramifications of poorly designed space and user interface?

    (a) Reduced interpretation speed
    (b) Reduced accuracy
    (c) Job related injuries
    (d) All of the above
    (e) None of the above

9. What is one of the causes of veiling glare?

    (a) The room's color and tonal value
    (b) Ergonomic chairs
    (c) Air conditioning
    (d) All of the above
    (e) None of the above

10. Considering airflow in a reading room to reduce the risk of airborne disease spread, airflow should preferably:

    (a) Be from the floor upward
    (b) Be from supply vents on the ceiling and returns on or near the floor (downward flow)
    (c) Occur sideways with supply vents on one side of the room and returns on the other
    (d) Flow from the ceiling down with returns also on the ceiling (downward and upward flow)
    (e) Negative pressure with flow around the doors.

Chapter 22
Enterprise Distribution

Dawn Cram

Contents

22.1 Introduction

Medical imaging distribution encompasses imaging of various formats and workflows. Over 30 clinical specialties perform medical imaging in some capacity. The purpose of imaging extends well beyond diagnosis and may be for evidentiary, procedural, or image-based clinical reporting reasons. Medical image distribution is continuously becoming more complex, and capabilities to deliver accurate image content, in the context needed by

> **FURTHER READING: Enterprise Imaging Governance: HIMSS-SIIM Collaborative White Paper**
>
> Roth CJ, Lannum LM, Dennison DK, Towbin AJ. The Current State and Path Forward For Enterprise Image Viewing: HIMSS-SIIM Collaborative White Paper. J Digit Imaging. 2016 Oct;29(5):567-73. https://doi.org/10.1007/s10278-016-9887-8. PMID: 27473474; PMCID: PMC5023528.

D. Cram (✉)
Healthcare Development Advisory Services, The Gordian Knot Group, LLC,
Fort Lauderdale, FL, USA
e-mail: dcram@gkhit.com

healthcare providers, have become highly dependent upon the upstream processes of identification, capture, labeling, indexing, storage, utilization, and validation. The purpose of this chapter is to introduce enterprise image distribution concepts and the infrastructure elements necessary to facilitate a comprehensive and patient-centered experience.

22.2 The Evolution of Enterprise Image Distribution

Traditionally, clinical care specialists throughout the healthcare spectrum relied on radiology and cardiology specialties for both the acquisition and interpretation of imaging studies. Clinical care specialists, once thought of as the **consumers** of medical imaging, have evolved to imaging **producers** and in many scenarios serve both roles. For this reason, image distribution has extended in technical complexity, requiring multidisciplinary methods of accessibility, image management, distribution, and support for different clinical workflows.

Whereas the radiologist's general workflow has mostly remained consistent, the incorporation of imaging from specialties such as pathology, dermatology, ophthalmology, wound care, emergency services, and endoscopy requires IIPs to extensively understand integrations and interoperability across upstream and lateral systems. It is equally important to understand the effects and requirements for deploying intuitive imaging platforms to all care specialists who utilize imaging in their medical practices.

Adding to the complexity, the advent of value-based care models has led to the use of traditional radiology imaging modalities in non-radiology specialties. Ultrasound imaging is a prime example, as its use spans almost every medical imaging specialty. In these cases, radiology has become the consumer of the imaging performed in other specialties, and availability of the images, diagnostic result reports, procedure notes, or clinical visit

HYPOTHETICAL SCENARIO

A dermatologist will primarily utilize the electronic medical record (EMR) for clinical care. Therefore, a dermatologist's most intuitive workflow for accessing the images acquired in the dermatology department, such as clinical photographs, is directly through the EMR. However, an ophthalmologist's most intuitive workflow for accessing diagnostic images may be from an ophthalmology PACS, and they may need the ability to reference the dermatology photographs via the EMR in conjunction with the ophthalmic diagnostic imaging.

FURTHER READING: CMS Value-Based Programs

https://www.cms.gov/Medicare/ Quality-Initiatives-Patient-Assessment-Instruments/Value-Based-Programs/ Value-Based-Programs

reports may be necessary for radiologists to appropriately interpret studies. Additionally, proper distribution of images leads to appropriate care/study interpretation. Minimizing unnecessary imaging and insurance denials are additional benefits.

Ironically, some debate still exists regarding what constitutes an "image." Industry-working groups such as the HIMSS-SIIM Enterprise Imaging Community have formed to collaborate and aid colleagues in defining this and similar topics. Medical image definitions can be additionally muddled by vendor content support variances, and industry standards organizations, such as Integrating the Healthcare Enterprise (IHE), where a "Medical Imaging Domain" does not exist and profiles may be categorized under domains with little logical connection. For example, the waveform content module falls under the patient care device domain, but the encounters-based imaging workflow (EBIW) and web-based image capture (WIC) profiles fall under the radiology domain.

22.3 Image Availability Notifications

When images are ingested by a DICOM archive, a DICOM image availability notification (IAN) should be triggered. The DICOM message is usually converted by the image archive to an HL7 Observation Results Unsolicited message (ORU).

Integrating the Healthcare Enterprise (IHE) suggests medical document management messages as alternatives. Some image archives will send a procedure update using an order entry messages (ORM) to relay image availability.

Conversion to an HL7 message is necessary either when the receiving system does not support the DICOM service to receive and process the message or DICOM services have not been implemented. IANs are used to inform systems, such as the upstream EMR, of an imaging study's availability in the archive. The messages require specific patient and exam information as expected by the EMR's interface. EMR interface validation criteria will also differ based upon the imaging study's workflow as being orders-based vs. encounters-based.

Fast Healthcare Interoperability Resources (FHIR) is a standard for exchanging medical data and images. Built on HL7 data format standards, it utilizes an HTTP-based, RESTful protocol. The more recent Imaging-Study domain resource incorporates DICOMweb service calls, such as Query based on ID for DICOM

> **KEY CONCEPT: FHIR**
>
> Fast Healthcare Interoperability Resources is a standard, developed by Health Level Seven International (HL7), for exchanging medical data across clinical information systems (See **Chap. 12**.)

Objects-RESTful Services (QIDO-RS) and Web Access to DICOM Objects-RESTful Services (WADO-RS), to query and retrieve images and image metadata. While some health information system and image archive vendors have begun FHIR development, widespread availability and adoption is anticipated soon. (See **Chap. 12** for more details.)

22.4 EMR Integration

The ability to distribute images throughout the enterprise is dependent upon the metadata captured during acquisition, the effectiveness of data synchronization across systems, and the storage and usage within the image archive and image viewers. How data is relayed back to a source system such as the EMR is a key differentiator in the ability to provide a fluid, intuitive workflow for imaging producers and imaging consumers. Ensuring the filing of references and granularity of links will offer a highly accessible, **holistic image record** while minimizing the amount of interaction required from a care provider to locate and review medical images.

22.4.1 Orders-Based Distribution

Traditional orders-based workflow with an EMR is an "order placer-filler" data flow. The EMR, being the source system, "places" the order for fulfillment. In the case of imaging studies, the order is typically "filled" utilizing another system such as a Picture Archiving and Communications System (PACS) or other image archive. It is important to note that the ordering system generates an order number, which may or may not be the same as the accession number. The image archive sends the IAN to the EMR, usually upon "a configured" status change. When receiving the IAN, the message fields are evaluated by the EMR's interface for filing to the appropriate patient record. In an order-filler transaction, patient and exam **validation criteria** set in the EMR interface will typically include:

DEFINTION: MPI (eMPI)

Each data system or hospital within an enterprise will choose a unique identifier (medical record number) for a patient. But these numbers may not be the same across the enterprise. The enterprise Master Patient Index, often housed as its own data dictionary, reconciles these different MRNs.

- Patient MRN and/or MPI ID
- Patient last name
- Patient first name
- Patient DOB
- Exam accession number

Additional fields may be required based upon individual EMR configurations. In cases where a single image archive receives orders from multiple sources, the patient ID's assigning authority may also be necessary for an interface engine to know which ordering system to inform about image availability. In an orders-based workflow, the procedure code is typically not required since the EMR is aware of the procedure code associated with the placed order.

DEFINITION: Assigning Authority

The HL7 assigning authority value is a unique identifier of the originating, or source, system generating a patient's medical record number. The HL7 assigning authority maps to the DICOM Issuer of Patient ID (IPID).

KEY CONCEPT: Imaging Study Hyperlink

A link in the EMR that allows the user to launch the associated image viewer in the context of a specific exam, procedure, or encounter.

The image archive or PACS allows the customer to define the exam status that triggers the IAN. Some organizations choose to share image links across the organization once the exam is completed fully by the performing technologist. Other organizations may choose to wait until the exam has been interpreted by the imaging provider, such as a radiologist, cardiologist, or ophthalmologist.

TROUBLESHOOTING: Orders-Based Distribution

The imaging study's hyperlink is generally set in the EMR as a concatenation of the static viewer URL string, the dynamic accession number value, and the user name, which are already known by the EMR. Other configurations or image archive query/retrieve requirements may necessitate the study's DICOM unique identifier (UID). When DICOM MWL is provided, the Study UID may be generated either by the EMR or by the image archive and can be used to identify the study across the entire orders-based workflow. If the Study UID is generated by the EMR and the image viewer or archive requires it to locate the study, the value will already be present in the EMR but may be necessary to validate the imaging study from the IAN received. In this case, it is possible to have the imaging study's hyperlink generated by the EMR upon the appropriate status change, rather than having the archive send the IAN. However, if workflows are not consistently followed, such as sending images to the archive prior to changing the exam status to "end exam" or "unread," exam hyperlinks will be created without validation that the images exist.

22.4.2 Encounters-Based Distribution

For certain clinical specialties, such as dermatology, clinical photographs may be included as part of a clinician's assessment. At the time of scheduling the patient's appointment, it is unknown whether the patient will require imaging. During the clinic visit, the provider may image the patient as part of their evaluation. This represents an encounters-based imaging workflow. The photographs acquired are associated with the patient's dermatology visit rather

> **DEFINITION: Encounters-Based Imaging**
>
> Encounters-based imaging is defined "as being performed during a clinic visit or procedure when image content acquisition is not considered the purpose of the visit. There is usually no indication preceding the visit that imaging will be performed and imaging is at the sole discretion of the provider, as with dermatology photographs".

than an order. Distribution is addressed in the EMR by linking the images to the encounter record for the visit.

When imaging follows an encounters-based workflow, the PACS or image archive serves as both the order placer and filler. The EMR generates a unique encounter number, which links everything performed by the provider during the patient's visit, including clinical notes. The image archive can only inform the EMR of image availability if certain information about the encounter is stored within the archive and provided back to the EMR via the IAN. Since the EMR is unaware of the images, as an order does not exist, the IAN will serve as an unsolicited procedure record when filing to the EMR. In an encounters-based workflow, notification of image availability to the EMR is always required if a hyperlink to any imaging performed is expected and the images are stored in a separate archive.

Common validation criteria required for filing an unsolicited result to a patient's encounter in the EMR include:

- Patient last name
- Patient first name
- MRN and/or MPI ID
- Encounter (visit) number
- Encounter provider/encounter provider number
- Procedure code (built into EMR with associated description)

DEFINITION: Unsolicited Procedure Record

An exam or procedure which has been performed without the request coming from the source system managing a patient's electronic health record.

In an encounters-based imaging workflow, the procedure code provided will need to be recognized by the EMR. Determination of the procedure code(s) provided is dependent upon the capabilities of the image archive and/or interface mappings that exist between systems.

When employing this method, a specific DICOM tag value can be assessed, either globally or per imaging specialty. The value within the tag can then determine the procedure code to be applied using varied logic operators such as contains or equals. The DICOM tag assessed may vary across encounters-based imaging specialties, modalities and organizations.

In some cases, an organization may choose a more generic approach in filing to the patient's encounter

FURTHER READING: Orders-Versus Encounters-Based Image Capture: Implications Pre- and Post-Procedure Workflow, Technical and Build Capabilities, Resulting, Analytics and Revenue Capture: HIMSS-SIIM Collaborative White Paper

Cram D, Roth CJ, Towbin AJ. Orders-Versus Encounters-Based Image Capture: Implications Pre- and Post-Procedure Workflow, Technical and Build Capabilities, Resulting, Analytics and Revenue Capture: HIMSS-SIIM Collaborative White Paper. J Digit Imaging. 2016 Oct;29(5):559–66. https://doi.org/10.1007/s10278-016-9888-7. PMID: 27417208; PMCID: PMC5023529.

record. Either in the image archive or through interface mappings, a single procedure code per imaging specialty and modality may be applied.

HYPOTHETICAL SCENARIO

The DICOM tag used for ultrasounds performed across Health System A may be the Protocol Name Attribute (0018,1030). Health System B may instead use the Anatomic Region Sequence Code Meaning (0008,0104). Community Hospital C may not populate Anatomic Region Sequence and therefore classifies based on the Body Part Examined (0018,0015).

Another option exists where an organization may choose to file the unsolicited procedure record at the patient level. Although this will minimize the criteria required to file, doing so will result in several distribution challenges:

> **HYPOTHETICAL SCENARIO**
>
> All clinical photographs performed in the dermatology department are associated with a single procedure code with a description of "dermatology photos." All clinical photographs captured in wound care are associated with a description of "wound care photos."

- The date of imaging will reflect the date the unsolicited procedure record was filed, which may not be the date the images were acquired.
- The performing department may not be captured since there is no link to the patient's encounter record.
- Associated results found in visit, progress, or procedure notes will not be linked to the imaging record in the EMR.
- Providers will encounter challenges locating current and previous imaging.

It is important to remember that patient and encounter validation criteria can vary from organization to organization, even when using the same EMR vendor. Criteria rules are usually configured within the EMR's interface and are based upon the organization's validation policies.

22.5 Infrastructure Considerations

Regardless of the infrastructure deployed, distribution must provide each provider with all image content and tools necessary for clinical care.

22.5.1 Storage

Organization decisions will vary in determining where images are stored, which impacts distribution capabilities, and where complexities are addressed. Some organizations may deploy a single image repository tasked with storage and distribution of all imaging studies. Other organizations may utilize several specialty PACS and even incorporate direct EMR storage and/or an enterprise content management system. While a single-archive approach can offer simplification with EMR integration, it will introduce greater complexity to the image repository. When multiple systems are charged with storing images, distribution to and access from the EMR will require greater configuration and maintenance within the EMR to manage the varied image locations associated with each specialty, as each system may be sending image availability notifications to the EMR. In this case, the complexity could be moved from the EMR by deploying an enterprise viewer capable of managing appropriated distribution of image content from multiple archives.

In some cases, an organization may use an enterprise viewer accessing an enterprise image repository, such as a vendor-neutral archive (VNA), which houses a second copy of images from one or more primary archives. A common configuration for this type of deployment has each specialty PACS sending images upon some method of validation, such as a manual completion trigger by the performing technologist, or automatically through a reporting status trigger when the radiologist signs the imaging report. For more information on storage, see **Chap. 7**.

22.5.2 Viewer Accessibility

Many organizations have either deployed a virtual desktop infrastructure (VDI) or distribute enterprise applications through server-based computing (SBC) delivery applications. In server-based computing, applications are delivered to the enterprise from a server environment.

> **DEFINITION: Server-Based Computing (SBC)**
>
> A general term for technologies that manage, distribute, and run applications from a server, rather than on individual client desktops.

Servers can host multiple user sessions from a single operating system. Application distribution can be centrally managed to various user groups. SBC applications, such as Citrix XenApp, may be primarily utilized when remotely logging into an organization's wide area network (WAN). Although in some cases, access to most applications, including the EMR, is handled through SBC deployment.

SBC benefits include:

- Easier to manage deployment of needed application dependencies when they exist (Perhaps a viewer relies on various media players to present non-DICOM image content such as with .pdf, .wmv, and .mpg formats.)
- Easier application deployment and upgrades
- Supports image viewing access needs for a majority of providers when the application is a thin client

SBC challenges include:

- Level of image compression may not be identifiable.
- Quality issues with rendering of x-ray images such as computed radiography (CR).
- Constraints on importing and exporting images.
- Heavier server resources, such as CPU and RAM, are required.
- Integrated reconstruction software tools, such as a 3D reconstruction, may require high-speed graphics cards installed on the servers.

OUR EXPERIENCE: SBCs

- When web browser-based image viewers are accessed from applications such as Citrix XenApp, launching the request to the local desktop browser may be preferred. This will reduce the number of SBC servers required to support image rendering and can minimize potential challenges.
- Some viewers may support idle timeout differences by the client, and when utilizing SBC to deliver applications, the server running the application must also be set to the extended timeout. Delivering images to controlled locations, where a clinical need for uninterrupted image display over multiple hours, such as an operating room, can be accomplished by pointing operating suite PCs to specific Citrix servers with the adjusted login period.
- Desktop operating system-dependent applications are not supported.

When a virtual desktop infrastructure (VDI) is deployed, each user accesses their desktop from a virtual server environment. Each user's desktop session runs on a separate operating system, similar to virtually deployed servers. VDI can effectively support both thin- and thick-client applications. Input devices, such as dictation handhelds, are often not natively supported, requiring a connection broker that can impact performance.

DEFINITION: Virtual Desktop Infrastructure (VDI)

Technology that provides virtual desktops from virtual host servers. Examples of VDI include VMware Horizon and Citrix XenDesktop.

VDI benefits include:

- Upgrades and updates are to servers rather than individual PCs.
- Several VM hosts to manage and maintain vs. potentially thousands of desktop PCs.
- Eliminates the need for traditional desktop PCs – tablets and thin-client terminals can be deployed.
- Supports image viewing for a majority of providers.

VDI challenges include:

- Server resources, such as allocated CPU and RAM requirements, are greater than SBA.
- Each user requires their own image on the server for apps specific to the user. However, this can be minimized through user group images.
- Integrated reconstruction software tools, such as a 3D reconstruction, require high-speed graphics cards installed on the servers.
- Peripheral input devices, such as dictation handhelds, and removable media such as CD/DVD drives may not be natively supported.
- A single server issue can impact multiple users.

22.5.3 Logins and Permissions

Enterprise image distribution may be deployed through direct login, via EMR hyperlinks or a hybrid approach. Access permission must account for what the provider needs to see in the current context for optimal clinical care and the tools the provider requires.

When accessing images from EMR hyperlinks, two potential approaches may be configured. The first approach uses a generic system login, such as "EMRuser" and the second approach implements access through individual user accounts.

Generic system accounts, while seemingly easier to manage and deploy, can typically only offer minimal, view-only access. Additionally, auditing will require compiling from both the EMR and the image viewer(s) for a complete record.

If both the EMR and image viewer(s) authenticate through AD/LDAP, AD groups can be defined. Appropriate permissions per role can be assigned, including image access by specialty, context management, toolsets, and integrated applications such as image sharing and import. A complete audit can also be run, rather than piecing together with an EMR audit.

Biometrics, single sign-on (SSO) applications, and two-factor authentication should be considered if they can be supported by the imaging applications. Over 20 types of biometric technologies are available, with fingerprint and facial recognition being the most used in healthcare organizations. Proximity cards and readers may be deployed instead of biometrics, enabling identity management, SSO, and login ease.

There are three primary methods of two-factor authentication:

- Text message – Sending a text message or call to the mobile device on record as a second verifier
- Hardware key – A FOB which autogenerates a token or key every 30–60 s
- Authenticator apps – Smart device apps that work similar to a FOB, where the user is provided a key which is regenerated every 30–60 s

Some image viewers and other imaging applications, such as a PACS, may not support two-factor authentication. This may create issues if required by an organization's IT policies and/or architecture, as with VDI and SBC. For more information on security, see **Chap. 8**.

22.5.4 Encryption

When a clinician clicks an image hyperlink in the EMR, a URL string is constructed and transmitted over the network to the respective image viewer. This URL string requires authentication and encryption utilizing SSL or Transport Layer Security (TLS). A cryptographic algorithm, or cipher, determines the encryption and decryption of the URL string between systems, as transmitted over a network. The type and key length used will vary across organizations and depend upon:

- Method of encryption supported by the EMR
- Imaging viewers and PACS
- SSL or TLS support or constraints
- Deployed web servers and clients

Commonly used encryption algorithms offering a high level of security are Advanced Encryption Standard (AES) and Triple Data Encryption Standard (3DES). AES is currently the strongest cipher supported by SSL, while 3DES is being retired with expected deprecation in 2023. Generally, the greater the encryption key length, the slower the delivery. IIPs should work with their organization's IT teams and vendors to determine what is required from an organization IT security policy perspective and what is supported within the IT infrastructure and the applications.

22.5.5 *Auto-Routing and Prefetching*

Some storage systems are multitiered, with recent studies available on faster, more expensive servers, but older studies stored only on slower servers. Auto-routing and prefetching are methods by which the image storage system predicts which older examinations are likely to be needed and copies them onto the faster servers in anticipation of the consumer's request. As storage systems have become more economical, multitiered systems have become less common. They are even less prevalent in applications focused on enterprise distribution (see **Chap. 7**).

Some archives may be limited to retrieving from lower tiers based upon receiving an HL7 order message (ORM). This does not account for patient arrivals to clinics, which require prefetching to be triggered by patient registration events such as HL7 admission, discharge, and transfer (ADT) messages like ADT^A04s (patient registration) and ADT^A01s (patient admission) events.

Archive variations include triggering imaging study fetches automatically when a patient or exam-level imaging record request is received, while others require the provider to manually request the retrieval. Every effort should be made to ensure broad event support for triggering prefetching when a tiered storage architecture exists.

HYPOTHETICAL SCENARIO

- Bad: A patient diagnosed with multiple sclerosis arrives for a routine neurologist follow-up appointment. The neurologist locates the patient's last brain MRI performed 12 months ago. However, the exam has not been accessed for a year and is stored in the organization's lowest-tier archive storage. The neurologist clicks on a button presented within the enterprise viewer to retrieve the exam from archive and must wait 10 minutes for the retrieval to complete.
- Better: When the patient arrives and the image archive receives the ADT^A04 signaling the patient's registration, the archive retrieves all imaging studies ever performed on the patient to online storage.
- Best: When the patient arrives and the image archive receives the ADT^A04 signaling the patient's registration, the archive recognizes the patient's diagnosis of "multiple sclerosis." Based upon robust archive configuration rules, all imaging studies indexed with a specialty of neuro are retrieved from the lower-tier storage when a diagnosis of multiple sclerosis exists. The imaging studies retrieved to online storage range from MRIs of the brain and spine performed in radiology to EEGs and EPs performed in neurology.

22.6 Enterprise Viewers

Enterprise viewers are often browser-based thin clients with server-side rendering. This eliminates the need to download and maintain software on all clinical computers and workstations across the enterprise. However, server-rendered viewers may only validate their products against a few browsers, and most organizations have a default browser identified on their network for all web applications. If a conflict arises, some network management tools allow for specifying application browser exceptions based upon their executable (.exe). This becomes easier to manage when image viewers are deployed through SBC. Additionally, it is important to note that while server-side rendering reduces complexities in the distribution and access to an enterprise

FURTHER READING: Enterprise Image Viewing

HIMSS-SIIM Collaborative White Paper. Roth CJ, Lannum LM, Dennison DK, Towbin AJ. The Current State and Path Forward For Enterprise Image Viewing: HIMSS-SIIM Collaborative White Paper. J Digit Imaging. 2016 Oct;29(5):567-73. https://doi.org/10.1007/s10278-016-9887-8. PMID: 27473474; PMCID: PMC5023528.

DEFINITION: Codec

Short for coder-decoder. Devices or computer programs that compress data so that it can use less storage space or transmit more quickly. The coder compresses the data; the decoder is needed to reconstitute the original.

viewer, server resources such as allocated server CPUs and RAM required to render images will increase from more traditional thick- and thin-client applications. While low bandwidth between server and device will be less noticeable, latency issues may nevertheless be more pronounced.

Enterprise viewers that display native images require support of varied image formats, video formats, and codecs. This may be addressed through applications embedded or integrated media players and file extension apps. Ease of maintaining these formats is another advantage of server-side rendering.

Imaging performed across multiple specialties is increasingly ingested and distributed using the same archive and image viewer previously reserved for radiology. This evolution has required enterprise viewers to extend capabilities beyond simple view-only distribution. Many image viewers now support permissions-based content management such as image validation tools, QA workflows, and granular access permissions to archived images. Some offer additional tools supporting multidisciplinary collaboration.

22.7 Image Sharing and Exchange

Prior imaging studies performed external to an organization may be received electronically or provided on portable media. Most imaging specialties require access to import prior images delivered on portable media and associate externally received image records with the patient record. As organizations continue to adopt enterprise imaging strategies, management of external images has begun moving from individual imaging departments to centralized health information management (HIM) departments.

> **FURTHER READING:**
> **Considerations for Exchanging and Sharing Medical Images for Improved Collaboration and Patient Care: HIMSS-SIIM Collaborative White Paper**
>
> Vreeland A, Persons KR, Primo HR, Bishop M, Garriott KM, Doyle MK, Silver E, Brown DM, Bashall C. J Digit Imaging. 2016;29(5):547–58. https://doi.org/10.1007/s10278-016-9885-x. PMID: 27351992; PMCID: PMC5023527.

Image exchange between organizations can be facilitated with IHE Cross-Enterprise Document Sharing (XDS), Cross-Enterprise Document Sharing for Imaging (XDS-I/XDS-I.b), Cross-Community Access (XCA), and Cross-Community Access for imaging (XCA-I) profiles. These IHE profiles provide details of the workflows and transactions to exchange DICOM and non-DICOM image content and can provide the structure non-DICOM content needs for purposes of distribution. For more information on incorporation of external data, see **Chap. 20**.

PEARLS

- Different clinical specialties capture image content and utilize medical images in different ways, defining their unique access needs.
- To accommodate unexpected medical images, EMR interface teams must determine the validation criteria for filing an unsolicited procedure record to the EMR.
- The processes, methods, and configurations for pre- and post-capture, storage, indexing, and access permissions will impact the capabilities and constraints associated with enterprise image distribution.
- The information provided to the EMR when filing an unsolicited imaging procedure record will determine the provider's ability to efficiently locate images performed during a clinical visit.
- Organizations can leverage the IHE XDS profile internally to provide structure to non-DICOM image content.
- Performance and security of image distribution is impacted by the underlying infrastructure of all involved systems and applications.

Self-Assessment Questions

1. Which of the following clinical specialties is usually considered an imaging producer?

   (a) Radiology
   (b) Cardiology
   (c) Dermatology
   (d) All of the above
   (e) None of the above

2. Which message type(s) could be sent to notify an EMR of image availability:

   (a) ORU
   (b) ORM
   (c) IAN
   (d) All of the above

3. True or False: The purpose of enterprise image distribution is to provide the clinical care provider with access to radiology images:

   (a) True
   (b) False

4. When might an unsolicited imaging procedure record be sent to an EMR?

   (a) During orders-based workflows
   (b) During encounter-based workflows
   (c) During every clinic visit
   (d) None of the above

5. What is an example of a placer/filler workflow?

   (a) Orders-based workflows
   (b) Encounter-based workflows
   (c) Patient registration workflows
   (d) None of the above

6. Which of the following is *not* an image sharing approach?

   (a) VDI
   (b) XDS
   (c) XCA
   (d) CD

7. Potential challenges with server-based computing include:

   (a) The EMR cannot open images from the imaging study hyperlink.
   (b) The ratio of image compression cannot be seen.
   (c) Image links cannot be emailed to external providers.
   (d) None of the above.

8. Which of the following is *never* a function of an enterprise imaging viewer?

   (a) Interactive collaboration
   (b) Image distribution
   (c) Sending an IAN
   (d) Image sharing

9. True or False: Generic system logins configured in the EMR support role-based, image viewer access permissions:

   (a) True
   (b) False

10. Would you prefer to maintain a server-based enterprise distribution model or a thick client? Which do you think the physician-users would prefer?

Chapter 23
Customer Relations

Janice Honeyman-Buck

Contents

23.1 Introduction

Customer relations refers to technical support, training, application assistance, and troubleshooting. In some cases the person offering service and support is the single point of contact for the customer, and their experience sets their opinion of the system. Customers are often vocal in their opinion on social media and recommendations to colleagues. The imaging informatics professional (IIP) should be able to troubleshoot PACS, speech recognition, DICOM, and networking software and should have a working knowledge of the interfaces between imaging systems and other healthcare IT systems. The IIP should provide hardware troubleshooting for radiologists' workstations and software display of images throughout the enterprise.

J. Honeyman-Buck (✉)
Society for Imaging Informatics in Medicine, Leesburg, VA, USA
e-mail: honeymanbuck@siim.org

23.2 Customer Groups and Their Concerns

As an imaging informatics professional, **who are the customers?** After
all, this is not strictly speaking a business. Since images produced by radiology are used throughout the healthcare
enterprise and are a critical part of a
patient's healthcare, almost anyone
working in the hospital associated with
a patient can be a customer. In addition, since images are produced by
imaging equipment, modality vendors
can be considered customers. Finally,
with the proliferation of patient portals,
the patients themselves are customers
of the radiology services. One thing to
remember in all cases is that listening
to the customer is the most important skill for the support person to learn.

CHECKLIST: Active Listening

- Ask questions and respond to the
  speaker.
- Verify understanding and possibly
  restate the problem to confirm
  understanding.
- Pay attention to what is said and
  how it is said.
- Listen to the language of the caller
  to assess the level of knowledge of
  the caller.
- Adjust your responses to reflect
  your understanding of the caller's
  level of knowledge.

23.2.1 Radiologists and Other Imaging Physicians

Physicians require that their digital
tools be functional and efficient **at all
times**. Radiologists are expected to
read more studies in an era when studies contain more imaging data. Multi-
slice CT scanners and new MRI units
can produce literally thousands of
images, and the combination of the
increased number of studies and
increased number of images per study
makes a workload that is nearly impossible to manage. A radiologist workspace that functions correctly, including
the PACS workstation, the dictation
system, and the RIS/HIS/Decision support access, is absolutely critical to the
success of the interpretation process.
The IIP's job is to be sure this
need is met.

**CHECKLIST: Radiologists'
Work Areas**

- Meet with a small group of radiologists regularly (e.g., monthly) to get
  a "wish list" of things that could
  be better.
- Have your support team check the
  work areas and computers for
  proper functioning weekly.
- Be visible; sit in each reading area
  for an hour every week to see how
  things are going. By being there,
  the radiologists will see you are
  interested in their problems and
  will often tell you about issues
  before they become critical.

IIPs who come from medical backgrounds understand the **primacy of patient
care** and the urgency of correcting problems before they impact care. IIPs from

HYPOTHETICAL SCENARIO: Radiologist

Dr. Jones calls at 7:30 AM on Monday morning – the keyboard on her PACS workstation does not work. When she types, nothing happens and everyone needs their studies read, and this needs to be fixed immediately, and "why can't we keep these workstations operational?"; she doesn't have time for this kind of problem. As the IIP, you know that the keyboard has probably become unplugged from the computer. It will take 20 min for you to get to Dr. Jones' location, and that is too long for her to wait. If you ask her if the keyboard is plugged in, she will be embarrassed and perhaps more angry, a situation you want to avoid. Instead, try this. "Dr. Jones. I'm so sorry, this is entirely my fault. It will take about 20 min for me to get there, but I think if you help, we can fix this for you right now. Sometimes dust gets into the keyboard connector. If you would please unplug it, blow on it gently and plug it back in, it will probably work and I'll come down as soon as possible to make sure it won't happen again. Did that work? It did? Great! I'll be down shortly."

The IIP diffused the situation by apologizing, using the phrase "this is my fault" and then finding a solution that did not embarrass or talk down to the radiologist. The IIP recognized the fact that she could not get to the workstation location in a time frame that would meet the needs of the radiologist and worked out a solution on the spot that resolved the situation.

other backgrounds may need to adapt to a culture that demands an immediate response to IT issues that would be considered nonurgent in other businesses.

23.2.2 Clinicians

With digital acquisition and easy distribution of images, many clinicians now want to see their patients' images as soon as the study is completed. When and how they receive these images is a matter of policy and technology at each institution. It is common that

HYPOTHETICAL SCENARIO: Password Security

You, as an IIP, do a spot audit of the web-based image distribution system to see how it is working, and you are disturbed to see that one particular physician appears to be logged on from the medicine clinic in several different examination rooms. Since it is difficult for a person to "clone" themselves to be in multiple places at the same time, you investigate. You find that all the physicians in this medicine clinic have forgotten their usernames and passwords so they have decided to use one person's login. To save time, the clerk in charge logs into all the examination room workstations with the same login at the beginning of the clinic day. They know this is a violation of the security rules, but patient care comes first so they don't care. How would you deal with this?

clinicians will access patient studies using a **web application** which requires authentication for application entry (see **Chap. 22**). Passwords are ideal from a security viewpoint, but keeping track of them can be challenging for end users, especially when they are required to remember passwords for multiple systems.

Prior to implementing a web application, there must be a way to manage users and passwords, preferably using a **single sign-on system** at the institution. Forcing a group of people to remember many different passwords encourages them to write passwords on slips of paper, bottoms of keyboards, and other non-secure locations, which leads to frustration and outright anger. The best solution to a forgotten password is an automatic method for the user to reset their password using information known by the system such as an answer to a security question. Of course, a **24/7 help desk** must be in place to support end users who care for patients.

It is not uncommon for clinicians to have undergraduate computer science degrees and if given the appropriate access can solve many of their own issues such as setting up a loop to keep their workstation from going idle and timing out. Occasionally, clinicians are forced to call for help. Since the types of problems that might occur are difficult to anticipate, the best defense is a good offense. Proactively publishing a

> **HYPOTHETICAL SCENARIO: Timeouts**
>
> The head of surgery calls you to complain that the imaging application on the OR workstation not only times out but also logs the users off in the middle of surgery and demands a no-time-out login account for the operating rooms. You are concerned that if you fulfill this request, people will use that account in other locations. This could potentially lead to numerous computers that do not timeout after a reasonable amount of time, which is a clear security violation. On the other hand, security should not get in the way of patient care. How would you deal with this?

short **online tutorial** is an excellent solution to help the new users navigate the system. While vendor-prepared user guides are comprehensive and useful, many users just want to log on, find the patient, look at the images, and log off. An IIP may find it useful to create a link to a page of frequently asked questions (FAQs) and keep it updated as new problems arise. Most users are familiar with the FAQ idea and will try to work things out. Be sure to include an escalation method in case the FAQ doesn't answer their question. Since the web access will quickly become *mission critical* for the institution, it is likely there will be a backup or *business continuity plan*, and any downtime announcements with further instructions should be displayed when the system is unavailable (see **Chap. 29**).

Radiology departments are in competition for their patients, and the clinicians are the customers who determine where their patients go for

CHECKLIST: Clinician Outreach

- Visit your community medical association meetings as a guest speaker.
- Attend staff meetings for other practices or departments.
- Publish an occasional newsletter with information and tips for better viewing of images.

studies. Community or clinician **outreach efforts** in the form of educational programs on the services offered by radiology are an excellent way to **publicize image access** to referring physicians and to get feedback and ideas about improving the quality of image communications.

23.2.3 Technologists

Technologists are critical to the production of high-quality, correctly labeled, and accurately identified studies. In the days of analog-film radiology, if a technologist made an error on an imaging study, it was easy to correct with a grease pencil. Now, in the digital age, the incorrect image could simultaneously be in dozens of locations before the error is caught. It is important for the IIP to understand how technologists "see" the radiology operation. In general, the technologists deal with a patient, the technology that acquires the study, and the setup of a study, which can sometimes be simple or sometimes very complex. Technologists do not usually have a picture in their minds of the enterprise networks, the necessary computer interfaces that are implemented throughout the entire healthcare enterprise, and may not grasp the implications of the advantageous work going on behind the scenes. Rather, they are trying to deal with what is sometimes the difficult task of imaging a patient. Mistakes are bound to happen, which are occasionally difficult to recognize and correct.

For the radiology department to run smoothly, it is important that everyone understand how technology works together and how information flows, including the technologists. When they are educated about how

CHECKLIST: Technologist Outreach

- Schedule regular in-service times with technologists for education on systems and listen to concerns.
- Shadow technologists in various divisions to observe challenges they may have using the systems.

orders are turned into instances on a modality worklist and how the modality informs the RIS that a procedure step has been performed, the technologists will have an instinctive understanding of what is happening behind the scenes. Subsequently, when an unusual event takes place, they will be able to help troubleshoot the incident and contact the correct people to resolve a problem. Thus, **education** is the key to correct technologist interaction with imaging informatics technology (and to job satisfaction).

Even with the best integration and the best workflow, technology will occasionally fail. Some examples of workflow disruptions include scheduled and unscheduled downtimes, a portable modality disconnecting from the modality worklist, and a network failure. Technologists should be prepared to recognize when these scenarios occur and rely on well-documented downtime policies and procedures that make the process of doing their jobs as easy as possible (see **Chap. 29**).

23.2.4 Hospital IT

The IIP will most likely have a close relationship with, or be a part of, the hospital IT team as hospitals tend to centralize IT support. There is a close and critical interoperability requirement to enable correct functioning of PACS and hospital information systems. Historically, HL7 messages regarding orders are sent to radiology devices, and PACS while imaging studies and reports are transmitted throughout the institution. Just like the integration of the healthcare enterprise, it is important that the people who manage these systems speak the same language, **agree to transfer protocols**, and communicate information effectively. Cooperation on the communication of service and access issues can be crucial and essential to the successful integration and operation of all systems needed for patient care.

CHECKLIST: Working with Hospital IT

- IIP should be part of IT planning teams for all systems that send information to PACS or consume PACS products (images and reports)
- Hospital IT should be part of radiology planning for PACS, RIS, dictation, decision support, AI, and other radiology-centric systems that need input from hospital systems and provide images or reports.

23.2.5 Hospital Personnel

Anyone who is responsible for patient care in the healthcare enterprise may have permission to access radiology images and reports. Examples include:

- A physical therapist may need to see a shoulder diagnostic radiograph while treating a rotator cuff.
- A clerk on a patient floor may need to schedule a CT imaging study.
- A coder may need to access imaging reports to generate accurate codes for billing purposes.

HYPOTHETICAL SCENARIO: Hospital Personnel

A nurse from the neurology clinic calls; all the patients are there, but the doctors can't see any of their CT studies. PACS is down!!! Consider what over-the-phone solutions might make the CTs show up again. Perhaps someone has set a filter that only shows CRs or MRIs.

All these users have their own unique interfaces, needs, and levels of understanding of how the systems interact and at some point will need help from the IIP when the system does not work as expected. It is impossible for the IIP to anticipate the numerous scenarios in which people will misunderstand imaging informatics workflows. The IIP needs to ask the right questions in order to get the right information from a user, often starting from an ambiguous complaint. For example, a clerk may complain that the monitor doesn't work when actually the computer isn't powering on. Another example is that a clerk may position a computer monitor where patient health information is exposed. The IIP has to be the translator between the words used to describe issues or proactively recognizing other problems that are unintentionally created by end users and problem-solve these issues realistically. At the same time, the IIP has to instill soft skills into their practice in order to be successful. Some of the soft skills include:

- Good verbal and written communication
- A sense of **humor**
- A sense of **compassion**
- A real commitment to service
- Understanding of technical weaknesses in others
- **Respect** for other people and their knowledge levels

23.2.6 Vendors

Imaging vendors are a part of the big picture. Without imaging vendors there would not be any imaging studies. However, there may be instances when the interests of imaging vendors and IIPs conflict. For example, a vendor wants a sale and wants to continue making sales in an imaging department, while an IIP wants equipment that conforms to IHE protocols, produces the best quality images, and has a user interface that promotes optimized workflow while minimizing errors.

The IIP should be involved at the onset of any purchase or vendor interaction in order to set the standard expectation of IHE compliance and avoid conflicts. Additionally, the IIP needs to be aware of any changes a field service engineer proposes to any equipment prior to the change. There is nothing worse than coming into work and finding out that your CT modality had a field service change during the night and the technologists no longer see a DICOM modality worklist or the imaging studies acquired on the modality no longer send to the PACS, or the ultimate… the modality does not "see" the network anymore. The IIP needs to have a **close working relationship** with all vendors and field service engineers. No service or upgrades should ever be performed without prior knowledge of the IIP. Strictly stating and enforcing this rule fosters an excellent working relationship between both groups.

23.2.7 Patients

Patients are our most important customers. While the IIP may be a member of the healthcare team who rarely interacts with patients, there are times when patients may need to know more about imaging, imaging services, and their own images. The IIP is bound by HIPAA rules, cannot give out any health information, and needs to make patients aware of this from the beginning of their communication. However, the IIP may certainly guide the patient to the correct person to answer questions.

The IIP needs to be **sensitive** to the real problems that patients are experiencing. Most people simply do not understand the complexities of technology, disease, treatment, or hospitals and are only looking for help. They do not understand the **privacy rules** that have been created to protect themselves and their families and may become hostile when you can't help them for a very legitimate reason.

HYPOTHETICAL SCENARIO: Patients as Customers

Here are some common scenarios (these have all happened to me):

- Scenario 1: Mr. Smith calls to find out how to get one of those digital whole-body CT scans he saw on the early morning TV show that morning, and somehow the call was directed to you because your name was associated with digital CT scans.
- Scenario 2: Mrs. Jones calls because she wants all her brother's X-rays put on a CD so she can take them to another hospital.
- Scenario 3: Mrs. Brown is in the waiting room. She has some CDs of her neighbor's studies from another hospital, and she can't make them work in her computer at home so she came in to find someone here to help her. Her neighbor is not a patient at your hospital.
- Scenario 4: The webmaster forwards a message to you because she doesn't know who else can answer this question. The person has a son with cancer, and she heard that digital PACS can cure cancer and wants to set up an appointment.

In Scenario 1, I suggested that Mr. Smith call his physician to ask about getting an order for a scan. In Scenario 2, I explained that while we could do that, her brother would have to request it unless she was on his list of people who could act on his behalf because we had privacy rules. I explained to Mrs. Brown that her neighbor's studies were private, and I was not allowed to see them because of privacy. I responded to the person in Scenario 4 that if her physician didn't refer her to our hospital, that we had a physician "finder" service which could help her find the best doctor and gave her the phone number. I did not explain that digital PACS could not cure cancer because I did not want to further confuse her situation.

That's how I handled each scenario, but everyone will have to come up with their own responses as these unusual situations occur. There's really no right answer, just a sensitive, caring, thoughtful answer. The IIP should be sure that when she interacts with patients that she has compassion. The patient has a real problem, and even if he can seem unreasonable and may sometimes be angry, it is his situation and not the IIP he is attacking.

23.3 Tools of the Trade

Not all issues will have instant solutions, and in fact, much of the IIP's customer relation tasks will consist of keeping track of ongoing and recurring issues and creating documentation and educational materials.

23.3.1 Documentation and Education

A complete description of software available for writing documentation is beyond the scope of this chapter, but there are some good starting places for many of the things an IIP may want to provide.

Self-service portals encourage and empower users to solve issues without calling for support by providing system documentation as well as educational content about how to use the system. Self-service portal systems are widely available from a number of third-party vendors.

CHECKLIST: Self-Service

- FAQs
- Knowledge bases that can be queried
- Tutorials
- Step-by-step troubleshooting instructions

23.3.2 Ticket and Issue Tracking

Tracking and following up on outstanding issues is unmanageable without a well-designed system. This system should not be a color-coded set of post-it notes on a wall. Luckily, the IIP has excellent resources available to help solve the problem of keeping track of hundreds of tiny details. An Internet search will result in dozens of systems available for managing the support desk and prioritizing tickets. In addition, many of these systems provide the self-service options that will enable customers to solve the common and minor problems while allowing the IIP to focus on the most difficult issues.

23.3.3 Proactive System Monitoring

It would be ideal if IIPs were only contacted about suggested improvements to a system or even praise about how well the system is operating rather than complaints about systems that are nonfunctional. To get ahead of issues, a proactive monitoring approach can be used to identify

DEFINITION: Dashboard Display

A graphical interface that summarizes input from many sources into a small visual area that can be quickly understood. More detailed information is available by expanding individual elements of the dashboard.

errors before users are aware there is even a problem. These systems can provide the IIP with a dashboard that shows how things are working and identify if there is a weakness that needs to be addressed before it becomes a widespread issue. In fact, the IIP does not have to be watching the computer; the **monitor software** has the ability to page, email, or call the IIP if a problem is detected.

An open-source availability system has been developed exactly for this application and is available for download. Researchers and developers at the University of Maryland developed **Nagios Core** software to proactively monitor systems, networks, and infrastructure. Nagios can give the IIP instantaneous information and alerts about servers, switches, applications, and services. In addition to being able to proactively manage immediate problem events, periodic review allows the IIP to look for patterns of weakness in the network or in specific systems.

> **FURTHER READINGS: Nagios**
>
> https://www.nagios.org
> Towland C, Meenan C, Warnock M, Nagy P. Proactively monitoring departmental clinical IT systems with an open source availability system. 2007;20(Suppl 1): 19–124.

23.4 Final Thoughts

In addition to the technical skills required to manage complex PACS and imaging informatics systems, it is important that IIPs possess the ability to perform business-related functions. These include creation of written communications including reports, business correspondence, and procedure manuals as well as the presentation of data to imaging informatics consumers. It is essential that the IIP stay abreast of current trends and regulations in IT and healthcare. IIP support requires a culture that reflects the organization's values and enhances productivity.

The IIP needs to be aware of the customer relations side and be prepared to assist users who may not be technically savvy or who may not understand how the systems fit together. Education can certainly help, but tact, compassion, and understanding of the stress incurred by those who care for patients are important. Keep a notebook of the funny things people complain about; maybe someday you will write a book. Finally, look for tools that will proactively identify issues that would cause users to call with complaints in order to avoid problems before they happen. If the IIP makes themselves available by visiting areas where users frequently work, the users will know the IIP is passionate about their careers and will be less likely to complain. This can be a 5-min trip through the ultrasound department to say hello to the technologists or 5 min in a reading room, but that's all it will take to make the job easier. One last word, make sure you know your users and their names; it will make all the difference in your job and your job satisfaction.

> **FURTHER READING**
>
> Reed D, Cottrell D. Monday morning customer service; Cornerstone Leadership Institute; 2004

Self-Assessment Questions

1. Which of the following is a potential customer for an imaging informatics professional?

   (a) Patients
   (b) Radiologists
   (c) Vendors
   (d) Hospital IT
   (e) All of the above

2. If a patient has a question about how to access his or her images on the radiology Internet, the imaging informatics professional must teach the patient how to access the images from home:

   (a) True
   (b) False

3. Which of the following systems used by the radiologists would typically be supported by the IIP?

   (a) PACS workstation, email, and Internet
   (b) HIS interface, PACS workstation, and dictation system interface
   (c) Dictation system, Internet, Microsoft office, and email
   (d) HIS/RIS, dictation system, and turbo tax

4. Which of the following techniques might help keep the radiologists' work areas running smoothly and correctly?

   (a) Regulate exactly when each computer can be used and how it can be used so that no one can use it during a scheduled downtime and so you have complete control over its use.

   (b) Change the passwords on the reading room computers every morning at 6AM with an automatic reboot to enforce security.

   (c) Monitor the computers in the work areas for correct operation.

   (d) Purge all the images and databases from the PACS computers every morning at 7AM to be sure they start fresh each day.

5. What functions might be included in a self-service portal?

6. What business skills are likely to be expected in the IIP support person?

7. What advantages can you expect from proactive system monitoring?

8. What features does Nagios software perform to help the IIP?

9. What solutions can you put in place to help users who forget their passwords?

10. What types of outreach techniques might help improve communications with clinicians?

Chapter 24
User Training

Ann Scherzinger

Contents

24.1 Introduction

Training is an ongoing requirement of a successful PACS program. Staff turnover, workflow changes, upgrades, new systems, and general performance improvement initiatives should all trigger some formal staff training. Training opportunities must be provided if your organization desires maximum productivity, accurate information and consistent workflow from your informatics applications. The following discussion defines the common aspects of all training programs. Generally, these programs are performed sequentially; however, continual assessment of the program should be performed and may require redesign of an earlier component.

A. Scherzinger (✉)
Radiology-Radiological Sciences, University of Colorado School of Medicine,
Aurora, CO, USA
e-mail: ANN.SCHERZINGER@CUANSCHUTZ.EDU

© The Author(s), under exclusive license to Springer Science+Business Media, LLC, part of Springer Nature 2021
B. F. Branstetter IV (ed.), *Practical Imaging Informatics*,
https://doi.org/10.1007/978-1-0716-1756-4_24

24.2 Assessing the Need

24.2.1 Training Purpose

- The **why** of training – determines the purpose of the training:
    - New software and upgrades are obvious reasons for a training program, and a system implementation plan typically includes training phases.
    - New staff members, both within and outside the department, require access to a training program that allows them accurate and efficient use of appropriate information systems to do their job.
    - Workflow changes from new care programs often dictate training or retraining of staff. It is important for the imaging informatics professional (IIP) to be involved in any new program analysis to assure that workflow changes can be supported by the PACS.
    - Retraining related to a quality or process improvement issue is often required.
    - Performance review of an individual staff member may dictate retraining.
- **Who and what** to include in the training program:
    - The outcome of this portion of the needs analysis should be a list of users, their roles, and a description of those tasks, with appropriate performance measures, that each user or user role needs to perform.
    - For each user, obtain a list of their roles, their normal work hours and availability outside of their normal hours.

> **KEY CONCEPT: Purpose of Training**
>
> Training has one primary goal: better job performance. When assessing training needs, determine the why, who, what, where, when, and how of a training program.

> **FURTHER READING: Training**
>
> Training instruction is normally a human resources function, and literature related to training systems development can be found by searching topics such as performance-based training, skills training, and technical training.

CHECKLIST: Triggers for Training

- New software
- New staff members
- Software upgrades
- Workflow changes
- Result of QI process
- Remedial training

> **KEY CONCEPT: Role-Based Workflow**
>
> It is not uncommon for the role of a staff type to vary within a single department. For example, a technologist in CT may be required to schedule patients while those in X-ray may not.

- For new systems and system upgrades, the best way to determine the training tasks and audience is through review of a **workflow assessment** that was done by the project implementation team (see **Chap. 25**). That workflow was most likely done to assess equipment needs and placement and may not have the details needed for training. To be useful for training, it should describe the normal flow of data as well as decision points when the normal data flow is modified. A workflow document should be created for all user roles. A comparison of the new workflow with that of the existing will best indicate gaps: who and what should be included in the training plan.
- A specific **role-based workflow** analysis will best determine the training program for a new staff member. Review this role-based workflow with the staff member's supervisor to assure that it is accurate and current.
- New care programs can require from minor to significant changes in workflow or software. Here, it is important to identify both those within and outside the immediate area or department that will be affected by the change when developing the scope of the training program.
- Retraining related to a quality or process improvement can be treated similar to that of a new program, with the scope of training based on users and processes affected.
- The training program that results from a performance assessment can be focused on the specific performance issue. It is important to review needs with the staff member's supervisor and to determine and address issues in the user's environment that may contribute to the performance deficit.

> **HYPOTHETICAL SCENARIO:**
> **Adding a New Option**
>
> 3D visualization labs are commonly used to provide specialized analysis for selected studies. When a new lab comes on board, what users need to be involved in the workflow training besides those in the 3D lab?

- **Where** to train
  - The outcome of this portion of the analysis should be a list of training facilities available to your department, with a description of features and of the process for reserving these facilities.
  - Determine the facilities that are available for teaching at your site.
    Computer training classrooms:
    - How many workstations? Typically, classes should be no larger than 8–12 users.
    - What hours are classrooms available? When do the end users need to be scheduled?
    - Who will be responsible for loading the application or making it accessible?
    - Is a projection system or other audiovisual equipment available?

    Is there available equipment, unique to your system (scanners, printers, dictation equipment) that can be relocated for training?
    Is there an area that can be set up for follow-up training after the primary training occurs?

If **one-on-one training** is desired, is there a quiet location where this can occur without affecting normal workflow?

– Can all users come to a central location for training or will you need to provide some training in off-site facilities?

– Does your facility have the ability to support web-based training programs? Is there a **learning management system (LMS)?**

An LMS can monitor training use and performance of electronic or web-based learning.

Such systems may negate the need for a training room for updates or small workflow and process changes.

An LMS can provide opportunities for online, instructor-led sessions which can be useful for off-site education.

An LMS requires a major investment in time to create training modules unique to your organization.

- **When** to train
  – Determine how soon before "go live" the training sessions should occur. Users need time to practice skills prior to use. However, training too early will most likely result in loss of

DEFINITION: Learning Management System

System that supports the delivery, tracking, and management of training resources and user evaluations.

FURTHER READING: Effective Use of eLearning

Rudd KE et al. Building workforce capacity for effective use of health information systems: Evaluation of a blended eLearning course in Namibia and Tanzania. Int J Med Inf. 2019;131:103945

KEY CONCEPT: Simulation

Make use of the testing period for new software by having the users participate. Simulation of the live workflow by entering "real" patient information in a test environment will reinforce learning and point out workflow and systems issues not necessarily seen when using "test" patients entered by management or vendor personnel.

skills prior to go live. Group training often occurs just prior to the go-live simulation, and users can practice during the simulation:

Small changes or additions to workflow may be taught with on-the-job training, just prior to first use.

Users receiving one-on-one training prefer to be trained just prior to go live, with on-site support during the go live.

Coordinate all training with area supervisors. There may be other circumstances, such as the arrival of new imaging equipment or other staff commitments, which affect staff availability for training.

If a vendor is involved in training, determine when vendor trainers are available.

Create a user list to determine when trainees are available. Will the facility pay staff to come in off-hours for training?

Develop a **policy and procedure** plan to make training available to new users as they are added to an existing system.

24.2.2 Typical Training Methods

- **Train the trainers**
  - In this scenario, **vendor trainers** train department **superusers**, who then train the remaining staff. Normally superusers become a valuable part of the support for all users in their area, even after go live.

  > **DEFINITION: Superusers**
  >
  > Volunteers who become intimately familiar with the system and can train their peers, both during formal training and during routine use. First adopters often become superusers.

  - Staff chosen for this role should be comfortable with information systems, upbeat, and have a good rapport with the users they train. They will need to understand the workflow of the area and be able to communicate issues to the primary PACS support team.
  - This method requires a large time commitment from department staff. The superusers need to be given time off from their normal duties for training and to get a comfort level with the new system. Superusers need to become experts so that they do not pass on faulty information. Additional cost occurs if a superuser leaves the organization during the training period.
  - Train the trainers also works well for outpatient clinics and referring physician offices. A lead technologist or clinic nurse can be an ideal superuser and provide on-site PACS support.

> **OUR EXPERIENCE: Technologist Superusers**
>
> The superuser roles need not default to the chief technologists if they serve a primarily administrative role. It is best to have a user who works with the system and uses it daily.

- *Vendor training* of all staff
  - Typically, vendors include a set number of hours of training as part of the contract. If the new application is not a major change to workflow, the vendor could train the bulk of the users in the time that it takes to train superusers.
  - This method decreases the time commitment of your staff but may be more expensive and less flexible. This method also requires that provisions be made for training staff who are away when the vendor training takes place as well as off-site users who can't attend the group training.

- A unique issue arises when converting to a new vendor's PACS. Keep in mind that vendor trainers will not be able to relate to existing departmental processes during training and will not be able to help your users **translate old processes** to new ones.

OUR EXPERIENCE: Translation Table

When converting to a new PACS vendor, we found it useful to create a translation table for the training sessions. That way, the vendor trainer and the user trainee can see that "exam type" in one system is "procedure type" in the new system. This facilitated a transfer of skills from one system to the next.

- *IT staff as trainers*
  - Some sites have IT staff that can serve as application trainers. The vendor trains the staff pool in group sessions.
  - Such staff should have the skills to provide adequate to excellent training. However, they need to be pre-trained in the workflow of the department and are not normally available for guidance after go live.
  - Scheduling of IT staff normally must be done well in advance and may not be very flexible to modifications in the training schedule.
- **One-on-one** training
  - Individual training sessions should be used for some users, particularly those who are difficult to schedule (physicians), need customization of an application (radiologist for hanging protocols and standardized dictations), or need more detailed technical information (support staff).
  - Training typically takes place at the user's normal work area in 1-hour sessions just prior to go live.
  - Basic tasks are normally covered in the first session, and plans should be made for follow-up sessions to learn advanced application features or further customize the user's interface. Typically, this occurs after go live and after the user has had 1–2 months to work with the system.
  - Special arrangements may be needed for users that work off-site.
- Electronic and online media
  - **Virtual training modules** can be very useful for training hospital staff who have limited use of the system (e.g., review results in the clinic).
  - Electronic and online media provide a standardized presentation that is accessible at the convenience of the user. If developed in-house, it can be tailored for your organization.
  - A common use of the web facilitates the use of instructional videos that can be streamed on-demand. Placing instructional videos on servers that are internally hosted and behind organizational firewalls allows users to stream videos over the organization's intranet. Instructional videos can also be hosted on web-based commercial platforms. These, combined with some testing on an actual system, may be sufficient for many applications.

- An LMS can monitor whether the user has reviewed the module, prior to allowing access to a system for further training or testing.
- More sophisticated online simulations of workflows and system use can be created, but they require significant programming, the appropriate LMS, and continual modification as workflows change.
- An LMS can incorporate gamification as a method to motivate learners, although it has met with mixed success.

> **FURTHER READINGS: Creating a Virtual Training Platform**
>
> Devolder P, et al. Optimizing physician's instruction of PACS through E-learning: cognitive load theory applied. J Digit Imaging. 2009;22(1):25–33.
> Metzger J, Fortin J. Computerized physician order entry in community hospitals: lessons from the field. Available at: https://www.chcf.org/wp-content/uploads/2017/12/PDF-CPOECommHospCorrected.pdf. Accessed Sept 2020.

24.3 Design and Development

24.3.1 Training Adult Learners

- Training should be relevant. Adult learners need to know why the lesson material is important. Clearly define how the new knowledge is relevant to their job performance. Change is particularly difficult if the reason is not understood. Remember that medical personnel are motivated by patient service goals. It may help to relate the new application to service and your department or hospital strategic plan:
  - Adult learners are generally autonomous and self-directed. They have formed a concept of how they best learn and what their learning needs are. They may be resentful if they feel others are imposing a learning structure on them. Although the material to be presented may be dictated by the software change, users should be involved in planning how the training experience is designed. Classroom situations should be flexible in order to respond to the variety of adult learning styles.

  > **FURTHER READING: Adult Learning Theories**
  >
  > TEAL Center. 2011 https://lincs.ed.gov/sites/default/files/11_%20TEAL_Adult_Learning_Theory.pdf

  - Instructors will need to take into account the learners' foundation of prior experiences and existing knowledge. Adults have an acquired set of habits and biases that can affect learning and may make them resistant to change. This includes prior workflow processes, software terminology, and workplace experiences. Past experiences may facilitate learning if they can be connected to the current learning experience. However, they can be harmful if the training is attempting to effect a change and the change is not described.
  - Adults are receptive to learning information and tasks that they perceive will help them perform. Workflow and expectations are important. Be able to

answer how each step in the workflow will help provide a better result for the patient or fewer system problems with the patient record. Timing is important, as training too soon prior to a change will be met with little enthusiasm.

- Adults are problem-or task-centered learners. They are goal oriented. Clear learning objectives that are tied to specific tasks should be created and shared with learners to motivate their participation. The training environment should be as close as possible to the work environment. On the job, training is very effective but not always practical.
- Adult learning motivation is affected by external and internal factors:

     External motivations: to fulfill the expectations or recommendations of the job or an association (CME), to obtain a better job, or to provide service to the community.

     Internal motivations: to achieve higher job satisfaction, to improve self-esteem, and to learn for the sake of learning.

     Motivation is difficult to sustain if other adult learning principles are not followed during training.

FURTHER READING: Adult Learners

Knowles M, Holton E, Swanson R. The adult learner. New York: Elsevier; 2005. Russell SS. An overview of adult learning processes. Urol Nurs. 2006;26(5):349–52, 370.

24.3.2 Learning Objectives

- Create learning objectives for each task defined for each staff user role.
- Creating course objectives is a process by which abstract goals must be converted into measurable objectives.
- For workflow and software training, the goal is typically defined by a hospital goal. The measured objectives should relate to why the new system was purchased and the change tasks necessary to achieve the goal.
- The value of each objective is that both the learner and the supervisor will know what competency (skill or ability) the learner will acquire from the training.
- Basic concepts and rules of creating measurable learning objectives include:
  - A learning objective should define what the learner will be able to do following the training. Typically, objectives begin with the phrase "After attending this course the student will be able to…."

HYPOTHETICAL SCENARIO: Sample Learning Objectives

After attending this course, the student will be able to:
- Summarize the PACS workflow related to his/her role.
- Set column display preferences on the workflow screen.
- Schedule an inpatient exam appropriately.

– This is followed by an action verb chosen from those found in Bloom's cognitive taxonomy. Verbs range from those that describe the lower levels of learning such as knowledge of material, through mid-levels such as the application of learning to perform a task, to higher levels such as the synthesis of learning to formulate or evaluate new procedures.

> **FURTHER READING: Writing Objectives**
>
> Bloom's Taxonomy of Learning Domains. Available at: https://www.nbna.org/files/Blooms%20Taxonomy%20of%20Learning.pdf. Accessed Sept 2020.

– The verb is then followed by the specific task to be measured.

24.3.3 Select a Delivery Method

- Adult learners need to be accommodated with a variety of training strategies. Typically, three types of adult learners are identified.
  - The **visual learner** prefers documentation and presentations:
    - Provide written instructions, illustrations, charts, and graphs as appropriate.
    - Orient learners to the user manual by describing the table of contents.
    - The visual learner is typically well organized and may study by outlining. Present outlines or "cheat sheets" on how to perform tasks.
    - Use a variety of visual examples of task performance and outcomes, including errors that can occur.

    > **KEY CONCEPT: Cheat Sheets**
    >
    > Manuals typically are multipage and contain screenshots and lengthy text describing how to perform a task. Although useful for training, most users prefer to have single sheet with a brief list of steps and perhaps an icon representing the task button or field.

  - The **auditory learner** prefers verbal instructions and can remember what they are told:
    - Verbal repetition and discussions enable the auditory learner. Rephrase points and present questions in several different ways to stimulate discussion.
    - Jokes and anecdotes are appreciated and may stimulate memory.
    - Auditory learners find it difficult to work quietly for long periods.
    - Incorporate multimedia to vary the speech and aural texture of the presentation.
    - Ensure that the teaching location has adequate acoustics.
  - The **kinesthetic learner** remembers best by getting involved:
    - Has good motor coordination.

Provide many opportunities for hands-on use of the system.

A kinesthetic learner has trouble staying still for a long time. Often, he/she will go ahead of the lesson plan and miss some of the workflow detail.

Provide lots of scenarios to illustrate all facets of workflow. Allow the learner to practice rather than listen.

> **OUR EXPERIENCE: Your Class Consists of Auditory and Kinesthetic Learners**
>
> When this occurs, try having teams of students prepare each scenario and present it to the class. Students are more likely to listen when their peers are presenting, and you can incorporate questions, cautions, and pearls during the presentation.

24.3.4 Creating Materials and Documentation

- Training materials
  - Ask the vendor for training materials. At a minimum, they should have materials for new applications. If the vendor is doing the training, review all materials to make sure they are consistent with your workflow and the expectations you have of each staff role. Obtain electronic copies of training materials and cheat sheets. These can then be modified for your facility(s).
  - Review the materials against the adult learning styles discussed above to assure that you have a variety of presentation styles.
- Documentation
  - As part of any process change, upgrade, or new install, workflow and procedural changes will naturally occur. Documentation should be upgraded as needed to incorporate these changes.
  - The training program should begin with a review of the old workflow and tasks, which should be related to the old workflow. Make copies of the workflow for each of the staff roles being trained.
  - The organization's training manager should review workflow with the vendor and trainers prior to any staff training sessions. It is particularly important to review how the workflow will change. It would be ideal for the trainers to know the system that is being replaced as well. Relating the new application to similar tasks performed on the old system facilitates the transition.
  - As training occurs, it is likely that the workflow will be altered or enhanced. Modification of documentation and training sheets may be required and should be done prior to the next training session.
- Create testing materials that correlate with the learning objectives:
  - Review vendor testing materials. Typically, this testing consists of simulated scenarios that require the user to perform the appropriate steps in the application.
  - Confirm that the materials cover all common scenarios and workflow variations such as:

Points in the workflow that require a user to decide the appropriate action

Steps required to recognize or correct errors

- Validate that training and testing materials are consistent with the course objectives:
  - Each objective should have corresponding teaching and testing materials.
  - Do the materials cover the breadth of information needed to do the jobs?
  - What are the expectations for determination of readiness or passing the course?

24.4 Implementation

24.4.1 Schedule

- Create a training plan to include days, times, locations, and users being trained.
- The plan should be finalized at least 1 month in advance and made available to all users being trained as well as to the trainers:
  - Scheduling should be done by user role so that users only receive training on areas that are within their job scope.
  - Work with administrators and supervisors to determine a training schedule that is consistent with department operations. If staff are trained during their normal shift, insist that department operations are reduced during the training period.

  > **FURTHER READING: Learning Participant Roles**
  >
  > Transfer of Learning: A Guide for Strengthening the Performance of Health Care Workers. Available at http://reprolineplus.org/resources/transfer-learning-guide-strengthening-performance-health-care-workers. Accessed Sept 2020.

  - Third-party applications may require a separate training schedule and arrangements with the third-party vendor.
  - Follow-up, post go-live training may be required for advanced applications. Examples include advanced hanging protocol setup or third-party image processing applications.

24.4.2 Preparation

- Preparation of the site learning environment is essential to training success:
  - The goal of any training is to enable an employee to utilize the skills learned in the training sessions on their job. Transfer of learning happens best when an employee has appropriate ability, motivation, and environment factors in place [1, 2].
  - **Ability to transfer** is enabled by:

A match between the training content, environment, and the tasks learned

Availability of resources and decreased workload to enable study

Physical workplace design to enable use of new skills

Ability to immediately use the new skills on the job

- **Motivation to transfer** is affected by:

    Employees' desire to improve skills

    Trainer's style

    Expectations of the job

- **Environment to transfer** factors include:

    Organizational support and involvement from supervisors and peers.

    Establishment of specific goals and regular and follow-up feedback from trainers and supervisors.

    Defined match between department and organizational goals and the new learning material.

    Secondary influences seen to affect motivation and training success include employee disposition, attitudes, and the organization's learning culture.

    Review issues with the department administrator and supervisors to eliminate any environmental factors that may impede staff from learning and performing their new duties.

- Set up the training system:

    Set up your test system for training with all or a representative sample of the dictionaries on the live system. Many users will want to try scenarios beyond those planned for the training class. The more real that you can make the training system, the more relevant the training will be.

    Set up users with the roles and privileges that they will have in the live system. Eliminating extraneous options and screens in the training environment will reduce confusion when users transition to production.

    Have the trainers create the patients and studies required for their training scenarios. Scenarios should be as close to the job experience as possible. When training staff, make sure that there is time for the learners to construct their own scenarios and to make and correct errors.

- Create ongoing training and support materials:

    Knowledge retention depends on frequent use of information. Seldom-performed tasks benefit from electronic performance support systems [3].

> **KEY CONCEPT: Employee Motivation**
>
> An employee will consider training as important only if their supervisor does. A trainee should not have to worry about the work that is piling up while they are in training. Bring in extra staff or schedule downtime during training.

> **FURTHER READING: Employee Motivation**
>
> Perryer C, Celestine NA, Scott-Ladd B, Leighton C. Enhancing workplace motivation through gamification: transferrable lessons from pedagogy. Int J Manage Educ. 2016;14:327–335.

A study by Nguyen [4] concluded that end users preferred context-sensitive and online help features offered within the systems. In this survey, users preferred to click on a help button to open a window providing information on how to perform a task. Users also desired the ability to bookmark or print these help pages.

Traditionally cheat sheets should be laminated and placed near workstations for routine tasks and, perhaps more importantly, seldom-performed tasks.

> **OUR EXPERIENCE: Aiding the Transition**
>
> Many users adapt more quickly to a software application change if you can directly relate your new application to the system they currently use. Do this by creating workflow documents with screenshots of the old and new procedures.

24.5 Evaluation

24.5.1 Learning Cycle

- Most educational assessment tasks involve both formative and summative assessments:
  - **Formative assessment** monitors the learning progress throughout the learning cycle. The intent is to give rapid feedback to motivate learning and to give the teacher the ability to adjust the teaching process.
  - **Summative assessments** are performed at the end of a learning cycle. Often, they include an exam that measures what the student has learned and/or what the teacher has successfully taught. They can include on-the-job assessments as well.
- Both processes are necessary ways to monitor training activities in the workplace. They are useful only if they provide an accurate assessment and are used to enhance the training program.
- Assessment measures should be developed along with the training plan since they should be a measure of how well the goals of the training are achieved:
  - **Authentic assessment** practices became popular in the 1990s to assess whether the training received actually enhances job performance. A common scheme for authentic assessment of corporate training programs was developed by Donald Kirkpatrick [5].

> **DEFINITION: Authentic Assessment**
>
> Using real work tasks in the actual work environment to evaluate the success of training

- The **Kirkpatrick four levels** of evaluation included:
  - Level 1: Evaluation of reaction. How did the students like the program? Did it meet their needs? This is done by surveys that ask the users to evaluate the topics, materials, course design, and instructor. An inference is made that positive employee reactions to the training program motivate learning. This level of assessment is used to enhance training materials and course content but does not test whether any learning has occurred.
  - Level 2: Evaluation of learning. Both self-assessment by the users as to whether the program met their learning goals and skill testing of learners by the instructor during the training session are performed. Such exams can assess skill level at the time of the instruction but do not necessarily indicate whether those skills are retained on the job. A study by Ford and Weissbein [6] concluded that only 10–30% of such knowledge translated into on-the-job skills.
  - Level 3: Evaluation of the transfer of learning to the job. On-the-job assessment of skills learned is typically done by a supervisor. Assessments should be based around scenarios and requirements key to the learners' job. Results may be affected by supervisor distraction or by the type of work environment at the time of the review. Modern applications using computer-based performance testing can remove the bias of supervisor assessment for computer-based tasks [7].

> **FURTHER READING:**
> **Kirkpatrick Model, Four Levels of Learning Evaluation**
>
> https://educationaltechnology.net/kirk-patrick-model-four-levels-learning-evaluation/

  - Level 4: Evaluation of business process improvements that result from enhanced user training. Typically, this includes such enhancements as improved quality, production, sales, customer satisfaction, or reduced costs. This type of evaluation is most beneficial when justifying ongoing training program resources to managers. However, proper evaluation requires isolation of the contribution of training versus other process changes that may have contributed to the enhancement of these outcomes.

> **CHECKLIST: Skills Testing Metrics**
>
> 1. Were the correct tasks performed?
> 2. Were the tasks done in the right order?
> 3. Was the proper result obtained?
> 4. Was the task performed in a timely manner?

24.5.2 Financial Assessment

- Return on investment (ROI) analysis can provide a financial assessment of a training program:
  - ROI analysis is done to justify the cost of providing a training program by providing the management a monetary return on investment.

- Typical analyses build on the data collected using the Kirkpatrick model.
- Common metrics used include the benefit/cost ratio (BCR) or a traditional ROI. (For thoughts on the current status of ROI analysis, see [8]; see Deller, 2020 in Further Readings below)
- ROI analysis can be considered as Level 5 of evaluation. [9].

STEP-BY-STEP: ROI Analysis

1. Collect data from Kirkpatrick's Level 4.
2. Assess whether the application had a measurable result.
3. Isolate effects due to training.
4. Convert results to monetary benefits.
5. Determine the cost of training.
6. Compare the monetary benefits to the cost.

- Pros
  - Administration is able to see a tangible value to training.
  - Helps to point out where training activities are most effective for the organization's profit.
  - Allows one to justify an ongoing budget for training.
- Cons
  - Isolating the effects of a specific training can be difficult.
  - Calculating the benefits of the training can be very subjective.
  - Analysis can be very time-consuming, especially if the application involves many users or processes.
- In healthcare, competency testing [10] is done at four levels of assessment that correspond closely to those of Fitzpatrick. Studies however involve technical skills, problem-solving, and patient interactions that are beyond the scope of the standard PACS training environment.

FURTHER READINGS: Further Measures and Details of an ROI Analysis

Brauchle PE, Schmidt, K. Contemporary Approaches for assessing outcomes on training, education and HRD programs. J Indus Teacher Educ Fall. 2004;41(3).

Deller J. 5 easy ways to measure the ROI of training 2020. https://kodosurvey.com/blog/5-easy-ways-measure-roi-training Accessed September 2020.

Evaluating Training and Results https://managementhelp.org/training/systematic/ROI-evaluating-training.htm#roi

https://www.bptrends.com/publicationfiles/10-08-ART-UsingROItoMeasure-ResultsofBPI-Initiatives-Westcott-final.doc.pdf

24.5.3 Creating Assessment Materials

- Important considerations in creating **survey and testing materials** include:
  - Align exam/survey content with training course objectives. Make sure that you are testing what you want the student to learn.
  - The time devoted to testing a concept should reflect its relative importance.

> **KEY CONCEPT: Professional Competency Assessment Levels**
>
> - *Knows* (factual recall)
> - *Knows how* (describes procedure)
> - *Shows how* (performs in controlled setting)
> - *Does* (performs in real setting)

- The most common form of program evaluation is the survey. These can be effectively used for levels 1, 2, and 4 of the Fitzpatrick model.
- Survey implementation typically involves five steps:
  - Establish the goal of the survey. What do you want to know? For user satisfaction during training, this typically includes whether the training materials and presentation are clear and easy to follow, whether the learning environment is appropriate (proper lighting, visuals, and sound system), and whether the users feel the material is relevant to his or her job duties. For process improvement evaluation (Level 4), this may include patient or referral satisfaction surveys.
  - Plan the survey design:
    - What is the appropriate survey length and question format?
    - What are the response choices: yes/no and rating scale.
    - Are there biases in the design?
    - Do you have a budget to produce and analyze the survey?
  - Write the questions keeping in mind the training goals and keeping the wording simple. For Level 1, are you asking questions about training areas that you can actually change?
  - Test your survey on a few volunteers. They can let you know if items and responses are clear

> **FURTHER READINGS: Survey Development**
>
> https://dash.harvard.edu/bitstream/handle/1/8138346. Accessed Sept 2020
> https://psr.iq.harvard.edu/files/psr/files/PSRQuestionnaireTipSheet_0.pdf. Accessed Sept 2020

  and reasonable and if the survey is appropriately formatted. Modify the survey as appropriate.
  - Implement and evaluate the survey. Make sure that you allot enough time for respondents to thoroughly fill out the survey. Record the responses, looking for trends.

- Skill testing in Fitzpatrick Level 2 can be done by several means:
  - Each student is presented with a checklist of tasks to perform. Checklists are useful when a task can be broken down into a standard list of specific actions and responses. Checklists can be made to lead the student through a task, giving them a means to review the process. An instructor can monitor proper performance. The instructor often sees only the endpoint and not the path or time required for the student to perform the task.

FURTHER READING: Test Questions

Collins J. Education techniques for lifelong learning: writing multiple choice questions for continuing medical education activities and self-assessment modules. Radiographics. 2006;26(2):543–51.

Brame C. Writing good multiple choice questions (2013). https://cft.vanderbilt.edu/guides-sub-pages/writing-good-multiple-choice-test-questions/.

  - The student is given a written exam, often requiring the user to perform a software task correctly in order to determine the correct answer to a question. Questions can be constructed to alter the context of the real-world situation and assess the student's response. Questions must be carefully constructed to be clear and avoid bias.
- Fitzpatrick Level 3 on-the-job skill testing is more difficult to perform. Typical scenarios may include:
  - A supervisor reviews a worker's performance by observing the worker perform a task. Reporting relies on the supervisor's memory and can be influenced by the work environment at the time of the testing. Some days are just more hectic than others.
  - A department quality assurance program is established to review the timeliness and accuracy of system use. This is only effective if there is an accurate and easily accessible audit trail of which user has performed each task. This also requires the ability for a systems person to create summary reports of job performance measures such as number of studies performed, QA errors, or turnaround times for specific users.

24.6 Follow-Up

- A training and quality assurance program should be an ongoing process of teaching and evaluation.
- Use survey results to enhance the program for new users and new application training needs.
- Monitor user performance to assess when refresher or remedial training is required.

PEARLS

- User training is required before, during, and after any information system install or upgrade to assure productivity, data accuracy and quality throughout the hospital enterprise.
- Training programs should encompass well-defined learning objectives, training techniques that incorporate adult learning styles, and assessment strategies that provide feedback on training success and program enhancement.
- The transfer of skills from the learning environment to the real-life clinical environment requires opportunities for training during simulation and consideration of the environmental factors that may impede skill transfer.
- Monitoring and testing of job skills, with the opportunity for retraining, is required to assure consistent quality.
- It is difficult to perform a financial justification (ROI) of a training program. Therefore, training needs to be justified by improved quality of service.

References

1. Choi M, Ruona WEA. An update on the learning transfer system. Paper presented at the Academy of Human Resource Development International Research Conference in the Americas. Panama City, FL, 2008.
2. Holton EF, Bates RA, Ruona WEA. Development of a generalized learning transfer system inventory. Hum Resour Dev Q. 2000;11(4):333–60.
3. Gery G. Electronic performance support systems. Weingarten: Boston; 1991.
4. Nguyen F. EPSS needs assessment: oops, I forgot how to do that! Perform Improv. 2005;44(9):33–93.
5. Kirkpatrick DL. Evaluating training programs: the four levels. San Francisco: Berrett-Koehler; 1998.
6. Ford JK, Weissbein DA. Transfer of training: an updated review and analysis. Perform Improv. 1997;10(2):22–41.
7. Galloway DL. Evaluating distance delivery and e-learning. Perform Improv. 2005;44(4):21–7.
8. Phillips JJ, Phillips PP. Distinguishing ROI myths from reality. Perform Improv. 2008;47(6):12–7.
9. Westcott G. Using ROI to measure the results of business process improvement initiatives 2008.
10. Miller GE. The assessment of clinical skills/competence/performance. Acad Med. 1990;65(9 Suppl):S63–7.

Self-Assessment Questions

1. A good example of a learning objective for a training session on the QA module of a PACS system is: "At the completion of this course the user will be able to...

   (a) Define the image QA module."
   (b) Do image QA."
   (c) Successfully resolve typical image QA issues using the QA module."
   (d) Avoid creating image QA issues."

2. An important document which should be developed **prior to designing** the user training program is:

   (a) User workflow
   (b) Cheat sheets
   (c) ROI
   (d) Translation tables

3. A training method that provides the advantage of having departmental user support persons long after go live is:

   (a) Vendor training of all staff individually
   (b) Train the trainers
   (c) IT training of department users
   (d) One-on-one training

4. The type of adult learner who benefits most from illustrations and cheat sheets during training is:

   (a) Kinesthetic learner
   (b) Auditory learner
   (c) Visual learner
   (d) All of the above

5. An opportunity for training in a "real patient" environment is best provided during:

   (a) One-on-one training
   (b) Group training in a classroom
   (c) User presentations in the classroom
   (d) Simulation prior to "go live"

6. Formative assessments of learning progress are done to:

   (a) Motivate learners
   (b) Enhance training programs
   (c) Improve the teaching process
   (d) All of the above

7. What are four processes that should be included in a training program?

8. How are learning objectives used in the design of a training program?

9. ROI analysis of user training programs can provide:

   (a) Justification for ongoing training
   (b) An easy way to show training value
   (c) Resolution of user complaints about the system

10. An LMS allows:

   (a) Easy generation of user training modules
   (b) Methods for generation of training workflows
   (c) Management of user training progress

Chapter 25
Quality Improvement and Workflow Engineering

Matthew B. Morgan and Barton F. Branstetter IV

Contents

25.1 Introduction

Over the past decade, "quality" has emerged as its own discipline within radiology, with its own definitions and tools. Quality can be subdivided into quality control (QC), quality assurance (QA), and quality improvement (QI). These terms are often used loosely, but they do have specific meanings (see box).

M. B. Morgan (✉)
Department of Radiology, University of Utah, Salt Lake City, UT, USA
e-mail: Matt.Morgan@hsc.utah.edu

B. F. Branstetter IV
Department of Radiology, University of Pittsburgh, Pittsburgh, PA, USA
e-mail: BFB1@pitt.edu

© The Author(s), under exclusive license to Springer Science+Business Media,
LLC, part of Springer Nature 2021
B. F. Branstetter IV (ed.), *Practical Imaging Informatics*,
https://doi.org/10.1007/978-1-0716-1756-4_25

409

DEFINITION: Quality in Medical Imaging

The extent to which the right procedure is done in the right way, at the right time, and the correct interpretation is accurately and quickly communicated to the patient and referring physician.

FURTHER READING: Quality

Hillman BJ, Amis ES, Neiman HL. The future quality and safety of medical imaging: proceedings of the third annual ACR FORUM. J Am Coll Radiol. 2004;1(1):33–9.

DEFINITIONS: QA/QC/QI

Quality Control (QC)

A process for measuring and testing elements of performance at an **individual level**. For example, a radiologist corrects errors in a radiology report before signing it.

Quality Assurance (QA)

A process for monitoring and ensuring quality at an **organizational level**. For example, a department mandates standardized templates to minimize errors in reports.

Quality Improvement (QI)

A process for improving performance quality at an **organizational level in a systematic and sustainable way**. For example, a department implements a standardized report system with ongoing monitoring, feedback, and accountability.

25.2 Establish an Organizational Foundation

25.2.1 Leadership

- Set direction for QI with strong **patient focus**.
- Create **clear statements** of organizational mission and values and set operational objectives.
- Includes **systematic cycles** of planning, execution, and evaluation.

DEFINITION: Mission Statement Versus Vision Statement

A mission statement defines the purpose of a company, institution, or working group. Mission statements include current objectives and the approach to those objectives.

A vision statement, on the other hand, is aspirational – what do we want to become?

In other words, mission statements focus on today, while vision statements focus on tomorrow.

25.2.2 Key Staff Roles

- **Project champion** (sponsor) provides organizational oversight; sets the goals of the project; liaisons between the QI team, other providers, and leadership; and **evangelizes the need** for change/improvement. He/she should have organizational authority to provide resources, remove barriers, and resolve conflicts.

- **Project manager** (day-to-day leader) organizes and drives ongoing work, measurement, milestones, reporting, and follow-up. He/she serves as "key contact" and communicator. He/she should have strong organizational and leadership skills.

FURTHER READING: Project Management

Larson DB, Mickelsen LJ. Project management for quality improvement in radiology. AJR Am J Roentgenol. 2015;205:W470–7

- **Project supporters** provide perspectives and skills needed for the project. Examples include frontline clinical staff, data analysts, and IT support.

- **Project coach** is an expert in quality improvement methods (e.g., plan-do-study-act, six sigma) who advises and supports the team. This may be an internal expert or an outside consultant.

CHECKLIST: Readiness Assessment

- Is there QI understanding and leadership?
- Are the right people in the key roles, and do they understand the expectations?
- Are adequate resources dedicated to QI?
- Does the organization routinely and systematically collect and analyze data?

25.3 Project-Based Improvement

25.3.1 When to Initiate a QI Project

- Do it now if you haven't already (be proactive).
- Change in technology (e.g., introducing PACS, new PACS vendor, digital radiology, paperless workflow).
- New IT department.
- Major personnel change.
- Complaints from personnel about inefficiencies.
- Complaints from customers (better late than never, but you should avoid this reactive approach).

25.3.2 Identify the Problem

- A "problem" is any source of trouble in the workflow. Clearly define it. Make sure it is of high importance.
- Identify pain points.

> **DEFINITION: Pain Points**
>
> The problems that are most troubling to your users. Seemingly small issues can become pain points when they are encountered frequently, for example, needing two extra clicks to open an examination. If you read 200 cases in a day, that's a lot of clicks.

25.3.3 Form a Team

- Organize a dedicated team (see "Key Staff Roles" above) for a defined time period. This team is empowered to provide guidance, resources, and instruction and authorized to make process and organizational changes that improve performance in a sustainable way.

25.3.4 Identify Methodology

- **Plan-Do-Study-Act (PDSA)**
- Six sigma methods:
    - DMAIC = Define, measure, analyze, improve, and control.
    - DMADV = Define, measure, analyze, design, and verify.

FURTHER READING: QI Methodology

Plan-Do-Study-Act (PDSA) Worksheet|IHI – Institute for Healthcare Improvement. http://www.ihi.org/resources/Pages/Tools/PlanDoStudyActWorksheet.aspx.

FURTHER READING: Six Sigma

What is Six Sigma? A Complete Overview. https://www.simplilearn.com/what-is-six-sigma-a-complete-overview-article#

25.3.5 Observe Current Performance

- Survey
  - Relatively easy source of information.
  - May be formal (online or paper survey) or informal (division meetings).
  - Good for identifying pain points.
  - Low response rates (25–30% is typical)
  - Notoriously inaccurate – what workers **say** they do is often not what they *really* do:
    What managers say that their employees do is even less reliable.
  - Biased – people with "an axe to grind" and/or people who are most satisfied may be more likely to respond.
- *Direct observation*
  - **Visit the workplace** and spend time observing and taking notes.
  - Ask questions to deeply understand the process: what is done and why it is done that way.
  - Not quantifiable (but may not need to be).
  - Should be performed by someone who is familiar with the job (ideally someone who has worked in that job).
  - Convene and discuss observations, map out the process, and revisit the workplace to validate observations.

PERTINENT QUOTE: Survey Inaccuracy

If you asked a gorilla what he would like for his next evolutionary step, he would answer, "bigger muscles and longer fangs." He wouldn't ask for a larger cranial capacity. – Rudy Rucker

KEY CONCEPT: Prioritize

Prioritize observing people whose jobs are most time sensitive and expensive (radiologists, technologists), and identify processes tied to the main function of the department (obtaining and interpreting images).

- Time-motion study:
  - The most scientific approach
  - Provides quantitative data
  - Time-consuming

> **KEY CONCEPT: Time-Motion Study**
>
> A formal workflow analysis tool that measures the amount of time spent (and wasted) on every workflow step.

STEP-BY-STEP: Time-Motion Study

1. Videotape the worker doing their job.
2. Play the video and make a list of every workflow step that the worker performs, no matter how seemingly trivial (e.g., clicks the finalize button).
3. Replay the video again, using a stopwatch (or video timer) to measure the exact amount of time spent on each step.
4. The total amount of time allotted to each step should exactly match the total time working.
5. Analyze the process to discover bottlenecks and pain points.

25.3.6 Measure Performance

- Outcome measures (morbidity, length of stay, patient satisfaction, costs).
- Process measures (turnaround time, modality utilization rates, process adherence).
- Process mapping tools
  - Value stream mapping:
    aka Toyota Production System.
    Make a diagram showing the current steps, delays, and flow of information and personnel.
    Highlight bottlenecks.
  - *Run chart*
    Graph key workflow metrics such as number of undictated cases, average patient wait times, and employee over time (Fig. 25.1).
    Identify times where workflow efficiency is hindered.
    Measure before and after intervention.

25.3.7 Identify Problems and Causes

- Seek to discover and document the causes of problems that negatively impact performance.
- Use a **fishbone diagram** to show cause-and-effect relationships (Fig. 25.2).

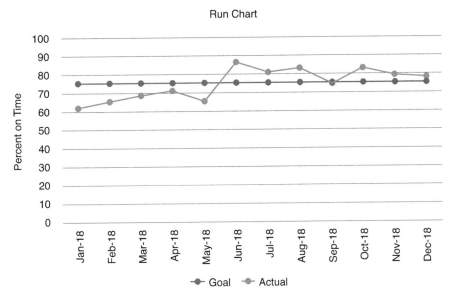

Fig. 25.1 Run chart. Desired measure (y-axis) is plotted against time (x-axis). Desired value is overlaid as a target threshold

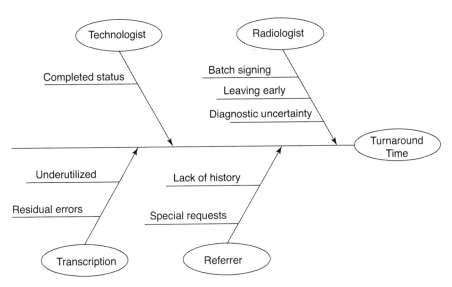

Fig. 25.2 Fishbone diagram. The desired outcome is placed on the right. Each contributing factor is a "rib," with potential causes listed along the rib

Fig. 25.3 Pareto graph. The problem is broken down into contributing factors, which are ordered by degree of impact so that the factors with the highest impact can get the highest priority

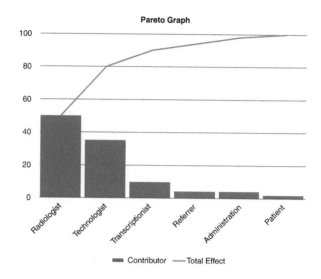

- Prioritize most important issues.
  - Pareto analysis:
      Assumes that 80% of delays are caused by 20% of workflow elements.
      Pareto graphs can focus attention on key workflow steps (Fig. 25.3).
  - Prioritization matrix:
      Quantify each pain point in terms of frequency, severity of impact, and feasibility of correction.
      Allow you to determine which projects to tackle first.
      Use "low-hanging fruit" (high impact, easy to fix) concerns to build employee confidence in the concept of workflow engineering.

25.3.8 Develop and Implement Solutions

- Use **iterative cycles** to test, refine, and validate changes (e.g., multiple PDSA cycles).

25.3.9 Sustain Improvement

- Establish regular measurement and feedback.
- Consider "handoffs" to enforce standards for changing personnel.
- When problems are encountered, stop and summon supervisors to investigate.
- Embed checks into the process.
- Make it easy to do it right.

25.4 Workflow Engineering

> **DEFINITION: Workflow**
>
> The steps that employees perform as they are getting their work done, and the relationships between those steps.

> **DEFINITION: Workflow Bottleneck**
>
> The most inefficient step in a process; the step that defines the maximum rate at which the entire process can proceed.

25.4.1 Workflow Enhancements

1. Customization

Workflow should be optimized for each working environment. Workflow that is optimal under certain circumstances may be inadequate with slight changes in working conditions. Optimization should be optimized at multiple levels:

- **User**: Knowledge workers should be able to adjust ergonomics of workspace, presentation/appearance of software, and communication tools, to reflect their own idiosyncratic needs.

- **Modality**: The workflow that is best for CT scanners differs from the workflows needed for digital radiographs. Similarly: inpatient vs. outpatient scanners; in-hospital vs. imaging center scanners.

> **FURTHER READING: Workflow**
>
> **Chapter 16** describes the specific workflow steps for radiology employees; this chapter provides information about measuring and redesigning workflow.

- **Division**: Workflows optimized for neuroradiology may not be optimal for musculoskeletal imaging.

- **Department**: Radiologists require workflows that focuses on "which scans require interpretation," whereas clinical departments focus on those patients who are currently in-house or currently in the clinic, regardless of whether the images have been formally reviewed.

- **Hospital**: Large academic centers have different workflows than small private hospital settings, whereas different hospitals may have local idiosyncrasies of hospital culture that define workflow.

- **Enterprise**: Geographic and cultural differences prevent us from taking a specific workflow from one institution and applying it to another institution without the addition of local modifications. Major software vendors often overlook the need for this level of customization.

- **Patient throughput vs. information throughput**: It is important to not only optimize the flow of patients through the department but also the flow of information.

2. Integration

Whenever a worker must change from one work environment to another, there is a disruption in workflow, the potential to introduce error, and a degradation in efficiency:

- Moving from room to room.
- Moving from one computer to another (from a scanner to a nearby computer or from the PACS workstation to a post-processing workstation).
- Switching between software applications on a single computer.
- The **integration of multiple software systems** (PACS, RIS, dictation, electronic health record) into a single, unified working environment is particularly important for radiologists.
- Integrating the Healthcare Enterprise (IHE) is a national initiative focused on improving the way computers share information through coordinating the use of established standards. Decision makers in imaging informatics should be familiar with IHE and **insist that software vendors comply** with the established standards.

CHECKLIST: Systems That Should Integrate with PACS

1. Speech recognition/dictation
2. Post-processing/advanced visualization
3. Clinical decision support tools (e.g., online knowledge bases)
4. Communication tools (phone lists, preliminary report tools, protocolling software)
5. Teaching files
6. Clinical data sources (RIS, HIS, EMR)
7. Clinical dashboards

3. Dashboards

- Dashboards combine key indicators from multiple systems into one unified view to support decision-making.
- Digital dashboards summarize the state of a complex work environment so that workers can remain aware of potentially overlooked events or unsuspected failures.

DEFINITION: Dashboard Display

A graphical interface that summarizes input from many sources into a small visual area that can be quickly understood. More detailed information is available by expanding individual elements of the dashboard.

- Dashboards are customized to provide different information to different workers (e.g., radiologists need to know how many unread cases are on the PACS, whereas IT personnel need to know if hard drives are becoming full).

FURTHER READING: Dashboards

Morgan MB, Branstetter BF, Chang PJ. Flying blind: using a digital dashboard to navigate a complex PACS environment. J Digital Imaging 2006;19(1):69–75.

- Dashboards can be developed by in-house software engineers. Some vendors are starting to incorporate dashboard features into their products.

4. Load balancing

Maximum efficiency can be achieved if the work can be distributed equitably between workers. It is undesirable to have some personnel overworked while others are idle. There are practical limitations on how much of the work can be conveniently distributed, but there are also software implementations that can assist with load balancing, and these should be investigated:

DEFINITION: Load Balancing

Ensuring that work is distributed optimally to avoid having some workers (or IT components) idle while others are overworked.

- Load balancing does not apply only to workers but to all resources in the enterprise, such as computer servers and networks.
- If possible, patients should also be load balanced between sites of care.

5. Asynchronous communication

Traditionally, knowledge workers have relied on communication models that require both parties to be available at the same time (such as a phone call). When workers can instead communicate at their convenience, each worker can minimize the disruption to their own workflow.

Examples in radiology:

- Radiologists communicating preliminary or unexpected results to referring clinicians.
- Technologists requesting protocol or other scanning information from radiologists.
- Electronic messaging software can be integrated into radiology and clinical workflows to support asynchronous communication.

DEFINITION: Asynchronous Communication

Two workers communicate asynchronously when they do not need to be simultaneously available. Thus, each worker can integrate the data into their workflow more efficiently. Email is the most familiar example of asynchronous communication.

FURTHER READING: Asynchronous Communication

Branstetter BF, Paterson B, Lionetti DM, Chang PJ. Asynchronous collaboration: an enabling technique for improved radiology workflow. J Digital Imaging. 2003; 16: 44–45.

6. Base case workflow design

Software systems are often designed such that any conceivable functionality is always immediately available. This creates confusing interfaces, because the most frequently used options are hidden in a sea of rarely needed features. Workflow should be designed to address the base case; this may result in rarely needed tasks becoming more difficult to access, but will save time on average.

7. Defined roles

- Each worker should have well-defined responsibilities.
- These responsibilities should cover all the needed tasks.
- Minimize overlap between workers' responsibilities.
- Failing to do this allows workflow gaps, and tasks may fall through the cracks.

DEFINITION: Base Case

The base case is the most frequent task that is performed. Workflow design should address the base case first and foremost, even if less frequently utilized workflows are made less efficient. For example, radiologists often use distance measurements – this function should be easily available, even if it would make more logical sense to have it in the same place as all the other PACS tools.

KEY CONCEPT: Workflow Gaps

"If it's everyone's responsibility, it's no one's responsibility."

For every task, make sure that there is a specific person who knows that they are responsible and can say "the buck stops here."

8. Redundancy

- Redundancy is critical in clinical personnel, just as it is in IT systems.
- Cross-training clinical personnel is essential to assure that all work can be performed regardless of scheduling (i.e., if only one individual knows how to perform a particular task, then the task cannot get done when that individual is unavailable).
- It is acceptable to have subject matter experts or superusers, but critical workflow-dependent knowledge should be shared.

9. Intuitive workflow design

- Make it easy to do the right thing – the path of least resistance should correspond to the desired workflow.
- Workers who must jump hurdles to perform workflow tasks will find workarounds that may subvert the intended workflow.

SYNONYMS: Intuitive Workflow

- Dummy proofing
- Mistake proofing
- "Path of least resistance" workflow

10. Appropriate workspace layout

- Often-used devices and computer should be placed near to each other.
- Minimize the distance that a worker needs to travel, especially for often-repeated tasks.

25.4.2 Workflow Bottlenecks

1. Extra steps

Small workflow inefficiencies are easy to overlook and may not be important for infrequent tasks. However, a small inefficiency that is repeated dozens of times per day is frustrating and inefficient.

Examples in radiology:

- Manual hanging protocols requiring the same step over and over again
- Unnecessary dictation steps (i.e., repeating the medical record number, patient name, type of exam, etc.)

Potential solution: work with vendors to eliminate extra steps.

> **HYPOTHETICAL SCENARIO:**
> **Small Inefficiencies**
>
> The radiologist needs to launch comparison cases on every patient because they don't launch automatically. The cost is only a single mouse click per patient, but if the radiologist reads hundreds of cases per day, it adds up.

2. Paper tokens

If your department needs to pass a piece of paper from person to person in order to continue the workflow, the paper can get lost, or workers can be idle waiting for the paper when they could instead be completing the next task.

- Potential solution: implement a "paperless workflow" to decouple radiologist and technologist workflows.

> **DEFINITION: Workflow Token**
>
> Reminder or indicator that a workflow task requires attention. Usually a physical object is passed from one person to another. Examples include paper exam requisitions and typed dictations to be signed.

3. Out-of-band tasks

- Workflow steps that are infrequently performed or are not part of the usual workflow are easily overlooked:
  - Example: Signing reports in a separate application (RIS) when the majority of the radiologist's time is spent in the image interpretation environment (PACS)
  - Especially true if more than one person shares responsibility for the task
- Potential solution: Implement a "digital dashboard" that tracks key indicators and facilitates task prioritization and task switching.

> **DEFINITION: Out-of-Band Task**
>
> A task that is not part of the routine workflow and must instead be performed while normal workflow is suspended. Workers often forget to perform out-of-band tasks.

4. Manual data entry

- Slow and prone to error (**fat-finger errors**).
- Example: Typing a medical record number into a scanner.
- Potential solution: Population of data fields should be automated (e.g., with IHE).

> **DEFINITION: Fat-Finger Error**
>
> Manual typing is inherently error-prone, especially when the data is numerical. Fat-finger errors are typographical errors that could be avoided by pre-populating data fields.

5. Interruptions

Although some are unavoidable, distractions and/or interruptions are a problem for knowledge workers who are performing complex tasks. At best, they reduce efficiency, and at worst, they may cause cognitive errors due to lapses in attention.

- Examples include phone calls, pages, and software alerts (e.g., email).
- Potential solutions:
  - Minimize workflow interruptions by assigning one worker to triage phone calls.
  - Implement asynchronous communication models where appropriate.

6. Task switching

- Moving between separate and/or isolated computers or software systems reduces efficiency.
- Potential solution: Integration of software and hardware decreases wasted movement.

7. Low signal-to-noise ratio

Though most often applied to the physics of image acquisition and display, the concept of **signal-to-noise ratio (SNR)** can also apply to a work environment:

- The complexity of a working environment can reduce the ability of knowledge workers to prioritize new information. An example of this occurs when urgent studies are "lost" in a long list of routine studies.

> **DEFINITION: Flag**
>
> Reminder or indicator that new data is available. Usually it is an auditory or visual cue within a software program. For example, "You've got mail!"

- Flags can be used to alert users to high priority tasks:
  - Workers must be able to trust that a signal to perform a workflow task is reliable. If a worker is sent on a wild-goose chase by an incorrect flag, that worker will learn to ignore the flag.

PEARLS

- Quality improvement (QI) is a process for monitoring and ensuring quality at an organizational level in a systematic and sustainable way
- A QI team should have the right people in the right roles to succeed.
- Direct observation is the most accurate and effective method to review a process.
- What people *say* they do is not necessarily what they *really* do.
- Any major change in technology merits a workflow analysis.
- The "Holy Grail" is the integration of all workflow onto a single workstation.
- Workflow must be customized to different individuals and different work environments.
- Integration of different software applications is particularly critical for radiologists.
- Frequently performed tasks by highly trained or highly paid individuals should receive the most attention when redesigning workflow.
- Interruptions and distractions are the largest barriers to efficient workflow.

Self-Assessment Questions

1. Which of the following is the **least** reliable method of workflow analysis?

    (a) Informal discussions
    (b) Formal surveys
    (c) Time-motion studies
    (d) Direct observation

2. Which of the following workflow problems should receive the most attention?

    (a) Low-frequency, high-time-commitment tasks.
    (b) Pain points.
    (c) Administrator workflow.
    (d) All of the above are equally important.

3. All of the following enhance workflow **except**:

    (a) Dashboards
    (b) Base case workflow design
    (c) Redundancy of key personnel
    (d) Paper tokens

4. Which of the following scenarios is most appropriate for asynchronous communication:

   (a) Alerting an emergency department physician to emergent radiologic findings.
   (b) Consulting a radiologist for an allergic contrast reaction.
   (c) Communicating the need for a 6-month follow-up examination.
   (d) Asynchronous communication is appropriate for all of the above.

5. Which of these changes should prompt a workflow analysis?

   (a) Introduction of new technology
   (b) Major personnel change
   (c) Complaints from personnel about software inefficiencies
   (d) All of the above

6. Imagine that your department installs digital radiography equipment that can perform X-rays five times faster than traditional equipment. You will have to redesign workflows for many different workers: radiologists, technologists, administrators, and even patients. Which of these is the most critical to take best advantage of your new equipment?

7. Describe how you would perform a time-motion study of a CT technologist.

8. If you were a gorilla, what would you choose as your next evolutionary step?

Chapter 26
Change Management and Acceptance Testing

Gary S. Norton

Contents

26.1 Introduction

Picture Archiving and Communication System (PACS) has become ubiquitous in the healthcare environment; many facilities have had a PACS for over 30 years. So, if you are looking at a chapter on change management and acceptance testing (AT), then it can be assumed that your PACS environment is about to change or has changed. Replacing or changing a PACS is a significant emotional event in any medical facility, and planning for how the change will affect the radiology staff and clinical users must be considered. Management protocols will need to be applied to the change process, the PACS acquisition, and the AT process, so that the transition to the new PACS is painless and runs smoothly.

G. S. Norton (✉)
Defense Health Agency, Integrated Clinical Systems, Program Management Office,
Fort Detrick, MD, USA

B. F. Branstetter IV (ed.), *Practical Imaging Informatics*,
https://doi.org/10.1007/978-1-0716-1756-4_26

An effective change management process will:

- Increase user buy-in
- Decrease implementation costs
- Shorten the implementation timeline

The acceptance test serves as an evaluation of the PACS performance, identifying deficiencies and the availability of the system. It can be used to certify contract compliance and as a payment milestone. It validates the interfaces to a facility's information systems and radiologic modalities, and checks the configuration and calibration of the PACS components. An AT is a technical evaluation of the system that demonstrates the clinical readiness for patient care. Additionally, the AT sets the baseline for a facility's quality control (QC) program that will monitor the PACS in the future.

> **DEFINITION: Acceptance Tests**
>
> Tests that determine whether predefined specifications and requirements have been met before deploying a new system. This includes operational and user acceptance tests.

> **FURTHER READING**
>
> Lewis TE, Horton MC, Kinsey TV, Shelton PD. Acceptance testing of integrated picture archiving and communication systems. J Digit Imaging. 1999;12:163–165

26.2 Change Management

Why do you need to change your PACS? *"Change happens!"* New leadership, hardware/software obsolescent, new software features, falling out of "love" with the vendor, expanded business opportunities, more modalities that require increased bandwidth. There are many reasons for an organization to change their PACS. When the decision to change has been made, it is time for the real work to begin.

> **FURTHER READING**
>
> Johnson S. Who moved my cheese? G.P. Putnam's Sons; 1998

26.2.1 Initiating Change

- Understanding the **project scope** is required to effectively start the change process, and the initial scope of the project should come from leadership. If just hardware or software obsolescence is the problem to be fixed, then engaging with your current PACS vendor to fix the hardware and software issues may be the entire scope of the project. If your organization has fallen "out of love" with your current vendor, then a new contracting effort must begin, and your organization's contracting/logistics office should be your first stop.

- Next, **build the team** to manage the project. Ideally, select a physician or **radiologist champion** to be the team leader. The current CIIP or an in-house project manager can act as the co-lead or vice-lead of the team, but the physician/radiologist champion will be the face of the project to the facility's leadership and other physicians in the community.
- The other team members should come from all the departments needed to complete the effort; other CIIP, department administrators, section team leaders, information technology experts, biomedical maintenance engineers, and facility contracting specialists are some of the knowledge base needed to change a PACS. Your facility may have different names for these departments, and there may be many subsections of departments involved (i.e., information technology may include experts from the data center, networking team, cybersecurity cell, and more).
- Additionally, the local PACS team will already have full-time jobs at your facility, so it's ok to hire a **PACS consultant** or consulting firm to manage changing the PACS.

Remember that the project's scope is at one point of the project management triangle, with cost and time at the other points. If one of the points changes, the other points are impacted. A change in scope could increase the project's cost and the time it takes to complete the project. If the timeline changes, the costs and scope are impacted. And if the costs are reduced, then the scope is impacted and the time to complete the project will change.

> **KEY CONCEPT: Project Management Triangle**
>
> Every project must balance scope, cost, and time. They are tightly interrelated, and you cannot optimize all three.

26.2.2 Managing Expectations

- After the team is built and the scope defined, it will be important to **communicate the vision** of the project to the primary users (stakeholders) at your facility. Identify stakeholders that use the PACS and how the PACS is used by the stakeholders (see **Chap. 25**). The emergency room, an outpatient clinic, and surgical suites/operating rooms will each use the PACS differently. There may be external clinics, across the street, or across town, and their needs should also be considered.
- Be prepared to change the scope of the project or redefine the project's approach when a unique workflow or obstacle is encountered. It is easier to alter the scope of the project now, rather than 6 months from now. The management team will need to be flexible and ready to identify external impacts to the project plan that have not been considered.
- The management team should develop a **regular meeting schedule**, and all team members need to be available for the meetings. Tasks should be shared by the team members; don't rely on a single person to gather all the information or write

everything. The stakeholders' unique workflows should be addressed. When obstacles are encountered, the management team should agree on how to correct them.

26.2.3 Accepting Change

- There will be **resistance to change** in your organization. Keep track of the resistance issues and address the issues during the management team meetings. How stakeholder workflows will be handled in the PACS should be discussed with the stakeholders, and stakeholder buy-in should be documented.
- The primary focus of all projects needs to be communication. Ensuring that the project progresses as planned, fixing the problems that occur, and making sure that users of the system are told about the small positive steps in the change process are important. Informed users will have a positive effect on the change progress.

26.2.4 Change Control Process

- Many organizations require that an integrated change control process be performed when sunsetting and/or deploying new enterprise-wide applications.
- Change requests should be recorded in writing. Many institutions use a standard template that include what is being changed, the reason for the change, testing documentation, approvals from leadership, date and time period for the change, and rollback procedures if the change is not successful.

> **DEFINITION: Integrated Change Control**
>
> An element of project management in which *all* system changes undergo a formal process of request, approval, management, and documentation. ICC is typically coordinated at an enterprise level.

- When required, the change control process includes presenting the change to a change control board, which is a group comprised of professional members who are responsible for reviewing, evaluating, identifying risks, approving, or rejecting the change.
- Communication of the change to the end users is very important, especially if the change incurs a downtime. Allowing the staff to prepare for scheduled downtimes makes the change go a lot smoother, especially when caring for patients (see **Chap. 29**).

26.3 Acceptance Testing

The "C" in PACS stands for communication. To function properly a PACS must communicate with the other information systems that are used in the department and the modalities that capture the images. In the digital world, all the orders, images, and reports are electronic information that is transmitted across a network. This section will discuss testing of the communication between the information systems and the interfaces to the modalities.

26.3.1 System Integration and Interfaces

- In most PACS implementations, the electronic medical record (EMR), hospital information system (HIS), and the radiology information system (RIS) are the primary sources of patient demographic and examination information.
- A robust, secure network connection between the EMR, HIS, RIS, modalities, and PACS is paramount; a PACS will not work efficiently without it.
- Most EMR/HIS/RIS/PACS interfaces will use the Health Level 7 (HL7) to communicate with each other. The EMR vendor, RIS vendor, and the PACS vendor should have HL7 **Conformance Statements** that describe how they use HL7 messages. The PACS will convert HL7 messaging to Digital Imaging and Communications in Medicine (DICOM) messages that are used to communicate to the modalities, and transmit and store images.

  > **FURTHER READING**
  >
  > Samei E, Siebert JA, Andriole K., et al. General guidelines for purchasing and acceptance testing of PACS equipment. RadioGraphics. 2004; 24: 313–334

- In addition to a HL7 Conformance Statement, the PACS and modality vendors will each publish a DICOM Conformance Statement that defines their connection information, to the data element level, which can be shared between systems.
- The PACS may also communicate with mammography imaging/reporting systems, separate billing systems, dictation/transcription systems, or speech recognition systems using HL7.
- Some facilities use **interface engines** or **network brokers** to handle the message traffic between the systems and the PACS, and the interfaces may be unidirectional (one way) or bidirectional (two way).
- It does not matter how many systems communicate with each other; the overall system throughput for a patient's examination from the time of order to archive must be tested to ensure that the data format has not changed.

  > **FURTHER READING**
  >
  > Lyche, DK, Romlein, J, Norton, GS, et al.: Benchmark testing of DICOM PACS, SPIE proceedings: medical imaging. PACS Des Evaluation Eng Clin Issues. 1998; 3339: 342–353

As part of the AT project, and to understand the interaction of the information at your facility, it is suggested that you map your PACS configuration and all the systems that touch it prior to beginning AT. Figure 26.1 is one example of the information data flow in a PACS-driven workflow (C. Head, personal communication, 2020).

KEY CONCEPT: AT Readiness

Every modality connected to the PACS must be calibrated and functioning properly to perform the acceptance test.

PACS Information Flow

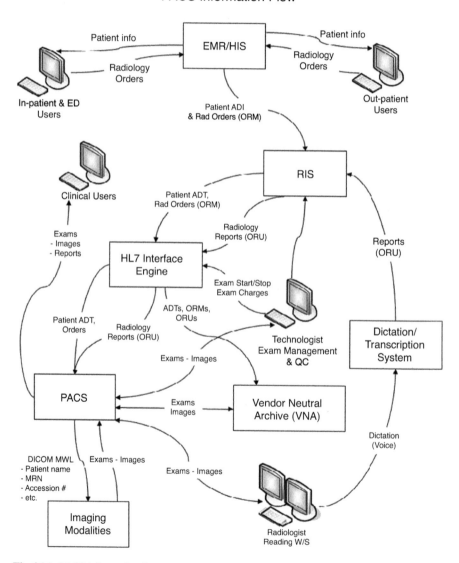

Fig. 26.1 PACS information flow

26.3.2 Modality Integration

DICOM is the key! Each modality vendor may have a slightly different approach to how they implement the DICOM Standard.

- DICOM connections between the modalities and the PACS are made of three elements:
  - IP address
  - Application entity (AE) title
  - Port number
- Some modalities are completely DICOM ready when purchased, and most modalities will have

OUR EXPERIENCE

It is important to make the AE title unique for each device and meaningful for your facility. Later, when you are trying to track an error, an AE title like "XMC-US01" is more useful than "650879."

DICOM Store and DICOM Print capabilities as part of their basic installation package. However, DICOM Modality Worklist (DMWL) may be a separate purchase option in the modality vendor's proposal, and depending on the age of the equipment, most modalities can be upgraded with DMWL.

- Non-DICOM modalities or modalities that have partial DICOM capabilities, but cannot be upgraded to achieve DMWL, can be connected to the PACS with a third-party interface box or broker. The broker spoofs the modality and can query the PACS or EMR for a DMWL. Some modalities may require the interface box to do a video capture

KEY CONCEPT: DMWL Data Elements

- *Patient name*
- *Patient ID*
- *Accession number*
- *Patient's date of birth*
- *Patient's sex*
- *Study description*
- *Modality type*

(screen scrape) or cine capture from the modality's console screen. Other modalities may be able to DICOM Store to the interface box, and the interface box can query for a DMWL and update the exam prior to sending it to the PACS.

- Both system integration and modality interfaces can be tested using thread tests. **Thread testing** allows the overall system to be evaluated for integrated functionality and throughput. Thread tests use clinical scenarios to evaluate the information and imaging stream from examination order, to acquisition, to display, to reporting, and to archive. Thread testing can be tuned to specifically follow the steps of a facility's information workflow and examine how a PACS interacts with that workflow.
- Historically, film digitizers and laser film printers were widely used to export or import examinations. If you still use film digitizers and laser film printers, you will need to validate their connections and functionality.
- CD/DVD burners may be used to export examinations and/or import examinations; document those connections and test the output.

This checklist shows the basic radiologic modalities and DICOM modality codes. Document each of the modality types to be connected to the PACS, the number of that specific type of modality, and validate that the individual modalities are functioning and testable. There are many other DICOM imaging types available (cardiology, radiation therapy, endoscopic, visible light, etc.); focus your testing on the modalities in your department.

CHECKLIST: Types of Modalities

Modality	Number of units	Testing complete
Computed radiography (CR)		
Radiographic/fluoroscopic (RF)		
Digital radiography (DR)		
Angiography (XA)		
Computerized axial tomography (CAT)		
Ultrasound (US)		
Magnetic resonance imaging (MR)		
Nuclear medicine (NM)		
Positron emission tomography (PET)		
Bone mineral density (BMD)		
Mammography (MG)		

STEP-BY-STEP: Thread Tests

Testing step	Variations and comments
Register a test patient in the EMR/HIS	There may be some network latency at each step in the test. Information may not appear instantaneously
Enter a test order for a CT of the head on a test patient in the RIS as a STAT. Verify that the patient and exam data is present on the CT scanner console's DICOM Modality Worklist (DMWL)	Order entry might be done in the HIS for inpatients and the RIS for outpatients. The patient's name, DOB, sex, MRN, study description, and the unique accession number are some of the data elements passed to a modality
Select the test patient and test order from the CT scanner console, verify that the data elements map correctly into the scanner's fields, and capture CT head images using a phantom	The examination requested may map directly into the CT console, or the technologist may have to select the correct procedure from the CT's predefined protocols
Post-process the test CT head examination. Send the exam to the PACS	Some PACS may require a QC step, at a technologist's PACS workstation or acquisition workstation, to validate that the examination is complete, and/or to place the exam in a "To Be Read" status, and/or to scan paperwork to be viewed with the images. The technologist may have to enter exam charges into the RIS or the exam complete message in the PACS to send the exam complete message to the RIS so the exam can be billed automatically

STEP-BY-STEP: Thread Tests

Testing step	Variations and comments
The test patient and the completed exam should appear on the radiologist's specific "To Be Read" worklist	*The worklist may be the "CTs To Be Read" worklist or a predefined subset: "CT Heads To Be Read," depending on the site's worklist build*
The exam should display as a CT head preset. Any historical exams on the test patient and/or dictated reports should also display with the uninterpreted new exam images	*The radiologists should work with the vendor's application specialist to establish a display protocol for each exam type. Verify that the display protocol presents (hangs) the images as defined*
There should be an indication on the radiologist's PACS desktop that an interfaced dictation system or speech recognition system is ready to receive the radiologist's dictation. Enter a test dictation (or notify the transcriptionist that the dictation is present)	*The indication may be a dictation window displaying the test exam's accession number*
The transcriptionist will select the test patient/test exam from the transcription system's worklist (speech recognition (VR) may or may not makes this step unnecessary)	*The radiologist's dictation may be placed in a wave file in the transcription system. The transcriptionist listens to the dictation and types the report. The report is sent back to the radiologist for verification. Alternatively, the transcriptionist acts as a correctionist after speech recognition*
After the transcription is complete, verify that the preliminary report is available with the images in the PACS	*Some PACS do not support this functionality; the preliminary report may only be available in the RIS or the EMR*
The radiologist will verify (final sign) the preliminary report in the RIS (may be simultaneous with speech recognition)	*Separate billing interfaces should be checked to verify that the report verification drops the interpretation charge*
Verify that the completed report is available at a clinical workstation with the images	*Some PACS have separate web viewing applications. Verify that the images and completed report are available via the web application*
Verify that the EMR/HIS displays the final report	*Check that the report is formatted correctly and that the data fields are correct*
Have the vendor or system administrator log into each downstream archival location to verify that the test patient's examination and report is available	*There may be some system latency in the archival process. Exams may not immediately move to the long-term or redundant archive*

26.3.3 PACS Components

The "A" in PACS stands for archive or archiving. Getting the patient and examination data from the information systems and the image data from the radiologic modalities is basically the same process, no matter which PACS vendor is used. The digital environment of PACS has allowed more efficient archive scenarios and enabled image archiving to multiple sites so that off-site disaster recovery storage is an easier option.

1. **Image Storage and Archive**

The primary purpose of a PACS Image Archive is to provide a secure location for the images and attending information to be stored and accessed. To test a PACS Image Archive, the configuration of the system storage architecture will have to be established prior testing:

- **Short-term storage** (STS) (also called the image cache) for recently acquired examinations awaiting interpretation, or examinations that are complete, but have not "aged" to the point where they are removed from the STS. The STS will also contain manually fetched or prefetched historic examinations that were retrieved from the next level of storage to be reviewed or compared to a recently acquired examination. Examinations in STS should be quickly retrieved for display.
- The **long-term archive** (LTA) is where all examinations are stored. Typically the PACS DICOM stores each examination to the LTA when a predetermined event flag has occurred. That event flag may be set immediately after an examination is written to the STS or when the examination is interpreted and the status in the PACS is complete. The LTA may use a network-attached server (NAS) or a storage area network (SAN) server for storage and backup. The LTA may also contain DICOM Structured Reports (SR) that are stored with the examination. Display speeds from the LTA may be slower than the STS.
- Redundant or **Disaster Recovery archive** is a long-term archive that is maintained separately from the LTA. The Disaster Recovery archive may be located across campus, across town, or out of state.
- **Vendor-neutral archives** (VNAs) and cloud storage have now replaced most LTAs and Disaster Recovery archives. Commercial VNAs are typically connected via the Internet and can be located anywhere an Internet connection is available, a facility may purchase their own VNA that resides in their data center, or it can be placed in an off-site commercial data center.

STEP-BY-STEP: Archive Tests
(G. Cohen, personal communication, 2005–2008)

Testing step	Variations and comments
Process and acquire an imaging study on a test patient and complete the exam in the PACS	*Archive testing will require system administrator or vendor level access privileges. Check and record the file size of the imaging study and the number of images in the PACS. Make note of the annotations and window/level settings made to the examination*
From the CIIP workstation, access the STS and verify that the examination on the test patient is present in the STS	*Check and record the file size of the examination and the number of images*
Access the LTA/VNA and verify that the examination on the test patient is present	*Check and record the file size of the imaging study and the number of images. (Compression algorithms will affect the file size. If the compression algorithm is 2:1, then the file size should be approximately half the original file size. Verify the presence of compression algorithms and the amount of compression used)*
Access the test patient's information on the EMR/HIS/RIS, and change the test patient's middle name. Verify that the name change on the test patient migrates through all the systems, so that the PACS, STS, and LTA/VNA have updated the test patient's name	*Verify that patient information is updated*
Have the CIIP delete or "age" the test examination from the STS. Verify that the test examination is no longer on the STS and verify that it is on the LTA/VNA	*The PACS vendor's representative may have to perform this step*
From a PACS workstation, select the test patient and fetch the test examination from the LTA/VNA. Verify that the annotations and window/level settings saved to the examination are present	*Verify that the number of images and annotations matches the information that was stored. Additionally, measure the time to display and verify that it meets your requirements and the vendor's specifications*

26.3.4 Workstation Functionality

The basic image manipulation functions of PACS workstations are virtually the same across vendors. Every vendor will allow a user to window/level, flip/rotate, zoom, invert video, and annotate an image. The PACS acceptance test needs to document the features that were purchased:

KEY CONCEPT: User Acceptance

Even though user interface functions may be similar, this does not mean that all PACS are the same. Ease of use of these tools is a major differentiator in user satisfaction.

- A workstation's functionality can be set to an individual's preference, and those preferences can be tied to the user's log-in. These functions are configurable, and **configurable functions** can be turned on or turned off. Testing a workstation's functionality is done to ensure that each of the functions is available.
- In addition to the image manipulation functions, historic examination prefetching/auto-routing and default display/hanging protocols must be checked.
- Extensive input from users, including mock readouts, is needed during functionality testing.

STEP-BY-STEP: Workstation Functionality Tests

Testing step	Variations and comments
Verify that the user is presented with a worklist/patient list and that the worklist is configurable according to vendor specifications	The user should be able to predefine worklists. Some facilities may just want a "CT To Be Read" worklist, or others may want to drill down to a more specific subset: "CT Heads To Be Read," depending on the site's preferences
Verify that the following are available for the user:	
Move the cursor across multiple monitors	The cursor should move across all screens of the workstation
Window/level all & individual images	The user should be able to window/level a single image or all images in a series
Digital magnifying glass	The user should be able to move/roam the image, increase the zoom, inverse video, and window/level inside the digital magnifying glass
Horizontal flip, vertical flip, and sequential 90-degree rotation of an image	
Inverse video	
Image roam	
Zoom	
View CT and MR scout w/ slice position indicators	
View CTs and MRs in stack mode.	
Display Hounsfield units & statistics	
Text annotations	
Image identification	
Undo last keystroke	
Save	
View full image header information	
Stack	
Cine	
Multiplanar reformatting	Multiplanar reconstructions (MPRs) and maximum intensity projections (MIPs)

STEP-BY-STEP: Workstation Functionality Tests

Testing step	Variations and comments
Verify that cursor focus acts as anticipated	Users may expect focus to shift whenever the cursor moves over an image, or may expect to click on the new image
Verify that presentation state can be saved	If a user adds annotations and rearranges the series or images, the new state should be saved, either automatically or manually
Verify key objects	Some PACS save key objects (e.g., images with annotations) automatically; others do so manually
Verify that point-to-point measurements are available (metric & inches)	To test this function, measure an object of known size and make sure metrics are correct
Verify that the workstation supports angle measurement	
Verify that the workstation supports area measurement	
Verify that the workstation supports perimeter measurement of objects	
Verify that a user can define and save image display protocols	
Verify that the display protocol allows a user to define image presentation order/number of images on screen	
Verify that the display protocol can be modality specific	
Verify that the display protocol can be body part specific	

26.3.5 PACS Monitor Testing

The American College of Radiology (ACR) and the American Association of Physicists in Medicine (AAPM) have recommended a set of standard testing to be done on display devices used for diagnostic imaging. TG270 replaces the TG18 report that was published in 2005. The test patterns in either TG18 or TG270 can be used for testing the monitor calibrations.

If your facility does not have physics support to check the monitor calibrations for the AT, you can contract with a physics group to do the monitor acceptance testing, or your medical maintenance department may have the capability. Remember that the Food and Drug Administration (FDA) along with the Mammography

> **FURTHER READING**
>
> American Association of Physicists in Medicine, Task Group 270: *Display Quality Assurance* 2019. https://www.aapm.org/pubs/reports/RPT_270.pdf

Quality Standards Act (MQSA) requires that a qualified medical physicist test the review workstation and perform acceptance testing on mammography softcopy display devices prior to clinical use.

PACS monitors today are primarily liquid-crystal displays (LCDs). Initially, cathode-ray tube (CRT) displays were used with PACS workstations. PACS/monitor vendors are no longer selling CRT monitors, and the installed base of CRTs has aged out of the PACS inventories. Organic light-emitting diode displays (OLED) are a technology that is growing, but has not been widely adopted. LCDs are dominant in the marketplace, so this section will focus on LCD monitors.

There are two types of LCD monitors being sold by PACS vendors: monitors with **internal photometers** and monitors without internal photometers. It is recommended that a calibrated luminance meter or laptop computer with luminance pod are used during the AT to validate the internal photometer measurements. The internal photometers come with software that records monitor readings at predetermined times, and readings are sent to the CIIP. Calibration issues can be discovered immediately and correctedversus the next time the monitor is physically checked.

Prior to beginning AT, basic information about each workstation should be recorded. The information should include:

- The workstation location
- The display manufacturer and model
- The pixel matrix
- The number of monitors on the workstation
- Installation date

Note: If the diagnostic workstation is constructed with an additional nondiagnostic grade monitor for EMR/HIS/RIS access of textual information, it does not need to be tested.

- Monitors with internal photometers are calibrated outside the PACS application. (The internal photometer application checks the monitor's calibration when the workstation starts or boots up and

> **FURTHER READING**
>
> **Chapter 27**, Imaging Quality Assurance, will provide information on monitor quality checks.

does not use the PACS application.) According to AAPM TG 270, a comparison of the internal meter and external meter should be evaluated upon acceptance testing and every 10,000 backlight hours. The TG270 or TG18 test images can be added to each workstation's hard drive, or the images can be added to test patient examinations in the PACS.
- The Society of Motion Picture and Television Engineers (SMPTE) created a test pattern that allowed users to visibly check the calibration of a monitor. SMPTE patterns are still being used today. The AAPM TG270-sQC (simple quality

control) test pattern is the SMPTE replacement and allows a user to scan grayscale patches and high-contrast bar patterns to evaluate luminance response characteristics around multiple gray levels over the entire luminance range.

- Since the monitor calibration and quality control software does not use the PACS display software, it is important to have a set of standard images available to test against. The AT team will need to coordinate with the PACS vendor. Either the AAPM TG-270 or the TG-18 image set can be loaded into the PACS as test images.

> **DEFINITION: Just Noticeable Difference**
>
> The minimum amount that the luminance can be changed for the human eye to perceive a difference. The JND varies with the current display luminance; a JND Index Curve is an element of diagnostic monitor evaluations.

STEP BY STEP: Monitor Tests
(J. Weiser, personal communication, 1993–2020)

Testing step	Variations and comments
Maximum luminance	*Using the TG270-sQC, TG270-ULN, or TG18-LN12-18 test image measures the maximum luminance in the center of the monitor (Check the documentation from your vendor and monitor manufacturer to establish maximum luminance)*
Minimum luminance	*Using the TG18-LN12-01 test image measures the minimum luminance in the center of the monitor*
Contrast ratio	*Max. luminance/min. luminance (the contrast ratio should be >250 for diagnostic monitors and >100 for clinical monitors)*
Contrast balance	*Display the TG270-sQC or TG-18QC (or a SMPTE) test pattern and look for the 5% and 95%. The perceived contrast difference between the 0% and the 5% should be the same as the perceived contrast difference between the 100% and 95%*
Luminance uniformity (done on each monitor)	*Display a flat field image, TG270-ULN or TG18-UL. Obtain luminance measurements of the four corners and the center of the monitor. The measurements should not vary more than 30%. Record the five luminance (cd/m²) readings for each monitor*
Workstation monitor uniformity (reported for each workstation)	*Display a flat field image, TG270-ULN, or TG18-UL. The center measurement of each monitor on a workstation should not vary more than 10%. Record the luminance (cd/m²) of each monitor*

STEP BY STEP: Monitor Tests
(J. Weiser, personal communication, 1993–2020)

Testing step	Variations and comments
Pixel dropout (large numbers of missing pixels could distract a radiologist during interpretation)	*Pixel dropout is indicated by dark specks in white images that do not change location when a different white image is displayed. Visually inspect the monitor for pixel dropout by displaying a white or light gray flat field. Refer to the manufacturers' specifications to identify the amount of pixel dropout that is acceptable on a monitor*
Visual evaluation of display noise	*Display noise is evaluated using the TG18-AFC test pattern. The test image is divided into four quadrants. Each quadrant is divided into 48 squares, with each square having low-contrast dots in random positions within the squares. The contrast-size values for the target dots are a constant in each quadrant, but the values are different for each quadrant. The image is viewed at a distance of 30 cm, at the normal ambient lighting conditions in which the workstation will be used. On a calibrated monitor used for primary diagnosis, the evaluator should be able to determine the location of all of the dots in three out of the four quadrants. On other calibrated monitors, the viewer should be able to determine the location of the dots in two out of the four quadrants*
Visual evaluation of display chromaticity	*In LCD monitors, the color tint of grayscale monitors can be affected by the spectrum of the backlight and by the viewing angle. Grayscale monitors used for primary diagnosis on multi-monitor workstations should be matched for tint at the factory, and sold and installed in matched sets in order to avoid perceivable differences in the tint of monitors on the same workstation. To perform this test, display the TG18-UN80 test pattern on the grayscale monitors. Note any perceivable differences in the relative color uniformity across the display area of each monitor, and between the monitors on the same workstation. The observer must be looking straight on at the monitor in order to reliably perform this test. Angled viewing will result in an invalid test*

STEP BY STEP: Sample Monitor Evaluation Worksheet

WORKSTATION #:_____

LOCATION:_____	TEST DATE: _____
Model#:_____	INSTALL DATE:_____

Place an "X" over nonrelevant monitors	Left Monitor	Right Monitor	Additional Monitor
Workstation Type	☐ *Clinical review*	☐ *Clinical review*	☐ *Clinical review*
	☐ *Diagnostic*	☐ *Diagnostic*	☐ *Diagnostic*
B/W or Color	☐ *B/W*	☐ *B/W*	☐ *B/W*
	☐ *Color*	☐ *Color*	☐ *Color*
Maximum Luminance (cd/m^2) (Using the TG270-sQC, TG270-ULN, or TG18-LN12-18 test image.)			
Minimum Luminance (cd/m^2) (Using the TG270-sQC, TG270-ULN, or TG18-LN12-18 test image.)			
Contrast Ratio (Max. Lum/Min. Lum)			
Contrast Balance (Is the perceived contrast difference between the 0% and the 5% the same as the perceived contrast difference between the 100% and 95%?)			
Luminance Uniformity (Measure the luminance of the four corners and the center of the monitor. The measurements should not vary more than 30%. Use TG270-ULN or TG18-UL.)	___ ___ ___ ___ ___	___ ___ ___ ___ ___	___ ___ ___ ___ ___
Workstation Monitor Uniformity (Measure the center of each monitor. The measurements should not vary more than 10%. Use TG270-ULN or TG18-UL.)	_____	_____	
Pixel Dropout (Count the number of missing pixels and refer to the manufacturers' specifications for the replacement recommendation. Use TG270-ULN or TG18-UL.)			

STEP BY STEP: Sample Monitor Evaluation Worksheet

Display Noise *(Using the TG18-AFC test pattern, visually inspect the monitor. The contrast-size values for the target dots are a constant in each quadrant, but the values are different for each quadrant. The image is viewed at a distance of 30 cm. On a calibrated monitor used for primary diagnosis, the location of all of the dots in three out of the four quadrants should be seen. On other calibrated monitors, the viewer should be able to determine the location of the dots in two out of the four quadrants.)*			
Display Chromaticity *To perform this test, display the TG18-UN80 test pattern on the grayscale monitors. Note any perceivable differences in the relative color uniformity across the display area of each monitor, and between the monitors on the same workstation. The observer must be looking straight on at the monitor in order to reliably perform this test. Angled viewing will result in an invalid test.*			
Comments			

26.4 Conclusion

Changing to a new PACS is initiated for many reasons. Emotional, operational, and financial impacts can be reduced by effectively managing the change. A well-defined change management process is critical to success. Understanding the scope of the change, building the right team, managing expectations, and performing an integrated change control process will serve you well throughout the changeover. The acceptance test of a PACS is an important evaluation of the PACS components, modality connections, network communications, and system performance. In addition to a system inventory, certifying contract compliance, and identifying deficiencies, an AT is a technical evaluation of a system that demonstrates readiness for clinical use and a baseline for a facility's quality control program that will monitor the PACS in the future.

"Change Happens" constantly in today's medical information/imaging space. Managing the change in our organizations and performing an acceptance test on the new PACS will make changing the PACS easier for you and your users.

Self-Assessment Questions

1. What is the first thing to be understood when change has been initiated?

   (a) User resistance issues
   (b) The scope of the project
   (c) Hiring a PACS consultant
   (d) All of the above
   (e) None of the above

2. What is the best way to manage user expectations?

   (a) The management triangle
   (b) Buy donuts for the staff
   (c) Communication of the project's vision
   (d) All of the above
   (e) None of the above

3. The best time to define the PACS acceptance test requirements is:

   (a) During user training
   (b) After the PACS is installed
   (c) In the request for proposal that the vendor responds to
   (d) All of the above
   (e) None of the above

4. The HIS/RIS/PACS and other medical information systems connect with each other using:

   (a) A robust, secure network connection
   (b) DICOM
   (c) HL7
   (d) All of the above
   (e) None of the above

5. A DICOM connections between the PACS and modalities include:

   (a) IP address
   (b) System license
   (c) AE title
   (d) Port number
   (e) A, C, and D

6. DICOM image sets used for evaluating workstation monitors are available from:

   (a) RSNA
   (b) IHE
   (c) SIIM
   (d) JCAHO
   (e) ACR/AAPM

7. PACS archives usually consist of:

   (a) Short-term storage
   (b) Long-term archive
   (c) Redundant or Disaster Recovery archive
   (d) All of the above
   (e) None of the above

Part VI
Operations

Chapter 27
Imaging Quality Assurance

Charles E. Willis

Contents

C. E. Willis (✉)
Department of Imaging Physics, University of Texas MD Anderson Cancer Center, Houston, TX, USA

© The Author(s), under exclusive license to Springer Science+Business Media, LLC, part of Springer Nature 2021
B. F. Branstetter IV (ed.), *Practical Imaging Informatics*,
https://doi.org/10.1007/978-1-0716-1756-4_27

447

27.1 Introduction

The goal of quality assurance (QA) is to maximize the efficiency of the imaging operation. Beyond the desire for efficient utilization of resources, QA is mandated in radiology by the American College of Radiology (ACR). Of course, compliance with standards of practice should not be the sole motivation for QA. Instead, QA should be a vehicle for providing the highest-quality medical care.

Automation allows digital acquisition of images, facilitates the marriage of patient demographic and exam information with images, and provides rapid distribution of images and reports throughout the healthcare enterprise. This same automation compounds the consequences of human errors (as only a computer can) and contributes to errors and delay of diagnosis. Dependence of the automation system on the human operator, the complexity of the human-machine interfaces, and an insufficient level of integration among disparate automation subsystems place the quality of our product at risk. Improvement of quality depends on aggressive quality control (QC) processes and comprehensive QA oversight.

DEFINITION: Quality Assurance (QA)

All activities that seek to ensure consistent, maximum performance from the physician and imaging facilities

DEFINITION: Quality Control (QC)

Activities that generate data indicating the current state of quality in the department

SYNONYMS: Quality Assurance (QA)

- Quality improvement (QI)
- Continuous quality improvement (CQI)
- Performance improvement (PI)
- Total quality management (TQM)

FURTHER READING: Quality Assurance

Reiner BI, Siegel EL, Carrino JA, editors. Quality assurance: meeting the challenge in the digital medical enterprise. Great Falls: Society for Computer Applications in Radiology; 2002.

27.2 QA of Digital Imaging

27.2.1 Errors in a Digital Imaging System

- Humans have a well-established propensity for introducing random errors.
- Automation, on the other hand, produces systematic errors.
- Humans use "inductive reasoning" and can work around machine errors. Machines do precisely as instructed, even when it is obviously wrong to a human.

> **KEY CONCEPT: Errors in Digital Imaging**
>
> Automated systems are not immune to errors. QA is a part of managing these errors.

- The human-machine interface creates a synergism that either makes up for the inherent deficiencies of humans and machines or aggravates the weaknesses of both parties.
- For example, increasing the complexity of the user interface increases human error exponentially.

27.2.2 False Sense of Security

- Electronic images are subject to deletion, **misassociation** of demographic and exam information, **misrouting**, and **misinterpretation**.
- Unlike film, the media that record electronic images are **impermanent**. Because of the huge capacity of electronic media, the loss of a single volume has greater consequences than that of a single film or even a single film jacket.
- Substandard electronic images can quickly be proliferated throughout the hospital, while an individual bad film can easily be controlled.
- Substandard electronic images can disappear without a trace, complicating repeat analysis. Film usage provided a telltale signature of repeated exams in a conventional operation.
- Systematically substandard images from an individual imaging system can avoid detection when multiple radiologists interpret images from multiple similar imaging systems. The tree gets lost in the forest!

27.2.3 Errors Inside and Outside the Digital World

- Improperly calibrated acquisition devices, inappropriate examination technique, operator typographical errors, and transcriptionist errors are examples of errors in the **translation of analog data** into the digital world.
- Errors that occur within the digital world include inappropriate lookup tables (LUTs), media failures, network failures, database failures, software bugs,

improper association of exam and image information, and image retrieval and distribution failures.

- Improperly calibrated display devices, such as soft-copy diagnostic monitors and laser cameras, are an example of errors that occur when trying to **extract analog images** for humans to use.

> **DEFINITION: Lookup Table for Display**
>
> A lookup table converts the pixel values of an image into brightness values for the display. Lookup tables are defined for each display monitor individually, so they can be used to ensure that an image looks exactly the same on every display.

27.2.4 Consequences of Well-Known Errors

- The same errors that are well-known in conventional imaging also occur in digital imaging systems; however, the consequences of the errors can be either more or less severe.
- While some mistakes can be readily corrected in the digital system, automation is not a panacea for bad practice.
- No algorithm exists to correct for patient motion, bad positioning, poor inspiration, incorrect alignment of X-ray beam and grid, wrong exam performed, or wrong patient examined.
- Image processing is a poor substitute for appropriate examination technique.

27.3 Processes and Products in the Imaging Department

27.3.1 Report Is the Product; Images Are Auxiliary

- If we intend to improve the quality of our product, it is important to identify the product and all processes that contribute to its creation.
- In an imaging department, the primary product is the physician's interpretation of the examination. In the most obvious case, this is a radiologist's report that may be communicated directly to the referring provider.

> **KEY CONCEPT: Radiologist Interpretation**
>
> The report is the primary product of the medical imaging operation. Images contribute to the interpretation process.

- The images themselves are an auxiliary product that enables the interpretation and may serve as reference, for example, as a therapeutic guide, but become less significant once the interpretation is documented.

> **SYNONYMS: Process Map**
>
> - Flowchart
> - Process diagram
> - Process chart

27.3.2 Process Mapping

- The sequence of processes that results in interpreted examinations is complex.
- Process mapping is a useful tool for identifying and understanding processes, as well as for **determining interference** with production.
- The details of process maps depend on the local clinical practice scenario as well as on the specific imaging systems and configuration.
- The intellectual exercise of constructing the process map is probably more valuable that the resulting map itself.
- Process mapping leads to **process reengineering** to improve the efficiency of production or the quality of the product.

> **DEFINITION: Task Allocation Matrix**
>
> A chart listing QC tasks indicating who is responsible for doing them and the frequency that they are performed

STEP-BY-STEP: Using a Process Map

1. List all the steps involved in producing and delivering the report of a medical imaging examination in chronological order.
2. At each step in the process, consider the possibility for an error to occur.
3. At each step of the process, consider the opportunity for detecting and correcting errors. These are QC checks.
4. Consider whether any steps in the process are unnecessary or redundant.
5. Revise the process map to include steps for checking and correcting errors and to eliminate unnecessary steps.
6. Compile the list of QC checks into a task allocation matrix.

STEP-BY-STEP: Creating a QC Task Allocation Matrix

Task	Responsibility	Frequency
Verify patient ID and exam info	Technologist	Each exam
Verify patient positioning	Technologist	Each view
Verify image quality – release or repeat	Lead technologist	Each image
Verify exam in PACS	Lead technologist	Each exam
Reconcile patient data/image counts in PACS	Informatics	Incidental
Report substandard images	Radiologist	Incidental
Erase cassette-based image receptors	Technologist	Start-of-shift
Test image receptor uniformity	QC technologist	Weekly
Clean cassette-based image receptors	Technologist	Monthly
Compile and review reject analysis data	QA coordinator	Monthly
Verify display calibrations	Clinical engineer	Quarterly
Review QC indicators	QA Committee	Quarterly
Verify receptor calibrations	Medical physicist	Semiannual
Verify X-ray generator functions	Medical physicist	Annual

27.4 Measurable Indicators of Quality of Imaging Services

27.4.1 Availability and Quality of Images and Reports

- The image quality can have an impact on the clinical interpretation.
- Making exams available to the radiologist is the gating event for diagnosis.
- The availability of prior exams and reports can influence the diagnostic efficacy of today's exam.
- Making the image and report available to the referring provider determines when indicated therapeutic actions can be initiated.
- The quality of the interpretation itself is the subject of active and ongoing efforts by the medical staff to monitor and improve diagnosis and treatment.
- National standards exist regarding the content of the report and communication of findings between radiologist and referring providers.

27.4.2 Physical Aspects of Image Quality

- The quality of a diagnostic image can be described by three broad characteristics – **contrast, resolution,** and **noise.**
- **Artifacts** are another broad category of features in the image that can adversely affect the diagnostic efficacy of the exam.
- Factors that influence the quality of the image include the fundamental capabilities and limitations of the imaging equipment; the condition of the equipment, such as how it is calibrated, configured, and maintained; and how the equipment is operated.

27.4.3 Ionizing Radiation Dose

- Another major consideration for modalities that involve ionizing radiation is the patient dose required to produce the image.
- Density, the usual aspect of conventional image indicating underexposure or overexposure, is an adjustable parameter in electronic imaging systems and therefore is not useful for monitoring exposure factor selection.
- Specific information about the amount of radiation used to acquire each image is contained in metadata accompanying the DICOM image.
- Some acquisition modalities have the capability to monitor and analyze this information.
- Data on patient dose is reported differently for different imaging modalities.
    - For CT, the Computed Tomography Dose Index (CTDI) is reported.
    - For fluoroscopy, the Entrance Skin Air KERMA (ESAK) and dose area product (DAP) are reported.

- For mammography, the mean glandular dose (MGD) is reported.
  - For radiography, a special exposure index (EI) is reported.
- None of the reported quantities is a direct measurement of patient dose.
  - Each one is an indication of patient dose to a **phantom**, or for radiography to the image receptor, with standard dimensions and characteristics that may or may not correspond to a specific patient.
- Interpretation of these data requires assistance from a **qualified medical physicist**.

DEFINITION: Qualified Medical Physicist (QMP)

An individual who is competent to independently provide clinical professional services in one or more of the subfields of medical physics

DEFINITION: Phantom

A test object intended to represent the patient in an imaging examination performed for quality assurance

HYPOTHETICAL SCENARIO: CTDI – A Phantom Problem

CTDI is not a direct measurement of radiation dose to the patient; it's actually a measurement of the radiation dose to a standard phantom in a standardized measurement geometry. The more that the patient's dimensions differ from the standard phantom, the less representative CTDI is of the patient radiation dose. For this reason, medical physicists developed a size-specific dose estimate (SSDE) to correct for patient dimensions. A further complication is that for some body parts, such as the head and neck, a 16-cm-diameter phantom is assumed in the CTDI, while others, such as the thorax, assume a 32-cm-diameter phantom. A CT examination of the CSPINE might report CTDI for a 32 cm phantom, but a combination head plus spine might report CTDI for a 16 cm phantom. This might not be the same for two different CT vendors or even on the same CT system, depending on how consistently personnel have configured their customized protocols.

27.4.4 Electronic Display Quality

- The quality of the electronic image depends on how it is displayed.
- Much of the QC effort in conventional departments was devoted to consistent automatic processing of photographic film.
- Recent standards address QC of multiformat cameras and laser film printers and electronic image displays.
- Electronic images depend on flat panel displays that degrade over time.

KEY CONCEPT: Radiation Dose Index Monitoring

Data reported by dose index monitoring systems provides only the basis for patient dose estimation. Interpretation of data reported by dose index monitoring systems requires the participation of a qualified medical physicist.

- Digital images can also be flawed if they use an inappropriate display **lookup table**.
- **Digital test patterns** can make display problems obvious.

DEFINITION: Digital Test Patterns

Standardized images with numerous shades of gray that can be used to test whether displays are performing optimally.

FURTHER READING: Digital Test Patterns

Bevins NB, Silowsky MS, Badano A, Marsh RM, Flynn MJ, Waltz-Flannigan AI. Practical application of AAPM Report 270 in display quality assurance: a report of Task Group 270. Med Phys. 2020;47(9):E920–8.

27.4.5 Repeated Images

- The percentage of images that must be repeated (**repeat rate**) is a gross indication of the quality of imaging services.

KEY CONCEPT: Repeated Images

Repeating images extends the time needed to complete an exam and delays interpretation. The imaging resource is occupied longer than necessary. It also requires additional radiation exposure to the patient.

DEFINITION: Reject

An image that is not useful for care of the patient. Includes test images and non-diagnostic images

---

DEFINITION: Repeat

Duplicate image obtained because original image was substandard or lost

HYPOTHETICAL SCENARIO: Repeat Rate

Without more detailed analysis, the repeat rate does not suggest specific actions that need to be taken to improve services. For example, in the early deployment of electronic imaging systems, dramatic reductions in repeat rates were reported and attributed to the electronic system's broader tolerance of overexposure and underexposure. An alternative explanation was that the technologists were using considerably higher doses than necessary to perform the examination producing images with much less noise that were more visually acceptable to the radiologist. Another possibility is that the technologists had no confidence that repeating the exam would result in improved images. It is possible that the technologists simply deleted many of the nondiagnostic electronic images to prevent them from being seen by supervisors or cluttering the PACS. Yet another plausible explanation is that in electronic imaging systems, the expedited availability of images becomes the number 1 priority, and image quality and patient dose are subordinated. A high reject rate, on the other hand, might result from inordinate emphasis on image quality.

27.4.6 Discrepancies in Demographic and Exam Information

- Patient demographic and exam information are associated with each image that is acquired.
- If the demographic and exam information in the medical imaging system does not match information in the radiology information system (RIS), then the image is classified as an **exception**.
- Exceptions may be hidden from view by physicians or may be tabulated in an area where they would not be normally viewed.
- Exceptions must be **manually corrected** to reconcile their data with the RIS.
- DICOM **modality worklist management (MWL)** reduces the number of exceptions but introduces new errors, such as misidentification.

27.4.7 Misidentification

- The image must also be accurately and unambiguously identified in order to be of immediate and future clinical value.
- In an electronic imaging system, misidentification of images should be treated as a **QA event**.
- Misidentified electronic images may be associated with the wrong patient or may be sequestered or otherwise unavailable for viewing, causing a delay in diagnosis.

DEFINITION: Exception

An image whose patient demographic and exam information disagree with the RIS. These images are usually quarantined until the discrepancy can be reconciled.

SYNONYMS: Exceptions

- Orphans
- Broken studies
- Penalty box

KEY CONCEPT: Exception Management

Reconciling demographic and exam information is a critical QC activity, often tedious and labor intensive.

FURTHER READING: MWL Errors

Kuzmak PM, Dayhoff RE. Minimizing digital imaging and communications in medicine (DICOM) modality worklist patient/study selection errors. J Digit Imaging. 2001;14(Suppl 1):153–7.

27.5 Mechanisms for Improving Performance in the Digital Department

An effective QA program is founded on **acknowledgment** of the errors that will occur; institution of **processes** to avoid, detect, and correct errors; and **enforcement** of these processes. **Documentation** of errors serves as the basis for root cause analysis and as an objective assessment of progress.

27.5.1 Selection of Indicators and Action Limits

- It is impractical to measure every possible indicator of quality.
- For this reason, specific indicators are selected that are expected to be sensitive to variations in quality of service, and these are measured periodically.
- The interval of measurement should be slightly more frequent than the incidence of corrective action.
  - If every measurement yields an inconsequential result, then the interval between measurements can be prolonged.
  - On the other hand, if every measurement dictates a correction, the interval should be reduced.

> **DEFINITION: Data Analytics**
>
> Collecting information, looking for patterns, and managing the information

> **KEY CONCEPT: Data Analytics**
>
> There is a wealth of information in an electronic imaging system including the transactions between clients of the network and the headers of the images themselves. Harvesting this information and interpreting it can provide valuable input to a quality assurance program. Automating this activity can reduce strain on personnel resources and highlight areas where quality improvement can be focused.

27.5.2 Timeline Analysis

- Most electronic imaging services have a radiology information system (RIS) that is an automated system for scheduling and tracking the progress of examinations.
- The RIS virtually documents the time when the exam is scheduled, when the patient arrives for the exam, when the exam is completed, and when the report is dictated, transcribed, and approved.
- **Interrogating the RIS** produces reports that can be analyzed to reveal the contribution each process makes to the overall turnaround time for an exam.
- Interpretation of the timeline can suggest modifications in resources to expedite the slowest steps.
- The image database may also provide data about receipt and viewing of images that can be coupled with RIS reports to identify areas for improvement.

27.5.3 Radiation Dose Index Monitoring

- Incidental patient dose monitoring has long been used to monitor the quality of imaging operations.
  - The electronic imaging system enabled more comprehensive dose monitoring.
  - Some newer digital radiography systems incorporate software to collect and report dose index information as well as reject analysis data.
- The priority for dose monitoring has increased in recent years.
  - Dose index monitoring in mammography is regulated by the Mammography Quality and Standards Act (MQSA).
  - Dose index monitoring is mandated by the State of California in CT. The Computed Tomography Dose Index (CTDI) is now part of the medical record for CT exams.

- The Food and Drug Administration (FDA) warned about potential adverse effects of fluoroscopy.
- The Joint Commission (TJC) who accredits hospitals has established a "Sentinel Event" involving high patient radiation dose in fluoroscopy.
- DICOM has established a **Radiation Structured Dose Report (RDSR)** information object for recording and reporting information necessary for estimating patient radiation dose.

> **DEFINITION: Food and Drug Administration**
>
> Responsible for protecting the public health by ensuring the safety, efficacy, and security of human and veterinary drugs, biological products, and medical devices and by ensuring the safety of the US food supply, cosmetics, and products that emit radiation

- Configuration of dose index monitoring systems and interpretation of the results require the active participation of a qualified medical physicist.
- For each imaging modality, data is collected to estimate the dose per image or per examination and is used to establish average values and confidence limits.
  - Doses outside of confidence limits are flagged for further analysis to determine whether excessive or inadequate doses were used for the examination.
- The American College of Radiology (ACR) has established a Dose Index Registry, so that hospitals can compare their data to the data reported by other and peer institutions around the United States.

> **DEFINITION: Dose Index Monitoring**
>
> The process of monitoring radiation dose used in diagnostic imaging procedures that use ionizing radiation, such as computed tomography (CT), interventional radiography (IR), projection radiography, and mammography

> **INTERNATIONAL CONSIDERATIONS: Dose Index Monitoring**
>
> Statutory regulations concerning dose index monitoring vary widely within and certainly outside the United States. MQSA is a US Federal statute; however, it is also followed in Canada. In Taiwan, an MQSA-like statute applies to mammography. The Joint Commission (TJC) is an American organization; however, through Joint Commission International (JCI), it promotes standards of practice in 100 countries.

> **FURTHER READING: RDSR**
>
> https://www.dicomstandard.org/using/radiation/

> **FURTHER READING: Dose Index Registry**
>
> https://www.acr.org/Practice-Management-Quality-Informatics/Registries/Dose-Index-Registry

OUR EXPERIENCE: Dose Index Monitoring

A large hospital decided to become an early adopter of a commercial radiation dose monitoring system. Although the system was intended to ultimately monitor all imaging modalities, it was initially applied to CT.

The imaging operation included CTs from two different vendors. Naming conventions for exam protocols was not standardized for the two vendors. Nomenclature for CT system station names was not systematic and uniform. Ad hoc attempts to map protocols to the dose monitoring database were incomplete and largely unsuccessful

The dose monitoring system hardware platform was sized at the minimum requirement for the software, rather than being scaled for the hospital's very large workload. Compounding the problem, an analyst indiscriminately routed all imaging examinations to the undersized dose index monitoring system server, including modalities that do not use ionizing radiation such as ultrasound and magnetic resonance imaging.

Even with frequent meetings, communication between the vendor and hospital personnel was poor, so that the vendor was unaware of the requirements of the hospital and the hospital was unaware of features of the product that could help or hinder implementation.

Reports produced by the dose index monitoring system were often discrepant from data obtained from other sources. The system reported dose by default in units of "effective dose," which was technically inaccurate and confusing.

KEY LESSONS LEARNED

- Institutions must shop for dose index monitoring systems with eyes wide open and by a committee of stakeholders. The stakeholders must include a radiologist, a technologist, an administrator, and a qualified medical physicist, and the group must be empowered by the institutional leadership.
- There are approximately two dozen commercial products for dose index monitoring. Although the products have become quite mature compared to the early days, they are not identical in capabilities or features.
- All stakeholders need to agree on the selection of a dose index monitoring system, and all must be committed to successful implementation and ongoing support of the system.
- An individual must be designated as the hospital "point person," with authority to make decisions and responsibility for the consequences. "Too many cooks spoil the broth!"
- The individual must have the support of hospital leadership to make the project successful.
- A qualified medical physicist must be involved in order to correctly configure the system and to interpret the results of the reports.

27.5.4 Reject Analysis

- Repeated examinations represent inefficiency in imaging operations and additional ionizing radiation exposure to patients.
- **Documenting the reason** for the repeated exam is best done concurrently with ongoing operations.
- Automation should facilitate documentation of repeated exams; in fact, some of the electronic imaging systems available today are designed to accommodate reject analysis.

FURTHER READING: Reject Analysis

Jones AK, Polman R, Willis CE, Shepard SJ. One year's results from a server-based system for performing reject analysis and exposure analysis in computed radiography. J Digit Imaging. 2011;24:243–55. https://doi.org/10.1007/s10278-009-9236-2.

Blado ME, Ma Y, Corwin RA, Carr, SG. Impact of repeat/reject analysis in PACS. J Digit Imaging. 2003;16(Suppl 1):22–6.

OUR EXPERIENCE: Reject Analysis

In 2002, the Texas Children's Hospital initiated a program for documenting rejected images. The demographic information was modified by the technologist supervisor, and the rejected images were archived to the PACS. Subsequent analysis of the reasons and responsibility for rejects had some surprising results.

The causes, frequency, and proportions of rejected digital images are comparable to those experienced in a conventional screen-film setting. Positioning errors cause about half of all repeated images. The group of technologists with the largest number of rejected images were agency techs, temporary employees who were unfamiliar with the equipment and pediatric patients. Their performance improved over time.

Another group of technologists with high repeat rates were supervisors! Further investigation revealed that supervisors were called on to perform technically difficult exams that frontline techs were unable to do. The supervisors also had a higher standard of quality for their own exams.

KEY LESSONS LEARNED

- Rejected images in a digital department are caused by the same errors as in a conventional department.
- Positioning errors are the biggest cause of repeats.
- Inexperienced technologists have the highest reject rates and therefore should be the focus of training and supervision.
- High reject rates can also be attributed to technically difficult examinations.

- Retakes need to be **assigned to categories**, such as positioning, patient motion, overexposure, underexposure, etc.
- It is important to record the exam and view being performed, the technologist performing the exam, and the imaging equipment used.
- In this way, remedial training or equipment service is indicated.
- The total volume of exams and views should be counted and used as the denominator in the reject rate.

27.5.5 Reliability Analysis

- In order to maintain continuity of clinical services, it is valuable to perform a reliability analysis of the electronic imaging system.
- In the analysis, **single points of failure** are identified.
- A local failure of one of these components has a global effect on other components of the system.

> **FURTHER READING:**
> **Reliability Analysis**
>
> Willis CE, McCluggage C, Orand MR, Parker BR. Puncture proof picture archiving and communications systems. J Digit Imaging. 2001;14(2 Suppl 1):66–71.

- Reliability of the entire system can be improved by building **redundancy** into the system.
- It is worthwhile to identify reasonable scenarios that involve the loss of components or utility services and to consider the effects on the imaging system.
- Planning and **rehearsing downtime procedures** (see **Chap. 29**) in advance of a catastrophe can ensure the availability of images for clinical operations.

27.5.6 Radiologist Image Critique

- **Radiologist feedback** is a driving force in effective QA.
- Feedback includes comments on both image quality and availability.
- This feedback is most effective when delivered contemporaneously.
- Electronic imaging systems typically do not provide mechanisms for such feedback.
  - To facilitate this feedback, codes can be developed for the radiologist's critique that can be dictated and transcribed into the RIS.
  - Another approach is to integrate instant messaging into the image viewer application to report quality or availability issues.

OUR EXPERIENCE: Radiologist Image Critique

A large hospital developed an in-house hospital information system that included a multitude of interfaces to disparate specialty information systems for pathology, the clinical laboratory, radiology, and many other services. As each individual information system was upgraded to a new software version, the new version had to be validated against the total integrated solution. The validation process became so expensive and labor intensive that the hospital sought a total hospital information system from a commercial supplier.

Despite extensive efforts to specify the requirements of the QA program for radiology in advance, at "go live," the QA program was completely nonfunctional. The integrated notification system for image quality problems and for misidentified and misassociated demographics was absent, and there was no longer a way to view unprocessed test images or to segregate test images from clinical images. In summary, a QA system representing about 5 years of development and functioning reliably for another 10 years was disconnected in an instant.

The priority for correcting "bugs" and "enhancements" was at the level of hospital operations rather than radiology operations, so that only vestiges of the QA system were restored 2 years after "go live." For example, image quality reports in the new system did not provide the IP address, AET, or station name of the device that produced the substandard image, complicating troubleshooting to the source. The new QA system maintained records of substandard images that had been corrected, but no information about the fault or corrective action.

KEY LESSONS LEARNED

- Accommodations for imaging QA must be fully integrated into hospital information systems. Imaging informatics professionals must facilitate provisions for QA.
- Provisions for QA should include automated direct communications between the radiologist and the technologists who produce the images and qualified medical physicists who can troubleshoot and correct the images.
- Radiology administrators and chief radiologists must be educated about the critical need for QA so that they can effectively advocate for integration of imaging QA into the hospital information system.

27.5.7 Training and Orientation

- An effective QA program must incorporate training and orientation programs.
- Applications training provided by the vendor is not sufficient.
- Local policies and practice must be developed, and these must be communicated to human operators of the system.

- These policies must be documented, reinforced periodically, and strictly enforced.
- **Clinical Competency Criteria** checklists are helpful in standardizing and documenting basic proficiency training.
- It is important to recognize that one size does not fit all: Training should be tailored for technologists, radiologists, referring providers, clinical engineers, and imaging informatics personnel.

27.5.8 Service Support

- Any QA program is incomplete without considering service support.
- Like conventional operations, the electronic department must plan for **service interruptions**.
- It is important to build in redundancy in the electronic components, which may be more expensive than their conventional analogs.
- To **minimize downtime**, it is wise to maintain a stock of on-site **spare parts**, especially for displays and long-lead items for devices that are heavily utilized.
- When a hospital has competent biomedical engineering staff, it is worthwhile considering first-call participation in service events.
- **Preventive maintenance** (PM) is always preferable to unscheduled maintenance.
  - In this regard, calibrations should be performed on-schedule.
  - Operators also have a responsibility to perform PM tasks: They should clean and inspect equipment and document what they do.
  - PM should be scheduled at the convenience of the clinical operation, not of the service provider.
- In an electronic department, software upgrades should be regarded as major service events where downtime is indeterminate and proper function must be reverified.
- **Notification** of users when a service outage occurs and when service is restored is critical to maintaining confidence in service support.

27.6 Roles and Responsibilities for QA

27.6.1 Radiologic Technologist

- In addition to performing the examination, the technologist, or technologist supervisor, in an electronic department has to assume responsibility for the delivery of all images to the physician.
- This implies a process and mechanism for verifying arrival of all images and a mechanism for detecting and correcting errors in delivery.
- In a department with a large workload, the QA activity may demand one or more dedicated QC technologists.

In an electronic department, the RT is responsible not only for performing the exam and producing acceptable images but also for assuring the delivery of all images to the referring provider for viewing.

27.6.2 *Imaging Informatics Professional*

- Involved in collecting and analyzing QC data, i.e., data mining
- Assist in correcting errors
- Support clinical operation teams in the exchange of medical images, imaging reports, and other medical data
- Can assist in automating QC processes
- Assist in training of personnel on the use of automated systems
- May be involved in troubleshooting and service support

27.6.3 *Qualified Medical Physicist (QMP)*

- The medical physicist has comprehensive, practical knowledge of imaging technology and workflow and is the sole member of the team who has primary interest in the quality of the imaging operation.
- The department should utilize the qualified medical physicist as a QA resource.

27.6.4 *Radiologist*

- Active and enthusiastic support of QA by radiologists is absolutely required for an effective program.
- Radiologists control resources and priorities in imaging departments.
- Radiologists must demand accountability for image quality and availability.

27.6.5 *Radiology Administrator*

- Must appreciate value of QA in radiology operations
- Must allocate resources to the QA effort
- Must enforce QA policies and procedures
- Must arrange for training of personnel
- Must coordinate QA efforts

27.6.6 QA Committee

- Includes all stake holders in radiology operations (see above)
- Meets periodically to review QC data and QA incidents
- Codifies QA and QC plans, activities, and responsibilities in policies and procedures
- Commits resources to QA activities

PEARLS

- Knowledge by department personnel of the consequences of errors, nonjudgmental reporting systems, and a sense of personal responsibility for timely and accurate delivery of images are keys to effective improvement in digital services.
- If you do not measure performance, you have no means to gauge improvement, and you will be sorry in the long run.
- QA costs resources; you must believe that this investment is insignificant compared to the benefits.
- Collecting and analyzing QC performance data serve no purpose unless it is widely communicated and used to target resources for improvement.
- Hospital staff is only capable of providing the lowest level of quality that is tolerated by radiologists.
- Post-processing is a poor substitute for appropriate examination technique

Further Reading

1. Adams HG, Arora S. Total quality in radiology: a guide to implementation. Delray Beach: St. Lucie Press; 1994.
2. American College of Radiology Position Statement. Quality control and improvement, safety, infection control, and patient education concerns. Available at: http://www.acr.org/SecondaryMainMenuCategories/quality_safety/RadSafety/general/statement-qc/safety.aspx. Accessed 23 Oct 2008.
3. Andriole KP, Gould RG, Avrin DE, Bazzill TM, Yin L, Arenson RL. Continuing quality improvement procedures for a clinical PACS. J Digit Imaging. 1998;11(3 Suppl 1):111–4.
4. Jones AK, Heintz P, Geiser W, Goldman L, Jerjian K, Martin M, Peck D, Pfeiffer D, Ranger N, Yorkston J. Ongoing quality control in digital radiography: report of AAPM Imaging Physics Committee Task Group 151. Med Phys. 2015;42(11):6658–70.
5. Papp J. Quality management in the imaging sciences. 2nd ed. St. Louis: Mosby, Inc.; 2002.
6. Willis CE. Quality assurance: an overview of quality assurance and quality control in the digital imaging department. In: Quality assurance: meeting the challenge in the digital medical enterprise. Great Falls: Society for Computer Applications in Radiology; 2002. p. 1–8.

Self-Assessment Questions

1. Who has the first opportunity to detect and correct errors?

   (a) Radiologist
   (b) Qualified medical physicist
   (c) Imaging informatics professional
   (d) Radiologic technologist
   (e) Radiology administrator

2. Who is the person who has the last opportunity to detect and correct an error before it can affect patient care?

   (a) Radiologist
   (b) Qualified medical physicist
   (c) Imaging informatics professional
   (d) Radiologic technologist
   (e) Radiology administrator

3. Who sets the standard for quality in an imaging operation?

   (a) Radiologist
   (b) Qualified medical physicist
   (c) Imaging informatics professional
   (d) Radiologic technologist
   (e) Radiology administrator

4. Which of the following is *not* a measurable indicator of quality?

   (a) Availability of images and reports
   (b) Single points of failure
   (c) Ionizing radiation dose
   (d) Repeated images
   (e) Exceptions

5. What is the single best method for understanding radiology operations?

   (a) Reliability analysis
   (b) Reject analysis
   (c) Task allocation matrix
   (d) Policies and procedures
   (e) Process mapping

6. List three sources of errors in an electronic imaging operation.

7. List three types of QA data that could be obtained by an imaging informatics professional by data mining of the RIS or image database.

8. A radiologist is complaining about the appearance of images on his electronic display. What are three possible causes? Explain how you would isolate and troubleshoot the problem.

9. From the text above, compile a list of ten components of a QA program.

10. List three characteristics of electronic images that make electronic QC different from conventional screen-film QC.

Chapter 28
Disaster Recovery

J. Robert Huber Jr. and Edward M. Smith

Contents

J. R. Huber Jr. (✉) · E. M. Smith (Deceased)
Medical Imaging Information Technology, Johns Hopkins Medicine, Baltimore, MD, USA
e-mail: Jhuberj1@jh.edu

© The Author(s), under exclusive license to Springer Science+Business Media,
LLC, part of Springer Nature 2021
B. F. Branstetter IV (ed.), *Practical Imaging Informatics*,
https://doi.org/10.1007/978-1-0716-1756-4_28

469

28.1 Introduction

Disaster Recovery and Business Continuity have an array of meanings. While the concept of Business Continuity is to ensure operations and core business functions remain working during an unscheduled downtime or disaster, the goal of disaster recovery is to return an organization to full, pre-event operations with minimal disruption, damage, or economic impact. New threats such as Ransomware are encrypting data and preventing organizations from access to their own data regardless of the physical state of their production and disaster recovery infrastructure.

The success of disaster recovery procedures relies on proper planning, budgeting, staffing, and technology in order to resume normal clinical operations after a catastrophic event. Disaster recovery is much like a form of insurance; your organization will pledge a fair amount of fiscal and personnel resources for a scenario that you hope never occurs. The commitment toward creating comprehensive policies, procedures, documentation, testing, and deployment practices is a great deal of work, but someday, having an effective disaster recovery plan in place will be a life saver. While there is a core list of best practices to follow, disaster recovery is an agile process that must be updated, tested, and re-evaluated on a regular basis.

28.2 Disaster Recovery

28.2.1 General

- Disaster recovery (DR) has been essential in health care for many years, but with the move to a digital environment, organizations must rethink their legacy analog DR protocols, procedures, and infrastructure.
- DR for healthcare providers are required under the Health Insurance Portability and Accountability Act (HIPAA) as well as accreditation organizations like the Joint Commission.
  - HIPAA security regulation requires backup disaster recovery of **retrievable exact copies** of patient data.
- DR is required due to:
  - Component failures—high probability
    - Server, storage system, or media
    - Data corruption
    - Human error
    - Virus
    - Internal or external system breach
  - Catastrophic events—low probability

> **DEFINITION: Disaster Recovery**
>
> A set of policies, procedures, processes, and systems put in place to enable the restoration and recovery of vital data and infrastructure following a natural or man-made catastrophic event.

- Major power failure due to severe ice or snow storms
- Fire, flood, hurricane, tornado, earthquake, etc.
- Terrorist act
- Ransomware

- Although DR is mandatory, it does not sufficiently provide real-time electronic protected health information (ePHI) that clinicians need during an unscheduled downtime. That is what business continuity planning is for.
- In order to provide uninterrupted patient care, business continuity procedures must be closely coupled with DR to provide a satisfactory level of continuity of care.

> **DEFINITION: Business Continuity**
>
> During a temporary downtime, business continuity provides access to the ePHI until the systems are fully restored to normal operating conditions (see **Chap. 29**).

> **KEY CONCEPT: Disaster Recovery Versus Business Continuity**
>
> Business Continuity is a backup system that gets used during brief planned or unplanned downtimes. You expect to use BC on a regular basis.
>
> Disaster Recovery is a complete recovery of all data and infrastructure from the ground up, assuming everything got destroyed. You hope never to need DR.

28.2.2 Planning

28.2.2.1 Critical Infrastructure

- Identify the critical systems in your enterprise. These systems can also be referred to as "**Mission Critical**" and are necessary for the business to operate.
- Financial, communication, and clinical systems such as PACS generally make up this category.
- Newly added or upgrade systems should be reviewed and matched against established criteria to determine if they are mission critical and require DR planning.
- A **test environment** should be used to test all application upgrades and integrations as well as new applications prior to clinical use.

> **DEFINITION: Mission Critical Application**
>
> A mission critical application is software or a suite of related programs that must function continuously in order for a business to operate.

- If economically feasible and information technology support is available, mission critical servers should be clustered or virtualized and direct attached storage (DAS) eliminated in favor of higher-redundancy storage solutions.

> **FURTHER READING: Mission Critical Application**
>
> https://searchitoperations.techtarget.com/definition/mission-critical-computing

28.2.2.2 Identify DR Scenario(s)

- Catastrophic—low probability:
  - Physical facility
  - Weather disasters
  - Power grid
  - Ransomware
- Isolated—high probability:
  - Limited to individual systems
  - Local sites and facilities
  - Human error
- Data Types
  - It is important to identify what data you are protecting when planning your organization's DR response.
    - ePHI
    - Financial records
    - HR records
    - Inventory
- **Service Level Agreements (SLA)**
  - It is imperative to have both internal and external SLAs negotiated and documented.
  - Internal SLAs should be negotiated and ranked against other mission critical systems.
  - Generally, the recovery process is implemented by a single enterprise team with input from individual departments. Therefore, it is necessary to have restoration and recovery options agreed upon well before a declared event.

> **DEFINITION: Service Level Agreement (SLA)**
>
> The promise made by a vendor that their machines or software will rarely malfunction. It is expressed as a percentage of time that the system is working (e.g., 99.9% of the time).

  - Require that all hardware and software vendors provide an SLA that is enforceable and contains **monetary penalties** if they do not adhere to the commitments in the SLA.
    - Downtime for the life of the contract is most favorable for the vendor.
    - Downtime per event is most favorable for the healthcare institution.

Table 28.1 Downtime associated with various SLA contract terms

SLA (%)	Downtime for life of 10-year contract	Downtime per year	Downtime per month	Downtime per event (on average, one per week)
99.0	3.7 days	88 hours	7.3 hours	1.7 hours
99.9	88 hours	8.8 hours	44 minutes	10 minutes
99.95	44 hours	4.4 hours	22 minutes	5.1 minutes
99.99	8.8 hours	53 minutes	4.4 minutes	1.0 minutes
99.995	4.4 hours	26 minutes	2.2 minutes	0.5 minutes

The longer the time period, the more flexible the agreement is for the vendor. But users experience frustration on a per-event basis!

- Planned downtimes are excluded from the SLA.
- The penalties associated with the SLA should be increased for each time the vendor fails to meet the SLA.
- The period over which the downtime is calculated for the SLA must be clearly specified as illustrated in the following table (Table 28.1).

- **Disaster Recovery as a Service (DRaaS)**
  - Replication of the production environment by a third party.
    - Useful for organizations without a DR budget or technical expertise to manage their own plan (e.g., Microsoft Azure can be used as a DRaaS).
    - SLA agreements are necessary.
    - Data Security and Privacy must be assured
- Using enterprise backup and disaster recovery solutions (e.g., Commvault and Veritas) accelerates the return to normal business operations.
- Virtualization is the process of creating a virtual presentation of items such as applications, servers, storage, and networks (e.g., VMWare, Microsoft Azure, and Amazon AWS).

28.2.3 Resources

- **Staff**
  - Clearly defined roles and responsibilities are paramount to ensure continuous operations in the case of a DR event.
  - Example DR team structure:
    - Manager of Security and Disaster Recovery
    - Disaster Recovery Coordinator
    - Information Security Analysts
    - Data Security Administrators
  - Example of team responsibilities to include:
    - Administer access to various production applications
    - Ensure security compliance to existing logon and password syntax standards
    - Monitor access activities for midrange applications

- Maintaining response, recovery, and restoration protocols for functions and systems
- Develop and execute comprehensive test plans for all aspects of recovery
- Assist other areas of the business in developing both disaster recovery and business contingency plans
- Designate a central authority and team in advance to direct the DR procedures during an actual unscheduled downtime event
  - *Onsite/Offsite Scenario(s)*
    - In-House team:
      - Depending on the size of the organization an in-house team to manage DR and continuity of business operations may be the most effective solution to swift and efficient data restoration and services.
      - Consider the best staff to strike the right balance for structure, roles, and responsibilities for in-house teams.
    - Offsite team:
      - Outsourcing the management and storage of DR.
      - Consider outsourcing management of your long-term storage (Tier 2) as well as BC to a Storage Service Provider (SSP).
      - Can be the most cost-effective solution and minimizes the use of physical and personnel resources of a healthcare facility.
      - Negotiation of SLAs and regular testing are necessary when an offsite team is leveraged.

28.2.4 Budget

- IT budgets have been steady or increasing since 2019. Nevertheless, many organizations find it difficult to justify the cost of a robust DR solution.
  - As healthcare information advances toward a completely digital environment, paper and film-based information approaches extinction. The costs associated with digital system redundancy can be quite costly.
  - During the budgetary process, organizational leadership must consider and decide how long their care teams and patients can tolerate system outages. This will assist in calculating costs and allocating funds for the acquisition of DR system components.
    - There are both **tangible and intangible costs** to mission critical system downtimes!
  - Mission critical system downtimes can have suboptimal impacts on:
    - Patient care
    - Productivity
    - Finances
    - Public relations

- Downtime Insurance:
  - Hospitals and enterprise health systems should have downtime insurance, especially in an era where virtual catastrophic events like ransomware attacks directed at health systems are becoming more common.
  - It is a form of "**risk management insurance**" similar to other insurance policies carried (e.g., should your organization encounter a ransomware attack, it could be financially devastating).
  - Compare the costs of using an in-house team to manage and support the DR platform vs. using DRaaS solutions to decide which option is best for your site.
  - Mandating specific procedures and deploying additional precautions to provide DR solutions and an acceptable level of BC will add to the operating costs of the digital environment.

FURTHER READING: Downtime Costs

Smith EM. The cost of downtime and risk management insurance. Enterprise Imaging and Therapeutic Radiology Management; 2009.

28.3 Execution of Disaster Recovery

28.3.1 Testing Scenarios

- Testing scenarios should include the restoration of:
  - Hardware
  - Network connectivity
  - Operating systems
  - Interfaces
  - User access
  - Data
- All scenarios should include bidirectional data flows (to and from ancillary systems).
  - Electronic Medical Record (EMR) systems with ePHI should include interface testing for order and result messaging in a healthcare environment.

> **KEY CONCEPT: Interface Engine**
>
> Interface engines handle the messages between mission critical systems. Interfaces may be unidirectional (one way) or bidirectional (two way).

28.3.2 In Practice

- Hopefully you will not be using your DR plan regularly, but what *should be* done regularly are DR drills (practice, practice, practice).

DEFINITION: Penetration Testing

Simulate an attack on a network to determine vulnerabilities.

SYNONYMS:

Penetration Testing

Vulnerability assessment
White hat attack

- Perform regular penetration testing and failover testing to expose network vulnerabilities and **single points of failure (SPOFs)** in your DR infrastructure.
  - Eliminate SPOFs in the infrastructure including routers, switches, application gateways and interfaces, etc.
  - It is best practice to ensure the systems in your infrastructure are updated regularly with security patches. This process will help to stop exploits like Trojans and Ransomware from installing on your systems.

FURTHER READING

Kent K, Souppaya M. Guide to computer security log management. 2007.

- If your data retention policies require it, backup information contained on legacy systems using tape or other media and store securely.
  - Although most organizations are using discs and cloud storage devices for primary storage, inexpensive (but slow) magnetic tape can still be used for backup and recovery purposes.
  - At some institutions, databases are backed up to magnetic tape; however, magnetic disk is faster, minimizes or eliminates downtime, increases data integrity, and may decrease cost in the long run **IF** the backup is transmitted to a secure datacenter or outsourced to an SSP.
- Back up information in a second secure datacenter preferably at a site 100-plus miles from the primary site.
  - Rent space and functionality at a Tier 3 or Tier 4 datacenter.
    - Acceptable, but expensive since hardware and software must be purchased and datacenter services must be leased.
  - Store data in multiple datacenters owned by healthcare facility and utilize grid storage technology—Applicable for Fibre Channel Forwarder (FCF) only.

HYPOTHETICAL SCENARIO

Significantly distancing your backup DR system and backup storage applications will serve you well if your area is hit by a significant natural disaster such as an 8.0 magnitude earthquake or EF5 tornado.

- Create redundant paths for data transmission in case a single provider experiences an unexpected downtime.

- Alternate backup power sources including:
  - Uninterruptible power sources that must be checked weekly
  - Automated emergency power generation capability
    - Both ensure functionality during an unexpected and extended electrical downtime.
- Have an **incident response plan**.
  - Review and update regularly to ensure that all systems currently in use are well thought out.

HYPOTHETICAL SCENARIO: Redundancy

You may need to employ multiple vendors.
- Vendor A uses broadband service for primary Internet connectivity.
- Vendor B uses cellular service as a redundant means of Internet connectivity.

- If disk is to be used as the backup medium, typically the database would be stored in a storage attached network (SAN) and a complete backup would be made each week and a backup of all changes to the database would be made each day.
  - SAN separates the storage system from the rest of the local area network (LAN).
  - Improves application disaster recovery.
  - Copies of the backup would be transmitted daily off-site to a secure datacenter or security services processor (SSP).
- For databases having a large volume of daily transactions or for an institution that is approaching a paperless environment, periodic backups (replications or point-in-time) during the day (asynchronous) or real-time backups (synchronous) would be preferable. This would be in addition to the disk backup protocol described above.
  - Daily and weekly copies of the database MUST be kept off-site in a secure and accessible location.
  - Longer data retention policies should be considered to mitigate the risk of ransomware. As this threat becomes more prevalent it will be necessary to have older copies of data as the ransomware threat can remain dormant for a period of time before discovery.
  - Cloud locations are becoming a desirable location (e.g., Microsoft Azure is HIPAA compliant).
  - A copy of the database should be restored on a test server to ensure its integrity at intervals established by the healthcare facility. Do not restore a backup or DR copy of a database on a clinical application server until its integrity is determined. If the database is corrupted, it will disrupt clinical operations.

28.4 Protection

28.4.1 Standards of Practice

Having a solid DR architecture in the healthcare environment is vital in order to protect patient data. Part of DR practices is deploying policies and procedures that protect all systems in the organization. Taking proactive steps toward mitigating threats in the first place will protect all systems, including your DR systems.

- Organizations encourage their employees to adhere to practices that protect against threats such as malware, viruses, and ransomware. These include:
  - Never click on links that you do not trust or are unverified
  - Never open untrusted email attachments
  - Download content only from trusted sites
  - Always avoid giving out your personal data
  - Use mail server content scanning and filtering
  - Never use unfamiliar USBs
  - Make sure your software and operating systems are updated
  - Avoid using public Wi-Fi but if you must always use a VPN
  - Use reputable antivirus and anti-malware software
- To mitigate threats to the organization as a whole, filter email messages prior to mailbox delivery.
  - Anti-phishing
  - Attachment scanning
- Educate the user base in best practices regarding files shares, websites, and email attachments.
  - All of these are ingress points to your system and the threats can be reduced with user education.
- Each of these best practices is important but when used in conjunction with each other the sum level of protection can be greater than the parts.

> **FURTHER READING: Ransomware Guide**
>
> Cybersecurity &Infrastructure Security Agency; https://www.cisa.gov/publication/ransomware-guide

28.4.2 Cyber Monitoring of Threats

- Check industry websites for new "in-the-wild" threats.
- Many software and internet vendors will proactively monitor and report on specific threats to their products.
- It is the responsibility of the health organization to compile and parse these threats to manage the organization's level of vulnerability.

> **DEFINITION: In-the-Wild Threats**
>
> Exploits propagating in real-world computers and not just in test labs.

28.4.3 Protecting Critical Data on DR Systems

- Actively scan for known vulnerabilities. Block and monitor known applications and protocols that can be used to access data (e.g., RDP and SMB protocols).
- Centralized log gathering tools are ways to quickly gather information from the enterprise to efficiently scan for abnormal behavior and known threats.

> **OUR EXPERIENCE: Segmented Network**
>
> Problem: Outdated Operating Systems (OS) on modalities can be challenging and could potentially expose vulnerabilities. Modality vendors are not always quick on the draw to update the OS on their modalities, and let's face it, hospital leadership probably will not go for the frequent replacement of expensive modalities either. That could be rather costly!
>
> Solution: Placing imaging modalities and devices on a segmented network away from the main network to restrict network traffic to and from the network segment. This will allow for a timely isolation response to potential threats.

- These tools help to identify abnormal behavior and isolate infected systems.
- Segment modalities and other nodes that contain older operating systems away from the main network using routing and firewall policies.
- Implement intrusion detection at the organization's perimeters and internal firewalls.
- At a minimum, critical data must be **backed up daily** and preferably multiple times during the day depending on the frequencies of new entries, "writes or changes" to the database.
  - If a database is corrupted all of the entries since the most recent backup will have to be re-entered after the database is restored from the most recent backup or point-in-time replication. This can be both time consuming and costly at best, especially as an institution becomes paperless.
- There are several protocols for backup:
  - The least desirable approach is to make a backup on tape each night while the system is not clinically operational, label it and take that copy to a secure offsite location. Three copies of the backup would always be retained and rotated:
    - Daughter copy: Current day's backup
    - Mother copy: Previous day's copy
    - Grandmother copy: The prior day's copy to the mother copy

28.5 Validation

28.5.1 Testing Scripts

- Every plan and scenario must be documented.
  - It is recommended that testing scripts include:

- Initial plan and scenario, including all systems and data to be restored
- Processes for restoration
- Control sheet for processes
- Expected results

OUR EXPERIENCE: Expected Results

At the end of the clinical day, imaging studies should be encrypted and backed up to Tier 3 storage as well as DR storage at an off-site location or to a storage service provider.

- Start and End time of restoration process
- Results, for example, Success or Failure
- Lessons Learned
- Sign-Off from DR team and business unit
- All access to DR copies of studies should be periodically audited and the integrity of these studies should be verified.

Disaster Recovery Tactical Workarounds

- A comprehensive disaster recovery plan incorporates the regular practice and up-to-date workaround documentation for system components that may fail:
  - It is necessary to develop viable workarounds for end users in order to provide continuity of care.
  - Validate that the storage capacity on the modalities is large enough to store imaging studies in the event the modalities are unable to send to PACS for an extended period of time.
  - Work with your clinical engineering team to find a method of exporting studies to an external storage medium in the event the storage space on the modalities are running low and unable to send to PACS or long term storage.

KEY CONCEPTS: THE IT RESILIENCY TRIO

There are three corresponding terms in the context of IT resiliency:
- **Fault Tolerance**: Individual components that are resilient to failure
- **High Availability**: An entire system resilient to failure
- **Disaster Recovery**: Restoring systems and vital infrastructure following a natural or human-induced disaster.

  - Hard-wire at least one of each type of critical modality to a DICOM compliant laser printer should the infrastructure fail.
  - Should the EMR become unavailable or prior studies are not available on Tier 1 or Tier 2 storage, arrange to retrieve the necessary studies from Tier 3 storage using a general-purpose viewer.
  - Prior to starting a surgical procedure, download all necessary imaging studies to a computer in the surgical suite. The surgeon most likely used imaging for surgical planning.

- Document and practice manual procedures and record keeping for incidents where electronic data is temporarily unavailable.
- These processes should include updating the electronic data when that data becomes available and can include manual entry, scanning, and optical character recognition (OCR) technologies.

Periodic Validations

- Scheduled Downtimes
  - Maintenance and system upgrades for DR systems are needed to keep systems in pristine condition and to provide assurances that when an organization encounters and unscheduled downtime, the DR Systems will engage as expected.
  - Reasons for scheduled downtimes might include:
    - Upgrades
    - Software patching
    - Application enhancements
  - Ideally, scheduled downtimes should be held to a minimum whenever possible.
  - When needed, scheduled downtimes should be performed at a time with the least impact on clinical operations.
  - Consider performing **failovers** to the secondary and redundant systems before performing preventative maintenance to decrease disruptions to clinical care.
- Unscheduled Downtimes
  - DR systems are essential to protecting against data loss in order to restore ePHI should a catastrophic unscheduled downtime occur.
  - At some point, your clinical systems will most likely encounter an unscheduled downtime.
  - Maintaining imaging department downtime procedures is essential to all imaging departments because it is not a matter of if, but when you will experience an unexpected downtime
- See **Chap. 29** for more information on Downtime Procedures.

OUR EXPERIENCE: Emerging DR Technologies

New technologies such as Microsoft's DFS Replication (Distributed File System) and SQL Always-On with clustering services are fantastic tools in the DR toolkit that limit the impact of required maintenance procedures. Support for these types of technologies should be negotiated with vendors prior to installation.

KEY CONCEPT: System Downtimes

Periods of time when computer system, applications, server, or the network is not functional. It is a Joint Commission requirement that backup systems must be in place for system downtimes, such as DR, Failover, and Data backup systems.

28.6 Documentation

28.6.1 Enterprise Level

- The healthcare organizations should maintain a full DR and continuity of business plan.
  - This plan can be a higher-level overview of the process but should include the following:
    - Team structure
    - Roles, responsibilities, and contact information
    - Vendor information
    - SLAs, roles, responsibilities, and contact information

28.6.2 Department Level

- Documentation should include all mission critical systems unique to that department. For example, radiology in a healthcare environment would list the PACS system as critical.
- This plan should be a more detailed view of the individual departments' roles and responsibilities. It must be a more granular view of the process.
- The department plan should include the following:
  - Individual roles, responsibilities, and contact information
  - Chain of command and escalation procedures
  - Detailed testing and validation procedures
  - Contact at the enterprise and vendor for sign-off and resumption of business activities.

FURTHER READING: Options for Disaster Recovery

Smith EM. Fee-per-study storage: the outsourcing option. ADVANCE for Imaging and Oncology Administrators; 2006. p. 45–50.

Smith EM. Advantages of outsourced storage surpass expenses. Diagn Imaging. 2008:S-1–5.

HYPOTHETICAL SCENARIO: Healthcare Ransomware Attack and Steps to Rebuild Your PACS

Ransomware is a type of malicious software that infects computer systems resulting in encrypted data. Owners of the encrypted data are unable to access their data until some sort of demand is rendered, usually monetary. Ransomware can infect a single computer, application, or can be distributed network wide.

Ransomware assaults have the potential of bringing health systems to their knees and are likely to remain a prominent threat to the healthcare industry. Why? Patient data sells for more than any other type of data on the black market. If you do not think it could happen at your site, think again. At the time of this writing, there have been over 172 ransomware attacks on healthcare organizations since 2016, despite best practices in security. Costs are estimated at more than $157 million. Q3 of 2019 saw an estimated 350% increase in ransomware attacks.

From an imaging informatics perspective, a possible consequence is permeation of malware throughout an enterprise network and infection of workstations, servers, and imaging informatics applications such as PACS. Health system leadership will face a series of difficult decisions including whether to pay the ransomware pirates. A benefit of payment is the possibility of resuming normal operations quickly, although this is not certain. If the decision is not to pay, your only option may be to wipe your systems clean and rebuild your systems from scratch. This could involve:

- Setting up a scaled down version or a temporary PACS. Consider using your test PACS server if it was not compromised. The upside to this approach is radiologists and other providers are no longer beholden to viewing imaging studies at the modality. The downside is that a temporary PACS server is a "from this point forward" solution. Prior imaging studies will not be available.
- Be prepared to ask for on-site vendor assistance. Your vendors may cut their virtual ties to your systems during the malware cleanup process. This is to maintain the integrity of their systems.
- Once the temporary PACS is no longer needed, a reverse migration of data from the disaster recovery archives to your clean PACS rebuild will be required.

KEY LESSONS LEARNED

- While rebuilding your primary PACS, have your temporary PACS solution assume the identity of your primary PACS server configurations. This will save you from having to change the destination configuration settings on all your modalities and other devices.
- Develop a mechanism to save the radiologist preliminary reports so that other providers can review the reports when radiologists are not available. Additionally, radiologists will want to later review these preliminary reports when all systems are back online. As rebuilding a PACS is a laborious and time-consuming effort, returning to normal operations will take some time.
- Schedule regular downtime drills with the imaging staff so they remain familiar with downtime processes.
- Maintain data integrity as a top priority, even on your disaster recovery archives. It will make the reconciliation process much less burdensome.
- Be prepared to have a reconciliation ultramarathon. It may take considerable time for you to reconcile the patient data contained in your EMR, RIS, PACS, long-term archives, and other third-party applications.

28.7 The Future of Disaster Recovery

What is the future of Disaster Recovery and Continuity of Business? We all wish we had that blue print but when pondering future disaster recovery features, some areas and suggestions may be prescient.

28.7.1 Filling the Disaster Recovery Skills Gap

- Virtual in-house on-demand training modules. Organizations are creating their own learning modules to provide their workforce the most current training materials and reference guides.
  - It is fairly common for IT professionals to migrate to different areas of the enterprise. This has the potential for high turnaround and hiring less seasoned personnel with a lack of institutional knowledge.
- Organizations are seeking real-time dynamic detection and protection from unwanted cyber intrusions. IT and Certified Imaging Informatics Professionals (CIIPs) are required to proactively learn the methods to keep DR systems as secure as possible.
  - IT Directors and Managers need to make sure their DR system team members have opportunities to take courses to stay current in DR technology.

28.7.2 The Disaster Recovery Return on Investment

- Organizations are still hesitant to increase the disaster recovery budget when having to justify the return on investment (ROI).
- Organizations need to complete a thorough analysis of the potential cost of a disaster or data breach.
- Organizations need to think of the intangible costs as well such as **patient leakage costs**, the devaluation of their brand, and negative public perception.
  - Example: A single breach in 2019 cost a hospital system $8.19 million due the number of records accessed.

DR Is Similar to Life Insurance

"Without a doubt, the most significant hurdle we face in implementing a Disaster Recovery strategy is the lack of ROI, as people draw to things that have an immediate return on investment. Similar to life insurance, DR has no immediate return on investment, as the disaster may never happen."

Chris Colotti (2018). https://www.dataversity.net/future-disaster-recovery/

28.7.3   Shift from "Recovery" to "Continuity"

- Focus will be on how to fundamentally protect data.
  - ePHI
  - Financial records
- It is no longer enough to just recover the systems that support the organization. Seamlessly transitioning back to normal operations without disruption in patient care is the ultimate goal.
- Proactive protection processes will overtake the recovery processes for many organizations.

28.7.4   Real-Time Adaptation to Threats

- The need for an agile response to immediate threats to compliment the planning and security of data and systems has increased significantly in recent years and the demand for actual real-time response and mediation is vital in medical imaging informatics.
- Artificial Intelligence (AI) as a data analytics tool to predict threats and estimate damage assessment is becoming widely used across the digital medical imaging industry.

PEARLS

- Disaster recovery is a set of policies, procedures, processes, and systems put into place to facilitate the restoration and recovery of vital data and infrastructure following a natural or man-made catastrophic event.
- Mission critical systems are those necessary for the business to operate.
- Internal and external Service Level Agreements (SLAs) are vital and should be negotiated and ranked against other mission critical systems.
- Resource allocation for DR system management and deployment must continuously be evaluated and updated.
- Document and practice various testing scenarios to keep DR systems and procedures polished.
- Protect the data in both the production and DR system environment.
- Create tactical DR mission critical system workarounds for the clinicians and end users.
- Documentation for DR systems must be maintained regularly.

Self-Assessment Questions

1. Who should have the responsibility of declaring a disaster event?

   (a) Self-assess the situation and declare based on your observations
   (b) A central authority defined by your organization
   (c) The IT manager
   (d) A committee of IT managers and directors

2. What are two (2) reasons a disaster may be declared?

   (a) Component failure and a catastrophic event
   (b) More than 50% of IT staff out due to illness
   (c) Virus or malware found on a single component
   (d) Results are missing from PACS due to an interface error

3. What types of systems in your organization should be identified for disaster recovery purposes?

   (a) All infrastructure including test and development systems
   (b) Only network equipment used for data flow
   (c) Mission critical systems your organization needs to operate
   (d) Only video conferencing equipment and cameras

4. What are the two (2) types of disaster recovery scenarios

   (a) Really bad and moderate
   (b) Catastrophic and isolated
   (c) Monday mornings and days before a holiday
   (d) Corrupt records and accidently deleted files

5. What is DRaaS?

   (a) Disaster Recovery as a Service. A way for your organization to leverage a third-party reproduction of your critical infrastructure usually at a more manageable cost than hosting your own team.
   (b) Disaster recovery as a Side Job. A way to make a little extra income.
   (c) Disaster recovery as a Sith. A way for your data to harness the power of the dark side.
   (d) Disaster recovery as a Substitute. Used instead of following commonsense steps to secure your data in real-time and for future recovery.

6. It is important to have clearly defined roles for IT staff in a disaster recovery event.

   (a) True
   (b) False

7. Practicing good disaster recovery prevention will include but is not limited to?

   (a) User base education
   (b) Actively scanning your infrastructure for known vulnerabilities
   (c) Centralize log gathering to look for abnormal behavior
   (d) All of the above

8. You can best protect against Ransomware by doing the following:

   (a) Do not open untrusted email attachments
   (b) Never click on links that you do not trust or are unverified
   (c) Make sure your operating systems are updated with the latest security patches.
   (d) All of the above

9. To validate your disaster recovery documentation is essential. All of these best practices to document *except* for:

   (a) Initial plan and scenario, including all systems and data
   (b) Test data from a specifically chosen patient
   (c) Control sheets for defined process(es)
   (d) Sign-off from business unit and DR team

10. The future of disaster recovery is moving from just a reaction to an event to:

   (a) Understanding "these things happen" and moving on.
   (b) Making sure you have your music downloaded for the long hours of recovery ahead.
   (c) Keeping your resume updated just in case.
   (d) A real-time adaptation to threats using agile responses and leverage new technologies such as AI to predict potential threats.

Chapter 29
Downtime Procedures

Sylvia Devlin

Contents

29.1 Introduction

Digital images are used across a wide range of medical specialties and acquired throughout the medical enterprise through use of encounter-based workflows. Health Information Technology (HIT) applications and systems used to acquire and view medical images are considered mission critical in healthcare and require uptime solutions to guarantee optimal system availability. As system failures are inevitable, every imaging informatics professional (IIP) must be prepared for downtimes. Downtime procedure planning, development of digital imaging downtime policies and procedures, and periodic downtime drills will help promote patient safety and continuity of care during system downtime events.

> **DEFINITION: Downtime**
>
> A period of time when a digital information system, an application server, or the network are unavailable or fails to provide its primary function, resulting in data communication interruptions.

S. Devlin (✉)
Medical Imaging Information Technology, Johns Hopkins Medicine, Baltimore, MD, USA
e-mail: sdevlin4@jh.edu

© The Author(s), under exclusive license to Springer Science+Business Media, LLC, part of Springer Nature 2021
B. F. Branstetter IV (ed.), *Practical Imaging Informatics*,
https://doi.org/10.1007/978-1-0716-1756-4_29

489

29.2 Downtime Considerations and Scenarios

All imaging systems incur both scheduled and unscheduled downtimes. Scheduled imaging system downtimes occur periodically to deploy patches and updates needed to keep the systems working at peak performance. Best practice is to upgrade less frequently and deploy patches only when necessary. Unscheduled system downtimes are due to unforeseen events that are caused by software corruptions, hardware and network failures, cyberattacks, or catastrophic environmental issues such as heating, ventilation, and air conditioning (HVAC) failures, fires, floods, or earthquakes. It is critical to remember that any digital imaging system downtime could result in patient care delays.

> **KEY CONCEPT: Types of Downtime**
>
> Both scheduled and unscheduled downtimes are inevitable in any digital system. Careful planning minimizes the negative impact.

29.2.1 Scheduled Downtimes

- Done for routine system patch deployment, maintenance, and upgrades.
- Can be scheduled for a time that is least disruptive to patient care teams.
  - Collaboration and communication with affected clinical care teams is essential to determine the best time.
- When planning scheduled downtimes, it is critical to understand the amount of time required for upgrades and patch deployments.
- Consider times when you can buffer the downtime window just in case extra time is needed. Better to come back on-line ahead of time rather than go longer than promised.
- Effectively communicating the scheduled downtime to system end users is imperative (see **Chap. 31**). Use of a standard downtime communication template is recommended and should include the following:
  - Identification of the system
  - Purpose of the downtime
  - Impacted users
  - Date of downtime and duration
  - Personnel available for support during the downtime and their contact information
- Determine the best way to disseminate the scheduled downtime information:
  - Email scheduled downtime announcement to system end users.
  - Post the downtime announcement ahead of time on the application splash screen to remind users of the approaching scheduled system downtime. (But be careful not to slow down or frustrate your users, lest they start to ignore your messages!).

- Departmental or application-based dashboards.
- Scheduled downtime procedures and protocols require periodic review and updating.

29.2.2 Unscheduled Downtimes

- Occurs when a system fails unexpectedly.
- Two distinct downtime procedures and protocols are required: one for business hour downtimes and the other for after hours. Downtime support will be different for each instance.
- Ensure that the IIPs have all relevant information needed to support an unscheduled downtime in soft and hardcopy formats. Depending upon the type of downtime, softcopy versions may not be accessible.
- Keep all information needed to support unscheduled downtimes readily available. Remember that unscheduled downtimes may occur when support personnel are not onsite or are off duty.
- Unscheduled downtime procedures and protocols require periodic review and update.

29.3 Planning for Downtimes

Planning for scheduled and unscheduled downtimes requires cooperation and collaboration among technical, operational, and clinical teams. Well-defined decision criteria are necessary to facilitate a seamless transition to downtime operations. Preplanning for potential adverse events that could occur during a scheduled downtime will enable the IIP to have external resources readily available if needed. But being able to seamlessly transition from normal operational processes to downtime operations requires careful planning to get ahead of unforeseen challenges. It is imperative that all clinical staff become well versed and comfortable using downtime tools and workflows so they can remain focused on patient care. Downtime mitigation strategies include the following:

HYPOTHETICAL SCENARIO

The PACS goes down unexpectedly. No images are transmitting. Should you transition to a backup system that could require the efforts of unprepared external personnel? Should you contact a radiologist to come into the hospital at zero hours to read emergent stroke studies? (Which radiologist reads stroke studies?) Having a plan and answers to these types of challenging questions ahead of time will help you successfully navigate the downtime chaos.

A. **Risk assessment and mapping**. The imaging informatics systems and applications used in the clinical setting require periodic review of technical and operational processes. This involves identification and quantification of all risks associated with the delivery of patient care during system failures. It is important to have a firm understanding of end user workflows during normal operations in order to create alternative yet equivalent workflows that can be deployed during a system downtime. The goal is to ensure that your end users are comfortable transitioning from normal operations to downtime workflows without disruptions in patient care.

B. **Performing a comprehensive review of all imaging informatics devices that connect to the hospital network**. This step should include an inventory of all modalities, clinical workstations, diagnostic workstations, and laptops. It is important to include static IPs, application entity titles (AETs), ports, and other external Information Technology (IT) infrastructure products related to the imaging systems. Access to this inventory must be accessible during a downtime event that prevents access to digital storage devices.

> **KEY CONCEPT: Information Technology Products and Infrastructure**
>
> All products and systems that could cause or could be affected by an unplanned downtime. Examples include modalities, workstations, information systems, network switches, and Internet.

C. **Creation of a downtime committee comprised of essential stakeholders is helpful**. A downtime committee facilitates process improvement initiatives and is ideally comprised of those stakeholders directly impacted by downtime operations. The benefit of regularly scheduled downtime committee meetings is the creation of a forum where policies, risk assessments, and downtime strategies can be discussed and continuously refined. Downtime committee members could include the following:
   - Radiologists
   - IIPs
   - IT staff
   - Executive leadership
   - Emergency department providers

D. **Change management processes aim to mitigate risk and the suboptimal impact of planned changes in infrastructure and operations**. Change control tasks and pre-release activities associated with the rollout of a new or upgraded system include release notes, testing documentation, quality control checks, and back-out processes. The goal of change management is to identify the actions required for the implemention of specific changes, the coordination of those changes, and the impact the change will have across the organization. Change control often involves a Change Control Board, which is a formal chartered group responsible for reviewing, approving, or rejecting system changes (see **Chap. 26**).

E. **Additional downtime mitigation strategies include the following**:
- Incorporating a **rollback plan** just in case unpredicted issues arise during the upgrade or failover process.
- Performing system and data backups prior to upgrades. Completion of these tasks prior to changes to the system will ensure that if a system rollback is necessary, the system will return to its previous state.
- Maintenance and upkeep of comparable diagnostic workstations in the event of hardware failure. This practice avoids reading workflow disruptions as it provides the ability for radiologists to easily relocate to an equivalent **hot spare** diagnostic workstation. It is also helpful to keep standby peripheral equipment available such as monitors and microphones for quick and easy replacement.
- Performance of periodic scheduled failovers of your Hospital Information System (HIS), Electronic Medical Record (EMR), Radiology Information System (RIS), Picture Archiving and Communication System (PACS), and voice recognition systems. **Intentional failover exercises** which transition to your secondary systems will expose any deficiencies that can be addressed while the primary systems are running without issue.
- During downtimes, it is helpful to ensure that IT support staff are physically on-site to assist end users with any operational issues and aid your remote support, such as vendors, by providing hands-on assistance.
- Maintain an updated contact list for all stakeholders including clinicians, IIPs, IT, hospital leadership, and vendor support. This should include both office and personal telephone numbers.
- Maintain an updated inventory of all system identification and configuration settings. Note that after-hours vendor support personnel may not be as familiar with your site as the support teams you work with during normal business hours.
- Define an escalation process and identify key staff who should be contacted in the event of an extended scheduled or unscheduled downtime.
- Request that system vendors provide references for other customer sites that are similar to your facility's size, workflows, and technology products. This provides the opportunity to ask these reference sites about any downtimes they have incurred, and discuss lessons learned from those experiences.

> **DEFINITION: Escalation Process**
>
> Defines who to contact next when the first point of contact does not respond in a timely manner. The sequence of individuals is an escalation policy.

29.4 Business Continuance

To minimize digital imaging downtimes, business continuance planning is essential. The premise of business continuance planning is to mitigate **single points of failure** (SPOF) in the diagnostic imaging ecosystem. Should a failure in any one function occur, an identical second function should be readily available to reduce disruptions in service.

Part of the planning phase should include an assessment and identification of every SPOF with the qualification that the more critical the function, the higher the priority to create redundancy for this function. Proactively asking the right questions to those on the frontlines during normal operation uptimes will provide a comprehensive understanding of what is needed and what resources healthcare providers can use during a system downtime. Consider how long your end users can tolerate having a system downtime before risks are introduced to patient care. Redundancy for mission-critical system elements including modalities, clinical and diagnostic workstations, HIS, EMR, RIS, and PACS will facilitate the continuity of care. Even small gaps in continuity can reduce healthcare outcomes and patient satisfaction scores, not to mention the morale of the healthcare workers. Disaster recovery (DR) planning is equally important (see

> **DEFINITION: Single Point of Failure**
>
> A single point of failure (SPOF) is an IT system element that can cause your entire system to stop functioning if that particular element goes bad. An SPOF can be hardware (e.g., a network switch), software (e.g., an HL7 interface engine), a facility, or even a person. Identifying and classifying SPOFs at the onset of planning will expose vulnerabilities.

> **DEFINITION: System Redundancy**
>
> The opposite of a single point of failure is system redundancy, in which every potential failure point has an equivalent fallback that can be quickly (or automatically) invoked. You should seek ways to replace SPOFs with redundancy.

Chap. 28). Unfortunately, catastrophic events are not uncommon, and if your data center is destroyed, the ability to restore your data and applications in a timely manner is vital. Proactive planning for disruptions in service by developing workaround processes to mitigate risks associated with operational disruptions is a critical element of modern high-quality healthcare.

29.4.1 Fault Tolerance

- **Fault tolerance** (FT) is the ability of a given system to continue functioning even if one of its components fails.
- FT systems minimize SPOFs and are designed to fail and recover gracefully should any components in the system fail.

- An example of FT design is two or more mirrored systems operating in tandem. A second server and database can be clustered with the primary server which allows the two servers to be synchronized. Should

> **DEFINITION: Fault Tolerance**
>
> The ability of a given system to continue functioning even if one of its components fails

the primary system fail, the secondary system detects the failure and simultaneously takes over with zero loss of service or downtime.
- A system that requires manual operator intervention in order to failover to a secondary server is not considered fault tolerant.

29.4.2 High Availability

- High availability (HA) solutions refer to the overall availability of a system including both hardware and software elements to support business operations.
- Digital imaging vendors offer continuance availability and architecture designs that promote system uptimes.
- Uptimes are often measured in percentages of availability per unit of time using "nines" as the unit base (e.g., 99%, 99.9%, 99.99%).
- Note that **uptime and availability** are not the same. Uptime refers to a specific component's ability to function. Availability refers to the capacity of the entire system to support business operations. An example is that a given system could have an uptime of 99.99% from the perspective of the server hardware but have only 99% availability due to frequent network service disruptions.

Due to advances in technology, vendors can more readily offer a four-nines uptime availability, which translates into approximately 1 hour of downtime per year. Although the four-nines option guarantee is an impressive standard, a higher availability option does exist. The holy grail of fault tolerance systems is the ultimate 99.999%, or **five-nines** availability rate. Should your organization choose this continuance availability solution, you would expect no more than 5 minutes of downtime per year. Although this option may sound appealing, pursuit of this standard may be impractical due to cost constraints. Before getting swept up in such hype, carefully consider how long your organization can tolerate having a system off-line before introducing risk to patient care and how promptly you would need your systems to recover from failures.

When planning your IT architecture, it is important to help leadership understand that both high availability and fault-tolerant designs are critical elements for ensuring business continuity and require consideration when purchasing high-end equipment.

29.4.3 Disaster Recovery

When the downtime is a result of catastrophic failures, a formal disaster recovery and contingency plan is required. Disaster recovery procedures aim toward protecting against data loss and alternative methods of image storage while the primary imaging system is down (see **Chap. 28**).

29.5 Policies and Procedures

Although downtime policies and procedures are specific to each organization, common elements include the following:

A. **Identification of all devices, systems, and end users engaged in patient imaging encounters:**

System	Examples of imaging service users
Hospital Information System (HIS)	Patient registration Imaging billing personnel
Electronic Medical Record (EMR)	Ordering providers Nurses Radiology technologists Radiologists
Radiology Information System (RIS)	Radiology technologists Radiologists
Imaging modalities	Radiology technologists Radiologists Emergency medicine (point of care ultrasound)
Picture Archiving and Communications System (PACS)	Radiology technologists Radiologists Providers from other specialties: – Emergency medicine – Orthopedic surgery – Neurosurgery – Fetal assessment

B. **Learn user workflow and describe the steps users would follow during a downtime event**. When composing the downtime procedures, take the time to speak with the end users to gain a firm understanding of how they use the system during normal operations and what they could use as a workaround when the imaging system fails. Creation of downtime templates, forms, and checklists of each system is beneficial. Downtime procedure templates provide a standard structure for each downtime scenario (Fig. 29.1). The steps should be kept in secure locations in soft and hardcopy formats and should be accessible to end users as well as support personnel. Should your facility experience a network outage or ransomware attack, referencing hardcopy formats may be your only option. Make sure the hardcopy downtime procedures are reviewed and updated regularly and accessible to all users.

C. **Maintain and incorporate a current list of contacts and system information into the downtime procedures**. Having contact and system information readily available during a downtime event will save time and effort (especially if the downtime occurs after hours when you are off-site!). Important information include the following:
   - Vendor support and after-hours contact information.
   - Your organization's site ID.
   - System configurations such as IP, AET, and port information.
   - The phone numbers and extensions for users impacted by downtime including radiology reading rooms, technologist control areas, and external critical department areas such as the emergency department.
   - Contact information for leadership and administration. Include both office and personal information just in case your downtime is after hours.

D. **Definition of a standard communication process which outlines how information will be disseminated to end users and stakeholders.** Usually this is deployed via email, application splash screen announcements, or other virtual mass notification technologies (see **Chap. 31**). The type of outage may dictate how the communications are broadcasted. For example, if your facility is experiencing a network outage, virtual communications will be unavailable, and your only communication options may be hospital overhead speakers or via telephone communications.

E. **Definition of an escalation processes for support and notification.** The downtime procedure should indicate who to contact if your support contact is unavailable or unreachable. Do not forget to include executive leadership. If you have a significant downtime, the Imaging Director, Radiology Medical Director, and other executive leaders may want to be made aware of the situation. Have their contact information embedded in your downtime procedures.

F. **Establishment of post downtime procedures.** These should be part of the downtime procedures documentation. Most roles will need to check that all data acquired during the downtime have been successfully reconciled such as patient demographic errors and all imaging data are back to normal state. Document the procedures in the same standard template format as your downtime procedures (Fig. 29.2).

G. **Scheduling of a postmortem analysis for unscheduled downtime events.** This process is used after unscheduled system downtimes and is intended to promote a comprehensive understanding of root causes. **Postmortem analysis** defines strategies to mitigate future unscheduled downtime events. Unscheduled downtime events are stressful, and it may be tempting to use the postmortem process as a vehicle to cast blame. When used constructively, utilizing a just culture philosophy, the postmortem process is quite valuable in identifying lessons learned. Some of the elements contained in a postmortem process include the following:
   - A record of what happened.
   - Time when system end users discovered the issue (this may be different than your vendor's time).
   - The impact the unscheduled downtime had on the department/institution.
   - The actions taken to resolve the unscheduled downtime.

- An incident report from the vendor which includes root cause analysis.
- Follow-up actions to prevent reoccurrence of the problem.

PACS Unscheduled Downtime After Hours	
During Downtime Procedures	
IIP:	1. Determine if isolated to one user, one hospital or enterprise wide
	2. Contact Vendor Support - Support telephone: Our Site ID: A123

	3. Use escalation process for support if needed. Start technical bridge call to include external resources if needed:
	   - Integration Services
	   - RIS Support
	   - Network

	4. Send virtual notification update to end users and enterprise

	5. Telephone system end users. Provide updates and answer questions:
	   - Radiology reading room:
	        or
	   - Radiologist reading after hours/off site: (Check on-call schedule)
	   - Tech control room:
	   - ED nurses' station:

	6. If deemed appropriate, failover to secondary node
	7. If PACS is still not on -line after 30 minutes, contact the on-call radiologist to return onsite to read emergent cases

	8. Notify hospital leadership if downtime persists > 30 minutes
	   - Imaging Director of Operations
	        ▪ Office:
	        ▪ Cellular:
	   - Radiology Medical Director
	        ▪ Office:
	        ▪ Cellular:

Radiologist	1. View study at modality
	2. Render preliminary reads for emergent orders
	3. Call STAT preliminary findings to ordering provider
Technologist	1. Enter patient demographics at modality
	2. Alert radiologist of STAT imaging studies
	3. Document all patients' name, MRN, study description on "PACS Downtime" form
ED Provider	1. Call technologist when patient needs imaging study
	2. ED Provider to come to modality to view image if needed
	3. Preliminary reports available via telephone or reading room visit

Fig. 29.1 Example of a PACS after-hours unscheduled downtime template

Post Downtime Procedures		
IIP	1.	Contact end users to confirm application is working as expected
	2.	Send out "All Clear" Communication
	3.	Gather downtime forms from technologists for reconciliation process
	4.	Check PACS for orphaned studies
	5.	Check with radiologists to ensure all studies have been reconciled appropriately
	6.	Perform reconciliations of broken studies
	7.	Schedule Postmortem Analysis (may take the vendor a few days to complete incident report)
	8.	Provide leadership with a Root Cause Analysis Status Report that includes an explanation and demonstration of how the problem can be mitigated in the future
Radiologist	1.	Reboot diagnostic workstation to reestablish integration
	2.	Perform diagnostic reads to confirm application is working as expected – let IIP know if working as expected or otherwise
	3.	Reconcile any preliminary reads – contact IIP if assistance is needed
	4.	Final sign studies read during downtime, so they are available in EMR
	5.	Resume normal operation
Technologist	1.	Create orders for all studies acquired during downtime in RIS
	2.	Track all studies to completed status in RIS so that studies appear on the radiologist reading worklist
	3.	Send all studies acquired during downtime to PACS
	4.	Confirm all imaging studies send to PACS from modality as expected
	5.	Check PACS to confirm studies and series display as expected
	6.	Complete downtime form and give to IIP
	7.	Resume normal operation
ED Provider	1.	Order any imaging studies that occurred during downtime
	2.	Confirm with technologist that order was received
	3.	Confirm that imaging studies and reports are available in PACS
	4.	Resume normal operations

Fig. 29.2 Example of a PACS after-hours unscheduled post-downtime template

DEFINITION: Just Culture

An adverse event reporting/debriefing system in which individual blame is de-emphasized and underlying systematic reasons for failure are addressed.

DEFINITION: Incident Report

Post-downtime report provided by the vendor that explains the cause of any unscheduled downtime.

29.6 Conclusion

System downtimes are inevitable. Therefore, creation and maintenance of downtime policies and procedures are critical for the continuity of clinical operations. Since imaging informatics professionals are essential during the downtime process, they are often solicited to assist with the creation of downtime procedures, support, and maintaining up-to-date documentation. The creation of effective downtime procedures can be perceived as an arduous and painstaking process. However, the impact of having established downtime procedures that are readily available during a crisis makes this painstaking process worthwhile. A well-defined set of policies and procedures coupled with a reliable IT infrastructure that includes high availability, fault tolerance, and disaster recovery architecture will minimize operational inefficiencies and ensure quality patient care and safety.

PEARLS

- Healthcare business continuance planning is critical as patients, clinicians, and healthcare systems require a viable workaround when primary systems fail.
- Downtime scenarios include scheduled and unscheduled downtimes. Resources and procedures are different for each downtime scenario.
- Planning is key to minimizing downtimes and includes due diligence, risk assessment, use of downtime committees, and change management processes to reduce risk.
- When scheduling a downtime event, consider times when you can buffer the downtime window, just in case extra time is needed. Better to come back online ahead of time rather than go longer than promised.
- Beneficial elements in health IT architecture design include high availability, fault tolerance, and disaster recovery.
- Elements common to the creation of downtime policies and procedures include the following:
  - Identification of all systems and users involved with patient imaging encounters.
  - Definition of the steps for users to follow for each system during a downtime event.
  - Maintenance of a current list of contacts and system information and incorporation of this information into downtime procedures.
  - Definition of a communication process which outlines specific information for dissemination to end users and stakeholders.
  - Definition of an escalation processes for support and notification.
  - Establishment of post-downtime procedures.
  - Completion of a postmortem analysis after an unscheduled downtime.

Further Reading

ACR-AAPM-SIIM Practice Parameter for Electronic Medical Information Privacy and Security. https://www.acr.org/-/media/ACR/Files/Practice-Parameters/Elec-Info-Privacy.pdf, Accessed 8/11/2020

Archiving, Chapter 6: Business Continuity and Disaster Recovery. https://siim.org/general/custom.asp?page=archiving_chapter6, Accessed 7/24/2020

Plan B: A practical Approach to Downtime Planning in Medical Practices. AHIMA. https://library.ahima.org/doc?oid=95715#.Xws6tNiSmUk, Accessed 7/11/2020

Ransomware attacks spike, cost healthcare orgs millions. https://www.medicaleconomics.com/view/ransomware-attacks-spike-cost-healthcare-orgs-millions, Accessed 8/11/2020

Securing Picture Archiving and Communication System. https://www.nccoe.nist.gov/projects/usecases/health-it/pacs, Accessed 8/11/2020

Self-Assessment Questions

1. Which of the following would *not* be considered a downtime type?

   (a) Hardware failure
   (b) Network outage
   (c) Printer failure
   (d) Software failure
   (e) Power outage

2. All the following terms are related to IT Architecture except:

   (a) Redundancy
   (b) IT Help Desk
   (c) Fault tolerance
   (d) High availability
   (e) Disaster recovery

3. What might you consider when developing strategies for minimizing downtimes?

   (a) Performing period system failovers
   (b) Risk assessment and mapping
   (c) Identifying vulnerabilities
   (d) None of the above
   (e) All the above

4. Who should be notified of a scheduled outage?

   (a) Hospital administration
   (b) House staff
   (c) Providers
   (d) All the above
   (e) None of the above

5. What clinical and technical roles would be considered to participate in a down-time committee?

   (a) Radiologist
   (b) Imaging informatics professional
   (c) Imaging leadership
   (d) Information technology
   (e) All the above

6. All are potential imaging informatics related downtime scenarios except:

   (a) EMR
   (b) PACS
   (c) Global pandemic
   (d) Network outage
   (e) Infrastructure failure

7. Which would be viable solution for communication during a network outage?

   (a) Email
   (b) Imaging application splash screen announcements
   (c) Telephone
   (d) VoIP notifications
   (e) Virtual mass notification technologies

8. True or false; hardcopy downtime procedures are not needed in the twenty-first century.

   (a) True
   (b) False

9. All elements are common when creating downtime policies and proce-dures except:

   (a) Identification of all systems and users used during imaging encounters
   (b) Casting blame and finger pointing after downtime events
   (c) Maintaining a current list of contacts and system information
   (d) Establishment of post downtime procedures

10. List several potential methods of communication for scheduled and unsched-uled downtimes.

Chapter 30
Policy Management and Regulatory Compliance

David E. Brown

Contents

D. E. Brown (✉)
Los Angeles, CA, USA
e-mail: David.E.Brown@kp.org

© The Author(s), under exclusive license to Springer Science+Business Media,
LLC, part of Springer Nature 2021
B. F. Branstetter IV (ed.), *Practical Imaging Informatics*,
https://doi.org/10.1007/978-1-0716-1756-4_30

30.1 Introduction

Policy management and regulatory compliance extend well beyond administrative management and touch all levels of an organization. The role of an imaging informatics professional is to be knowledgeable on organizational, local, state, and federal requirements and to assure that this area of responsibility is in compliance with these requirements.

30.2 The Health Information Privacy and Accountability Act (HIPAA)

30.2.1 Overview

- **The Health Information Privacy and Accountability Act of 1996** is a healthcare reform act adopted by the US Congress that required national standards aimed at protecting sensitive patient health information. Some of the regulations in HIPAA include:
  - Regulating the disclosure of sensitive health information without an individual's consent or knowledge
  - Provisions to protect against healthcare abuse and medical fraud
  - Requiring that personal health information be protected and kept confidential

  > **DEFINITION: PHI**
  >
  > Protected health information is any health-related data that is specific to an individual and thus could be used to identify the individual. There are 18 specific identifiers listed in HIPAA.

  - Standards for the management of protected health information (PHI)
- HIPAA is comprised of the following five titles:
  - Title I: HIPAA Health Information Reform
  - Title II: HIPAA Administrative Simplification
  - Title III: HIPAA Tax-Related Health Provisions
  - Title IV: Application and Enforcement of Group Health Plan Requirements
  - Title V: Revenue Offsets

30.2.2 Title II: Administrative Simplification

- **Title II specifically addresses the protection of PHI** and has significantly impacted how healthcare providers handle PHI throughout the United States.
- Title II focused on protecting against medical fraud and abuse by increasing efficiency and effectiveness of the healthcare delivery network by establishing requirements addressing the management of electronic healthcare information.

- Title II required that the Department of Health and Human Services (HHS) define national standards for administrative simplification.
- HHS defined **five rules addressing administrative simplification**:
  1. The Privacy Rule
  2. The Transactions and Code Sets Rule
  3. The Security Rule
  4. The Unique Identifiers Rule
  5. The Enforcement Rule
- The **Transactions and Code Sets Rule** specified standards for claims and payment information, including the International Classifications of Diseases (ICD) and Current Procedural Terminology (CPT) code sets.
- The **Unique Identifiers Rule** requires standard national identifiers for covered employers and providers. The National Provider Identifier (NPI) is a unique number for healthcare providers used in the administrative and financial transactions adopted under HIPAA.

CHECKLIST: The 18 HIPAA Identifiers

1. Names
2. Geographic subdivisions smaller than a state, geocodes (e.g., zip, county, or city codes; street address, etc.)
3. Dates; all elements of dates except year, unless individual is > 89 years (e.g., birth date, admission date, etc.)
4. Telephone numbers
5. Fax numbers
6. Electronic mail addresses
7. Social security numbers
8. Medical record numbers
9. Health plan beneficiary numbers
10. Account numbers
11. Certificate/license numbers
12. Vehicle identifiers and serial numbers (including license plate numbers)
13. Device identifiers and serial numbers
14. Web Universal Resource Locator (URL)
15. Internet protocol (IP) address number
16. Biometric identifiers (including finger or voice prints)
17. Full face photographic images and any comparable images
18. Any other unique identifying number, characteristic, or code

> **KEY CONCEPT: The Privacy Rule**
>
> To avoid interfering with an individual's access to healthcare or the efficient payment for such healthcare, the Privacy Rule permits a covered entity to use and disclose protected health information, with certain limits and protections, for treatment, payment, and healthcare operation activities.
>
> https://www.hhs.gov/hipaa/for-professionals/privacy/guidance/disclosures-treatment-payment-health-care-operations/index.html

30.2.3 The Privacy Rule

- The Privacy Rule went into effect in 2003 and established national standards on the **use**, **disclosure**, and **protection of health information.**
- The Privacy Rule pertains to protected health information (PHI) in any format, including **hardcopy** and **electronic** representations.

> **DEFINITION: Covered Entity**
>
> Any organization to which the HIPAA Privacy Rule applies, namely, health plans, healthcare clearinghouses, healthcare providers, and business associates of those entities

- The Privacy Rule generally requires that **covered entities**, which include health plans and most healthcare providers, provide individuals or those they designate access to their PHI upon request. This includes the right to inspect or copy as well as the transmission of a copy to a designated person or entity regardless of the date of service, whether the PHI is maintained in hard or soft copy (on-site or off-site), or where the PHI originated.

> **INTERNATIONAL CONSIDERATIONS**
>
> The European counterpart of HIPAA is GDPR (General Data Protection Regulations). GDPR emphasizes the following:
> - Opt-in consent for any use of patient data.
> - Strict digital security regulations.
> - The right to be forgotten – data must be deleted on patient request.

30.2.4 The Security Rule

- The Security Rule went into full effect in 2006 and sets standards for the management of protected health information in electronic format (ePHI), including confidentiality, integrity, and availability.
- The Security Rule includes standards and implementation specifications that are classified as "required" or "addressable."
  - **Required implementation specifications** must be implemented.

- **Addressable implementation specifications** require an assessment to determine if the addressable safeguard is reasonable and appropriate in the given environment. If the safeguard is determined to be unreasonable and inappropriate, then documentation is required to justify the decision. Equivalent alternatives must be considered in the assessment.
- During a HIPAA security audit, both required and addressable implementation specifications are examined closely by the Office for Civil Rights.
- The Security Rule identified three safeguards for compliance:
  1. **Administrative safeguards** include security management, assignment of security responsibility, risk analysis and management, information access management, security awareness and training, security incident procedures, data backup and recovery plans, and written security contracts with business associates.
     - **Security management** requires the implementation of policies and procedures addressing the prevention, detection, containment, and correction of security violations.
     - Assignment of **security responsibility** requires the designation of a **HIPAA compliance officer**, who is responsible for the development and implementation of security policies and procedures.
       - All personnel should know their HIPAA compliance officer's contact information, as well as contact information of the rest of the security team.
     - The security team may also include a privacy officer and a security officer.
     - **Risk analysis and management** includes risk analysis on factors for each system that could affect confidentiality, availability, and the integrity of ePHI.
       - Periodic risk assessments are required due to the dynamic nature of technology and environment.
       - Document HIPAA compliance capabilities for each system, including deficiencies and planned remediation. Describe measures being taken to reduce risks and vulnerabilities.
     - Review of information system activity is typically accomplished by using:

> **HYPOTHETICAL SCENARIO: Network Down**
>
> Suppose your entire network went down in the middle of the day and all of your downtime procedures were only posted on your company website. Would your staff know what to do?
> *Highly recommended*: Keep hardcopy manuals of downtime policies and procedures in key areas.

> **HYPOTHETICAL SCENARIO: Celebrity Health Records for Sale**
>
> Suppose an employee was selling celebrity health information from your facility to the tabloids. Would this be detected? Do you have a written policy on how to handle this breach?

- Audit logs
- Access reports
- Security incident track-ing reports
- Information access management includes policy and procedures on the establishment, modifica-tion, and termination of access for authorized personnel.
  - Information access authori-zation should provide appropriate levels of access based on job function.
  - Demonstrated competency with an application as mea-sured by competency tests should be required prior to providing access to the application.
- **Security awareness and training** is required for per-sonnel who works with or has exposure to ePHI and should be established as an annual competency. It is important to publicize any possible out-comes for an employee in the event of a security breach if it is determined that the breach is willful or significant in nature.
- Documentation of a **system backup policy** should include

KEY CONCEPT: Audit Logs

Audit logs should provide the fol-lowing information:

Who?	User ID of person looking at PHI
What?	Identify PHI viewed
When?	Date and time viewed
Where?	Unique PC station name that can be used to identify location

Note: The "Why?" will require follow-up with the employee or employee's supervisor

KEY CONCEPT: Server Security

- Are your servers located in a secure environment, protected from tampering and theft?
- Do you limit access to server rooms using key cards or proxy card readers?
- Is the room temperature controlled?
- Are the servers protected from electrical power spikes and outages?

patient data backups, database backups, and system backups. Include pol-icy of periodic checks for readability of backup tapes and other media.
- A formal, documented **disaster recovery and contingency plan** is required. Both catastrophic failure and system malfunction should be addressed.
  - Identify the disaster recovery manager and members of the disaster recovery team for each application, and include contact information in the disaster recovery and contingency plan.
- Business associates who have access to ePHI are required to sign a written security contract or other arrangement regarding the protection of ePHI.

CHECKLIST: Administrative Safeguards

1. HIPAA compliance officer and team selected and contact information known to personnel.
2. HIPAA compliance policies and procedures complete and up-to-date. Policies reviewed and updated on a regular basis.

Recommended P&P:	Master list of HIPAA-related policies and forms
	HIPAA policy approval process
	Confidentiality policy
	HIPAA violation inspection policy
	Minimum access information policy
	Minimum access job description documentation
	Privacy practices policy
	System and database backup policy
	Business continuity and disaster recovery policy

3. HIPAA compliance training of personnel performed on a recurring basis. Establishing training as an annual competency is recommended.
4. HIPAA compliance validation and documentation on all systems and applications containing PHI.
5. Signed contracts with business associates who have access to PHI assuring HIPAA compliance with regard to disclosure and protection of PHI.

2. **Physical safeguards** include facility access controls and security plan, workstation use and security, device media control, and data backup.
   - Physical safeguards must limit physical access to information systems containing PHI and the facility in which they reside while allowing proper access to appropriate personnel.
   - Document how physical access is limited to a system or application, including servers, workstations, and applications.
   - Workstation security includes the development of policies and procedures addressing appropriate workstation use and measures that can be taken to protect PHI.

> **DEFINITION: Physical Security**
>
> The physical environment around a computer system that prevents unauthorized access to equipment Examples include locks, security guards, video cameras, and biometric devices.

   - Safeguard against the **inadvertent viewing of PHI** by unauthorized individuals. Have computer monitors facing away from public view and use password-protected screen savers. Privacy screens are highly recommended in areas where unauthorized individuals may have the ability to view confidential information or PHI.

CHECKLIST: Physical Security

1. All servers should be located in a secure environment. Security includes limiting access to authorized personnel and controlling environmental factors such as room temperature and power sources.
2. Secure PCs and workstations located in public areas to safeguard against theft and the inadvertent viewing of PHI by the public.
3. Establish policy on the acceptable use of removable media including USB flash drives, CDs, DVDs, removable disk drives, and tapes.
4. Establish a procedure for the removal of PHI whenever a device is discarded or relocated to another area.
5. Establish a policy of requiring backups prior to the movement of equipment.

   - Device media control policies and procedures should address what is appropriate use of tapes, disk drives, removable drives, USB flash drives, CDs or DVDs, and any other devices or media that may contain PHI.
   - Document how PHI is eliminated prior to the disposal or relocation of electronic media containing PHI.
   - Data backup requires documentation on how a retrievable, exact copy of ePHI will be created. Data backup is an addressable item prior to the movement of equipment.

3. **Technical safeguards** include unique user identification, user account administration, emergency access procedures, audit controls, electronic data integrity, person and entity authentication, and transmission security.
   - User account administration requires that each user who has access to PHI have a unique user identification assigned. This provides a method for tracking individual users accessing PHI using audit logs.
   - User account administration establishes an approval process for account authorization and standard procedure for removing access when personnel leave or transfer to another work area. Accounts must be suspended for personnel taking an extended absence.
   - Review all user accounts periodically to identify dormant accounts that can be deactivated or removed. Establish a procedure for the removal of these accounts.
   - Automatic logoffs should be employed that terminate a user's session after a certain period of inactivity. This time can vary based on the function of the application. The inactivity period selected should be documented in policy and procedure.

CHECKLIST: Technical Safeguards

1. Establish unique user IDs for each application accessing PHI. Eliminate any generic user logons.
2. Establish account authorization procedure including the factors determining the appropriate assignment of user privileges.
3. Establish a procedure addressing the deactivation or removal of account access when personnel is transferred or terminated.
4. Document configuration settings of PHI-related components for each health information system, including automatic logoff intervals, password retries, password aging, etc.
5. Set up audit logging on all systems containing PHI and document pertinent information captured in the audit logs. Establish a procedure for backing up audit logs.
6. Establish policy addressing remote access of PHI including authentication of remote user or facility, and secure transmission of PHI between remote locations.

- Document emergency access processes for accessing a system or obtaining data when a system cannot be authorized in a normal manner.
- Audit controls should describe the procedure for recording and examining system and application activity. Include the name of the person reviewing the audit logs and document items captured in audit logs.
- Inform and remind employees of established auditing procedures on a routine basis. Annual review is recommended.
- Establish procedures for backing up audit security logs.
- Electronic data integrity includes establishing procedures that safeguard against the improper **alteration or destruction of PHI**. Identify users and user roles that have alteration and deletion privileges within an application or system.
- Person and entity authentication addresses authentication of remote users or entities accessing applications or systems containing PHI. Authentication should include user logon challenges, token keys, smart cards, security certificates, etc.
- Data transmission security includes integrity controls and the encryption of data that are exchanged between two remote locations.

30.2.5 The Enforcement Rule

- The Enforcement Rule establishes civil monetary penalties for HIPAA violations, including the processes associated with identifying violations and assigning penalties.

- The Privacy Rule is enforced by the Health and Human Services Office for Civil Rights (OCR).
- Non-privacy HIPAA rules are enforced by the Health and Human Services for Medicare and Medicaid Services (CMS).

30.2.6 The HITECH Act

- The Health Information Technology for Economic and Clinical Health (HITECH) Act was established as part of the American Recovery and Reinvestment Act of 2009 (ARRA).
- HITECH promoted the adoption of health information technology, specifically the use of electronic health records (EHR) systems.
- The **Meaningful Use of EHRs** focused on five goals:
  1. Improving quality, safety, and efficiency
  2. Engaging patients and families
  3. Improving care coordination
  4. Improving population health
  5. Enhancing privacy and security protection for PHI
- Expanded HIPAA regulations to include business associates and their subcontractors.
- Expanded regulations to include organizations involved with the transfer of PHI between entities such as health information exchanges (HIEs).
- Introduced the HIPAA Breach Notification Rule which required covered entities and business associates to **notify individuals** whose unsecured PHI had been compromised due to a security breach.
- Breaches that involve 500 or more individuals must be reported to the HHS secretary and prominent news media outlets serving the State or jurisdiction no later than 60 days after the event.
- Breaches involving less than 500 individuals must, at a minimum, be reported to the HHS secretary as part of an annual report of breaches incurred.
- Covered entities are required to have written policies and procedures on breach notification and must provide training to employees on these policies and procedures, including sanctions for noncompliant staff.

> **OUR EXPERIENCE:**
> **Cumulative Cost**
>
> The largest breach to date was one reported by Anthem Blue Cross Blue Shield in 2015. The ePHI of almost **79 million people** were exposed. The Office for Civil Rights determined that Anthem had not taken adequate measures to detect hacker intrusion. The breach resulted in a **$16 million** settlement with the federal government and corrective action plans. A class action suit from patients was settled for **$115 million.** The third settlement in this same breach was with State Attorney Generals for **$40 million**.

- "Unsecured PHI" is PHI that is not protected through a technology or methodology that renders PHI unusable to unauthorized individuals.
  - Encryption and destruction render PHI unusable, unreadable, or undecipherable to unauthorized individuals.

KEY CONCEPT:
Sanction Policy

Policy on security violations must be well documented, well known, and enforced. Sanctions can be as severe as employee termination when the violation is determined to be significant and intentional.

DEFINITION: Limited Data Sets

LDS are a HIPAA exception. They include partially de-identified data that excludes most (but not all) protected health information. Things like geographic divisions smaller than a state and dates can be included. LDS is permitted for research, public health, and healthcare operations if specific criteria are met.

- PHI is not to be used for marketing or sales purposes without prior authorization from the individual.
- Authorized use of limited data sets. Data use agreements must be in place before LDS can be shared.

30.2.7 The Final Omnibus Rule

- The Final Omnibus Rule went into effect in 2013 and updated the Privacy, Security, and Enforcement Rules, as well as enforcement defined under the HITECH Act.
- Business associates became directly liable for compliance with certain HIPAA regulations. PHI data transmission services, as well as individuals who offer personal health records to other individuals on behalf of a covered entity, are designated as business associates.

HYPOTHETICAL SCENARIO:
Online PHI

Masking PHI with text box overlays is inadequate for hiding PHI from search engines. Specific workflow steps are required to remove burned-in PHI from images. Guidance is available on the SIIM and ACR websites.

  - The **conduit exception** excludes courier services and Internet service providers as business associates. A conduit service should only provide data transmission, and should not routinely access PHI as part of its service.
- The Final Omnibus Rule defined a four-tier penalty structure:
  - Tier 1:
    - Covered entity unaware, reasonable adherence to HIPAA

- Fine: $100–$50,000 per violation
  - Tier 2:
    - Covered entity aware, was unable to avoid incident
    - Fine: $1000–$50,000 per violation
  - Tier 3:
    - Willful neglect, efforts to correct violation
    - Fine: $10,000–$50,000 per violation
  - Tier 4:
    - Willful neglect, no effort to correct violation
    - Fine: Minimum $50,000 per violation. Annual maximum $1,500,000
- Fines can be applied to each occurrence of a violation, even up to a daily basis. This could result in the penalty amount being multiplied by 365.
- Criminal penalty tiers:
  1. Covered entities or individuals who knowingly obtain or disclose can receive a maximum penalty of $50,000 and 1 year in jail.
  2. Obtaining PHI under false pretense can receive a maximum penalty of $100,000 and 5 years in jail.
  3. Intent to sell, transfer, or use PHI for commercial gain, personal gain, or malicious intent can receive penalties of $250,000 and 10 years in jail.
- Privacy protections regarding genetic information were included.

30.2.8 State, Local, and Organizational Regulations

State, local, and organizational regulations can be more restrictive than federal regulations. When these regulations are more restrictive, then they take precedence over HIPAA. At the time of this writing, there are 13 states that have regulations that are more restrictive than HIPAA including CA, CO, HI, LA, MD, NE, NV, NY, TN, TX, VA, WA, and WY.

30.3 Interoperability

30.3.1 ONC 10-Year Interoperability Roadmap

- In 2015, the Office of National Coordinator for Health Information Technology (ONC) published a 10-year interoperability roadmap which set the following goals:
  - 2015–2017: development of policies and systems focused on quality of care and health outcomes
  - 2018–2020: expansion of interoperability between health IT systems
  - 2021–2024: expansion to nationwide interoperability

- The Trusted Exchange Framework (TEF, 2018). The vision is to develop a technical framework that can develop into a national health information network.
  - The building blocks for the TEF are **qualified health information networks** (QHINs) that would be leveraged to establish standardized connectivity between health information exchanges.
- TEFCA Draft 2 (2019) specifies that the TEF and Common Agreement are distinct efforts and will be leveraged to create technical and legal requirements for sharing electronic health information across the United States.

KEY CONCEPT: Secure Image Exchange

Image sharing has its roots in film which involved sharing copies of X-ray films with other providers. In other words, the film copies were "pushed" to the other provider. With the emergence of PACS, film copies were replaced by CDs, and the "push" delivery model continued. Secure Image Exchange (SIE) vendors followed the same push model, which has limitations due to the absence of a common infrastructure to support the exchange of imaging exams between SIE networks. RSNA and Carequality have partnered to leverage image sharing using resources available on the Carequality interoperability framework. The current proposal diverges from the push model and focuses on a "pull" model. Participants would be able to pull exams from other providers on the exchange without having to engage that provider's support personnel. The approach requires trust agreements between participants before participating in the exchange.

  - The **Common Agreement** will focus on the governance needed to support the TEF including:
    - Minimum required terms and conditions (MRTCs)
    - Additional required terms and conditions (ARTCs)
    - Qualified health information network (QHIN) technical framework (QTF)
  - The Common Agreement aims to extend certain HIPAA requirements beyond covered entities and business associates to non-HIPAA entities by including these provisions in the agreement. Any entity that wishes to participate in the TEF will be bound by these agreements.
  - The ONC decided that a neutral organization in the industry would be the best approach to establishing the Common Agreement. As such, ONC sought applicants to become the recognized coordinating entity (RCE).
  - The Sequoia Project was designated as the TEFCA RCE in September 2019.
    - The Sequoia Project was previously involved with two significant nationwide initiatives: eHealth Exchange and Carequality. Carequality is a network-to-network trust used for the exchange of clinical documents. At the time of this writing, over 1 billion documents have been exchanged on the Carequality network.
    - In December 2019, Carequality, partnered with RSNA and the Sequoia Project, released a proposed *Imaging Data Exchange Implementation*

Guide Supplement which plans on leveraging the Carequality interoperability framework resources for the exchange of DICOM imaging exams.
- Successful implementation and adoption of this interoperability framework for imaging could result in a common infrastructure that is leveraged by imaging providers for the exchange of medical imaging data throughout the United States.

30.3.2 CMS and ONC Interoperability Legislation

- The EHR Incentive Program (2009), known as **Meaningful Use**, is a three-stage program that promoted the use of EHRs to:
  1. Stage 1: Capture and share data.
  2. Stage 2: Advance clinical processes through continuous quality improvement.
  3. Stage 3: Improve health outcomes.
- The CMS Interoperability and Patient Access final rule empowers patients by giving them access to their health information and the ability to use their information as they see fit. The new policies include:
  - **Patient Access API**: CMS-regulated payers will be required to provide patients with easy access to their claims and encounter information using a standards-based API. CMS specifies HL7 Fast Healthcare Interoperability Resources (FHIR) version 4.0.1 as the standard to be leveraged in API development.
  - **Provider Directory API**: CMS-regulated payers will be required to make provider directories available to the public using a standards-based (FHIR) API.
  - **Payer-to-Payer Data Exchange**: Implementation of a clinical data exchange between payers. Data to be exchanged is defined by the US Core Data for Interoperability (USCDI).
  - Improving the **Dually Eligible Experience** by Increasing the Frequency of Federal-State Data Exchanges aims at increasing the rate of enrollee data exchange for individuals who are eligible for both Medicare and Medicaid.
  - **Public Reporting and Information Blocking**: CMS will begin publicly reporting providers who may intentionally be limiting access to health information (aka information blocking). These include clinicians, hospitals, and critical access hospitals.
  - **Digital Contact Information**: CMS will begin reporting providers who do not maintain their digital contact information in the National Plan and Provider Enumeration System (NPPES).
  - Admission, Discharge, and Transfer (**ADT**) **Event Notifications**: Providers will be required to send ADT information electronically to another provider in support of patient care.
- The ONC 21st Century Cures Act Final Rule (2020) is designed to advance interoperability between systems, increase access to health information between medical providers, and provide patients with easy and secure access to their elec-

tronic health information. A driving force behind these efforts is to provide patients access to their health information using familiar technology such as apps that can be downloaded to their smartphones at no additional cost.

- Certification of application programming interfaces (APIs) to promote interoperability between healthcare solutions, including leveraging smartphone apps in a manner similar to the non-healthcare consumer market.
- Identifying standards to support the exchange of electronic health information, including:
  - Fast Healthcare Interoperability Resources (FHIR) release 4
  - SMART on FHIR
  - OpenID Connect
  - US Core Data for Interoperability (USCDI)
- Requires certified Health IT modules to support the *CMS Quality Reporting Document Architecture (QRDA) Implementation Guide* for reporting quality measures.
- Requires that certified Health IT modules export electronic health information (EHI) to allow for increased access and exchange of EHI between providers and patients.
- As part of the certification process, developers will need to indicate whether their product supports encrypted authentication and/or multifactor authentication.
- Defines information blocking as the practice of restricting access to electronic health information by healthcare providers, exchanges, or developers.
- There are eight exceptions that do not constitute information blocking:
  1. Preventing Harm Exception
  2. Privacy Exception
  3. Security Exception
  4. Infeasibility Exception
  5. Health IT Performance Exception
  6. Content and Manner Exception
  7. Fees Exception
  8. Licensing Exception
- The **Content and Manner Exception** was added to the final rule based on feedback from the healthcare community. The exception is allowed if the payer provides, at a minimum, content that is identified in the US Core Data for Interoperability (USCDI).
- **USCDI content** includes patient demographics, allergy information, health concerns, procedures performed, laboratory, medications, assessment and treatment plans, clinical notes, smoking status, immunizations, vital signs, implantable Unique Device Identifiers (UDIs) for implantable devices, care team members, and more.
  - USCDI version 1 specifies that an "Imaging Narrative" be included under clinical notes along with other narratives.
  - USCDI version 2 is currently available for public comment. Draft Version 2 includes the Diagnostic Imaging Order and the Diagnostic Imaging Report as part of its content.

– This exception also addresses requests specifying manner of EHI exchange. Market-negotiated terms for access and exchange of EHI are to be used. Requests can also be fulfilled in an alternative manner if the "actor" is technically not able to fulfill the request or an agreement cannot be reached with the requestor. It is stipulated that this approach is allowed as long as the Fees and Licensing Exceptions are satisfied (if applicable).

30.4 FDA Medical Device Regulation

- The US Food and Drug Administration (FDA) ensures the safety, efficacy, and security of human and veterinary drugs, biological products, medical devices, the national food supply, cosmetics, and products that emit radiation. The FDA is also responsible for advancing the public health by helping to speed innovations that make medical products more effective, safer, and more affordable and by helping the public get the accurate, science-based information they need to use medical products and foods to maintain and improve their health.
- The FDA's Center for Devices and Radiological Health (CDRH) is responsible for the regulation of medical devices and radiation-emitting electronic products.

INTERNATIONAL CONSIDERATIONS

- The European Union requires a CE (Conformité Européenne) mark on medical devices sold in the European Economic Area. Medical devices are classified into four categories (Claas I, IIa, IIb, and III). Class I and IIa are low-risk devices. Higher-risk classes require the engagement of a Notified Body to obtain CE status.
- China requires approval from China's State Food and Drug Administration. China uses three categories for risk (Class I, II, and III). Class I is the lowest-risk category.

- In Section 201(h) of The Food, Drug, and Cosmetic Act, a **medical device** is defined as an instrument, apparatus, implement, machine, contrivance, implant, in vitro reagent, or other similar or related article, including a component part, or accessory which is:
  1. Recognized in the official National Formulary or US Pharmacopeia or any supplement to them
  2. Intended for the use in the diagnosis of disease or other conditions or in the cure, mitigation, treatment, or prevention of disease, in man or other animals
  3. Intended to affect the structure or any function of the body of man or other animals and which does not achieve its primary intended purposes through chemical action within or on the body of man or other animals and which is not dependent upon being metabolized for the achievement of its primary intended purposes

- Some software functions are considered to meet the regulatory definition of a medical device and are subject to regulatory oversight.

- The FDA classifies devices according to risk. Medical devices are categorized into three classes:
  - **Class I** devices are considered low-risk devices for which general controls are sufficient to provide reasonable assurance of the safety and effectiveness of the device. Many Class I devices are exempt from 510(k) premarket notification. Examples of Class I devices would be radiologic phantoms or leaded aprons.
  - **Class II** devices are considered moderate-risk devices and require both general controls and special controls to provide reasonable assurance of the safety and effectiveness of the device. Premarket notification through the 510(k) marketing pathway is generally required for Class II devices. Examples of Class II devices include CT scanners or MIMPS (aka PACS). As of April 2021, the FDA has relabeled PACS to Medical Image Management and Processing System (MIMPS) to better align with the language of the 21st Century Cures Act.
  - **Class III** devices are considered high-risk devices and usually sustain or support life, are implanted, or present unreasonable risk of illness or injury. Premarket approval (PMA) is the process for scientific and regulatory review before Class III devices can enter the US marketplace. An example of a Class III device is an implanted cardiac pacemaker/defibrillator.

VIEW TO THE FUTURE: The Digital Health Center of Excellence

In 2020, the FDA established the Digital Health Center of Excellence within the Center for Devices and Radiological Health (CDRH). The goal is to focus on technologies that will advance healthcare through emerging technologies such as cybersecurity, Software as a Medical Device (SaMD), mobile medical applications, artificial intelligence, and machine learning. https://www.fda.gov/news-events/press-announcements/fda-launches-digital-health-center-excellence

KEY CONCEPT: FDA Cleared Versus Approved

Cleared: The 510(k) pathway is the most common way for medical devices to reach the US market. Some Class I and most Class II devices require Premarket Notification through the 510(k) program to demonstrate that the medical device is substantially equivalent to another legally marketed device, referred to as a "predicate device," which has already received FDA clearance or approval. Such devices are referred to as having been "cleared" by the FDA.

Approved: Premarket approval (PMA) is the process for scientific and regulatory review of Class III medical devices. The sponsor is required to provide valid scientific evidence demonstrating reasonable assurances of safety and effectiveness for the device's intended use. In order for such devices to have been "approved," the FDA must determine that the benefits outweigh the known risks for the intended use.

https://www.fda.gov/industry/regulated-products/medical-device-overview

30.5 Mammography Quality Standards Act

The Mammography Quality Standards Act (MQSA) of 1992 established national standards for both film-based and digital mammography, stating that all women should have access to quality mammograms for the detection of breast cancer in the earliest, most treatable stages.

STEP-BY-STEP: MQSA

1. Accreditation by body such as ACR
2. Certification by agency such as the FDA
3. Annual inspections by certifying agency
4. Three-year renewal of certification

30.5.1 Accreditation, Certification, and Inspection

- Accreditation is performed by an accreditation body (AB) approved by the FDA. Accreditation bodies include the American College of Radiology (ACR) at the national level and States that obtain FDA approval.
- New facilities will receive a provisional MQSA certificate. During the 6-month period, clinical images and phantom images must be submitted to the AB, as well as other required material.
- If the new applicant passes accreditation, the AB will notify the certifying agency and a full MQSA certificate will be issued by the certifying agency. A certificate is valid for a maximum of 3 years.
- Certifying agencies include the FDA at the national level and States that obtained FDA approval.
- Annual inspections are performed by the certifying agency or one of its agents.
- Random onsite visits may also be performed by the AB, as well as random clinical image reviews.
- Facilities must apply for reinstatement if their accreditation has expired, accreditation was denied, certificate renewal was refused, or the certificate was revoked.
- Changes in operational status must be reported to the AB. This include changes in ownership, address changes, personnel changes, and equipment changes.
- Application for accreditation is required whenever new mammography units are added to a facility.

KEY CONCEPT: Breast Imaging Center of Excellence (BICOE)

The American College of Radiology recognizes breast imaging centers that achieve excellence by seeking and earning accreditation in all of the ACR's voluntary breast imaging accreditation programs and modules in addition to the mandatory Mammography Accreditation Program.

https://accreditationsupport.acr.org/support/solutions/articles/11000068075-breast-imaging-centers-of-excellence-bicoe-revised-12-12-19-

30.5.2 Requirements

- Accreditation and certification require that certain standards be met regarding personnel qualifications, equipment standards, equipment performance, quality control testing, physics surveys and quality assurance testing, recordkeeping, reports to patients and physicians, record retention, medical outcome audits, consumer complaint mechanisms, and infection control. The ACR requires applicants to submit the following:
  1. Policies and procedures.
  2. Reporting mechanisms.
  3. Patient outcome data.
  4. Facilities must maintain **personnel records** documenting qualifications and current status of interpreting physicians, technologists, and medical physicists. Continuing education and continuing experience are required to assure that personnel maintain technical competence.
     - **Physicians** must be licensed to practice medicine in the State and be certified in the interpretation of radiologic procedures, including mammography. Physicians must have at least 3 months of documented training in the interpretation of mammography and a minimum of 60 hours of documented medical education in mammography.
     - **Technologists** must be licensed to perform radiologic exams in the State and complete 40 contact hours of documented training in mammography, including performance of a minimum of 25 examinations under the direct supervision of a qualified professional.
     - **Medical physicists** must be licensed or approved by the State and have certification in the appropriate specialty. A minimum of a Master's degree in medical physics is required. Documented training must include a minimum of 20 contact hours in conducting surveys.

> **KEY CONCEPT: Film Screen Mammography**
>
> Film screen mammography has largely been replaced by digital mammography systems in the United States and will most likely be phased out over the next few years.

  5. **Patient and Phantom Images** can be submitted electronically
  6. **Equipment performance evaluation** requires the submission of clinical images and phantom images for accreditation and certification review.
     - Mammography equipment evaluations are to be performed on new equipment or whenever there is a significant change to existing equipment, including replacing major components or equipment relocation.

30.5.3 Mammography Quality Control (QC)

Digital mammography requires weekly, monthly, quarterly, semiannual, and annual quality control (QC) testing performed by a medical physicist or a technologist under the supervision of a medical physicist.

- **Weekly**
  1. Cassette erasure test for two-dimensional (2D) computed radiography (CR) mammography modalities must be performed before clinical use.
  2. A phantom test must be performed to evaluate image quality.
- **Monthly**
  1. Compression thickness indicator
  2. Visual checklist
  3. Acquisition workstation monitor QC
  4. Radiologist workstation monitor QC
  5. Film printer QC (if applicable)
  6. Viewbox cleanliness (if applicable)
- **Quarterly**
  1. Facility QC review for 2D and digital breast tomosynthesis (DBT) units
  2. The tracking of repeat and reject rates review
     - If a change greater than 2% of images examined is demonstrated when compared to the previous quarter, then the reason for this change needs to be determined.
- **Semiannual QC** tests
  1. Compression force
  2. Film screening mammography: darkroom fog, screen-film contact, and compression device performance (if applicable)
- **Annual QC** tests include:
  1. Phantom image quality
  2. DBT Z resolution
  3. Spatial resolution
  4. DBT volume coverage
  5. Automatic exposure control (AEC) system performance
  6. Average glandular dose
  7. Unit checklist such as locks, detents, angulation indicators, and mechanical support devices
  8. CR photostimulable phosphor (PSP) imaging plates
     - Plate-to-plate uniformity
     - CR reader scanner performance
  9. Acquisition workstation (AW) monitor QC
  10. Radiologist workstation (RW) monitor QC
  11. Collimation assessment (DBT only)

12. Evaluation of display device technologist QC
13. Manufacture calibrations
14. Film printer QC (if applicable)

- Annual physics surveys and quality assurance testing are required to ensure continued compliance. These surveys are to be conducted by a medical physicist or by someone under the direction of a medical physicist.

30.5.4 Patient Results

- Content and terminology for patient results to patients and referring providers have been standardized and must include:
  1. The name of patient and second identifier
  2. The exam date
  3. The name of interpreting physician
  4. The overall assessment of findings
- Communication of mammography results must occur within 30 days of the exam or as soon as possible if the results are suspicious or highly suggestive.
- The overall assessment of findings must be stated as one of the following BI-RADS categories:
  1. Negative
  2. Benign
  3. Probably benign
  4. Suspicious
  5. Highly suggestive of malignancy
  6. Known biopsy-proven malignancy

> **DEFINITION: BI-RADS**
>
> Breast Imaging-Reporting and Data System is a reporting and QA tool owned by the ACR and used for mammography reporting. After the success of BI-RADS, similar systems have been developed for other anatomic regions, such as NI-RADS (neck), PI-RADS (prostate), etc.

- Mammography imaging studies and reports shall be maintained for a minimum of 5 years and no less than 10 years if no additional exams were performed at the facility. State regulations may require longer retention periods.
- Medical outcome audits must be performed on an annual basis. The audit will review the findings of all mammograms performed and will follow up on any mammograms with positive findings. A correlation with pathology results and the interpreting physician's findings is required. All audit data shall be reviewed annually by at least one interpreting physician. Breast information management software applications assist in compiling and organizing mammography outcomes and business analytics.

- Each facility is required to have an established mechanism for handling consumer complaints. Serious consumer complaints that are not resolved by a facility must be filed with the accreditation body.
- Each facility is required to have an established infection control program.

30.5.5 Full-Field Digital Mammography

- Full-field digital mammography (FFDM) can only be used at facility units that have been accredited and certified for mammography.
- Facilities must meet vendor recommendations in regards to quality assurance standards for FFDM equipment. Alternatively, facilities can follow the *ACR 2018 Digital Mammography QC Manual* using ACR Digital Mammography Phantoms.
- Personnel (interpreting physicians, technologists, medical physicists) must be qualified in FFDM, according to their respective roles. Personnel must have a minimum of 8 hours of initial training in digital mammography.

> **KEY CONCEPT: FFDM Resolution**
>
> The native resolution for FFDM images is much higher than standard CR/DR. A resolution of at least five (5) line pairs per millimeter is required to view breast tissue in sufficient detail. Thus, digital mammography devices such as display monitors, film printers, and film digitizers must be capable of supporting higher-resolution outputs.

- The FDA recommends that only FDA-approved monitors, printers, and film digitizers be used for digital mammography. Compliance with a QA program is required. In addition, any images produced by this equipment must pass image quality standards set by accreditation.
- Today with many mammography studies shared on digital media, the provision of printed hard copies is becoming obsolete. Therefore, the FDA no longer requires that facilities have access to a printer before mammography can be performed. The option to maintain a printer and/or the ability to print hard copy images is a decision left to each individual facility.

> **HYPOTHETICAL SCENARIO: Printing Mammograms on Film**
>
> If the facility chooses to retain a printer for mammography studies, it must be tested and approved by a medical physicist as acceptable for the printing of mammographic images.

- Film digitization is to be done for comparison purposes only. Digitized film cannot be used in primary interpretation, nor can it be used as a substitute for the long-term archiving of the original film.

- It is permitted to electronically transfer images if acceptable to the receiving party. The data are to be transferred in their original state or using lossless compression only. The transfer of lossy-compressed images is not permitted.
- The long-term archival of FFDM data must be in its original format or as lossless-compressed data. The long-term archival of lossy-compressed images is not allowed.

30.5.6 Digital Breast Tomosynthesis

- Accreditation is required for DBT. The FFDM and DBT components of a single modality unit are separate accreditations due to differences in the technology.
- Eight hours of new modality training for DBT are required for certification.

30.5.7 Breast Density Reporting

- Routine mammographic imaging of dense breasts does not always reveal potential cancer and may require additional imaging to complement the screen-film or FFDM procedure.
- At the time of this writing, 38 States and the District of Columbia have established regulations regarding breast density reporting in mammography reports.
- State laws vary from providing general information on breast density to informing patients about their breast density.

30.5.8 Proposed MQSA Update 2019

- The proposal includes updates regarding digital mammography technology, quality standards, and mammography results.
- A report summary in layman's language will be required.
- Breast density information is to be included in mammography results.
- Facilities that fail to become accredited after three attempts at accreditation would not be allowed to submit a fourth request sooner than 1 year after the last submission.
- The FDA and State Certification Agency would be allowed to directly notify patients, providers, and the news media when a facility does not comply with MQSA notification rules.
- Facilities that terminate mammography services would be required to provide mammography images and reports to patients and providers.
- Personnel records documenting training and experience must be provided by a facility upon reasonable request.

- Transfer of mammograms and reports to another provider or the patient within 15 calendar days after receiving request.
- Mammography Medical Outcomes Audits should include positive predictive value, cancer detection rate, and recall rate.

30.6 Imaging Informatics Professional Certification (CIIP)

The purpose of professional certification is to assess an individual's skill level with regard to imaging informatics. Certification helps employers identify individuals who have demonstrated a basic knowledge of imaging informatics and who would have the requisite skill sets needed to be successful in imaging informatics.

The section will focus on professional board certification administered by the American Board of Imaging Informatics (ABII).

30.6.1 Overview

- ABII was founded in 2007 by the Society for Imaging Informatics in Medicine (SIIM) and the American Registry of Radiologic Technologists (ARRT).
- Successful completion of the exam administered by ABII is required for an imaging informatics professional to become board-certified.
- Certified Imaging Informatics Professionals are awarded the designation "CIIP."
- ABII certification establishes a national standard of competency for demonstrated knowledge in imaging informatics.

30.6.2 Certification Exam Requirements

An applicant is eligible for examination based on a point system that summarizes prior education as well experience in the imaging field.

> **KEY CONCEPT: Separation of ABII from Teaching Entities**
>
> ABII is responsible for developing and maintaining a certification program and defers curriculum development to SIIM's Educational Committees and other parties interested in imaging informatics education.
>
> The development of the certification exam and the development of the educational curriculum are done independently by groups that are "firewalled" from each other to assure that test questions are not compromised. No educational body (including SIIM) can guarantee that their educational material will be representative of the questions found in the CIIP exam.

30.6.3 Certification Exam Preparation

There are many avenues for applicants to prepare for the CIIP exam, including the ABII TCO, the IIP Education Advisory Network Learning Objectives, imaging informatics textbooks, the *Journal of Digital Imaging*, other healthcare information journals and publications, the Society of Imaging Informatics (SIIM) website, other imaging informatics websites, IIP bootcamps, PACS administration vocational training programs, and university-affiliated programs.

> **FURTHER READING:**
> **CIIP Test**
>
> https://www.abii.org

30.6.4 Continuing Education

- Twenty-four CEUs must be earned every 2 years to maintain CIIP status.
- The Society of Imaging Informatics in Medicine (www.siim.org) sponsors many virtual educational opportunities with CEUs including online learning, webinars, and a virtual IIP bootcamp.
- The American Board of Imaging Informatics provides a list of education programs available from other educational providers on their website (www. abii.org).

> **INTERNATIONAL CONSIDERATIONS**
>
> The European counterpart of SIIM is the European Society for Imaging Informatics. EuSoMII is currently developing certifying examinations for physicians and IIPs similar to those available in the United States.

30.6.5 Ten-Year CIIP Recertification

- Ten-year recertifications require that the CIIP demonstrate ongoing maintenance and development of their imaging informatics skills and can be achieved in one of four ways:
  1. **The practice option** requires that the diplomat provide evidence of a completed imaging informatics project providing some form of quality improvement.

> **KEY CONCEPT: 10-Year Requirements**
>
> Demonstrating ongoing experience in the field of imaging informatics is an important metric that can be used to demonstrate the value of IIP certification to healthcare providers, vendors, and other employers of IIPs.

2. **The education option** can be satisfied in one of three ways:
   - Mentoring a non-CIIP
   - Preparing/presenting lecture(s) to non-CIIPs at a regional or national meeting
   - Serving on the ABII Examination Committee
3. **The research option** requires publication of research that is relevant to content found in the ABII TCO in a peer-reviewed journal as the first or second author.
4. **The examination option** is a retaking and passing of the ABII certification exam.

PEARLS

- Protected health information (PHI) is any information that can be used to identify a specific individual. This includes obvious PHI like patient name and patient ID number. It also includes more obscure information such as study accession number and study date and time.
- Establish well-documented procedures for creating user accounts on applications that access PHI. Also have a well-established procedure for deactivating accounts when users go on a long-term leave of absence, transfer to other work areas, or permanently leave the organization.
- Eliminate generic logons on all applications accessing PHI. Audit capability is severely compromised when the username is indeterminate.
- Have signed contracts with business associates assuring HIPAA compliance with regard to the privacy and security of PHI.
- HIPAA violations can result in fines up to $1.5 million dollars per violation. Significant breaches may include more than one violation.
- MQSA certification is required for all facilities performing breast imaging.
- Accreditation of digital breast tomosynthesis devices require separate accreditations of the FFDM component and DBT component before the device can be used for DBT.
- Content and terminology for breast imaging results have been standardized. BI-RADS is a commonly-used QA tool for mammography reporting.
- Professional certification in imaging informatics is administered by the American Board of Imaging Informatics. There are specific requirements for certification eligibility, and competency must be demonstrated by successfully completing ABII's certification exam.

Further Readings

American Board of Imaging Informatics. About ABII. https://www.abii.org/About.aspx. Last accessed 10/10/2020.

Carequality. Imaging data exchange implementation guide, version 0.2. https://carequality.org/wp-content/uploads/2019/11/Imaging-Data-Exchange-Implementation-Guide-v02.pdf. Last accessed 10/10/2020.

Federal Register. CMS interoperability and patient access for Medicare Advantage Organization and Medicaid Managed Care Plans State Medicaid Agencies, CHIP Agencies and CHIP Managed Care Entities, issuers of qualified health plans on the federally-facilitated exchanges, and the health care providers. 1 May 2020. https://www.federalregister.gov/documents/2020/05/01/2020-05050/medicare-and-medicaid-programs-patient-protection-and-affordable-care-act-interoperabilityand. Last accessed 10/10/2020.

Federal Register. HIPAA Omnibus final rule. 25 Jan 2013. https://www.govinfo.gov/content/pkg/FR-2013-01-25/pdf/2013-01073.pdf. Last accessed 10/9/2020.

Food & Drug Administration. How to determine if your product is a medical device. https://www.fda.gov/medical-devices/classify-your-medical-device/how-determine-if-your-product-medical-device#introduction. Last accessed 10/10/2020.

Food & Drug Administration. Mammography Quality Standards Act (MQSA). https://www.fda.gov/radiation-emitting-products/regulations-mqsa/mammography-quality-standards-act-mqsa. Last accessed 10/10/2020.

Food & Drug Administration. Digital breast tomosynthesis (DBT) system. https://www.fda.gov/radiation-emitting-products/facility-certification-and-inspection-mqsa/digital-breast-tomosynthesis-dbt-system. Last accessed 10/10/2020.

Food & Drug Administration. Regulations to Conform Medical Software Provisions in the 21st Century Cures Act. https://public-inspection.federalregister.gov/2021-07860.pdf. Last accessed 5/28/2021.

The Office of the National Coordinator for Health Information Technology. Connecting health and care for the nation: a shared nationwide interoperability roadmap. https://www.healthit.gov/sites/default/files/hie-interoperability/nationwide-interoperability-roadmap-final-version-1.0.pdf. Last accessed 10/9/2020.

The Office of the National Coordinator for Health Information Technology. Trusted exchange framework and common agreement (TEFCA) draft 2. https://www.healthit.gov/sites/default/files/page/2019-04/FINALTEFCAQTF41719508version.pdf. Last accessed 10/10/2020.

The Office of the National Coordinator for Health Information Technology. 21st Century Cures Act: interoperability, information blocking, and the ONC health IT certification program. https://www.healthit.gov/sites/default/files/cures/2020-03/ONC_Cures_Act_Final_Rule_03092020.pdf. Last accessed 10/10/2020.

U.S. Department of Health & Human Services. HIPAA for professionals. https://www.hhs.gov/hipaa/for-professionals/index.html. Last accessed 10/9/2020.

Self-Assessment Questions

1. HIPAA regulations focus on which type of personal information?

   (a) PCI
   (b) PHI
   (c) PHR
   (d) PII

2. There are how many direct HIPAA identifiers?

   (a) 6
   (b) 12
   (c) 18
   (d) 24

3. HIPAA regulations apply to which of the following?

   (a) Covered entities
   (b) Business associates
   (c) Subcontractors
   (d) All of the above

4. The primary officer responsible for ensuring that an organization meets HIPAA requirements is a:

   (a) HIPAA compliance officer
   (b) HIPAA privacy officer
   (c) HIPAA regulatory officer
   (d) HIPAA security officer

5. The Security Rule identifies three categories of safeguards for HIPAA compliance:

   (a) Administrative, legal, and technical
   (b) Administrative, physical, and technical
   (c) Legal, physical, and technical
   (d) Logical, physical, and technical

6. FDA medical device regulations specify that:

   (a) Class I devices require 510(k) premarket notification.
   (b) Class I devices require premarket approval (PMA).
   (c) Class II devices generally require 510(k) premarket notification.
   (d) Class II devices require premarket approval (PMA).

7. The Mammography Quality Standards Act (MQSA) establishes national standards for mammography and is regulated by the:

   (a) American College of Radiology
   (b) Centers for Medicare and Medicaid Services
   (c) Department of Health and Human Services
   (d) Food and Drug Administration

8. MQSA certification must be renewed

   (a) Every year
   (b) Every 2 years
   (c) Every 3 years
   (d) Every 5 years

9. Which of the following is a false statement?

   (a) Full-field digital mammography (FFDM) units must be accredited.
   (b) Digital breast tomography (DBT) must be accredited.
   (c) Both FFDM and DBT accreditations are required before performing DBT.
   (d) FFDM accreditation is not required for performing DBT.

10. Which of the following is true regarding mammography films that have been digitized?

   (a) Can be used for primary diagnosis and comparison studies and can be used as a substitute for film for long-term archiving
   (b) Can be used for primary diagnosis and comparison studies and cannot be used as a substitute for film for long-term archiving
   (c) Can be used for comparison only and not for primary diagnosis and can be used as a substitute for long-term archiving
   (d) Can be used for comparison only and not for primary diagnosis and cannot be used as a substitute for long-term archiving

11. The American Board of Imaging Informatics (ABII) administers a national certification exam for imaging informatics. The following designation is awarded upon successful completion of the exam:

   (a) CIIP
   (b) CISSP
   (c) CPA
   (d) CPHIMS

12. The American Board of Imaging Informatics (ABII) uses a seven-point system to determine applicant eligibility. In addition to requiring a minimum of seven points' total, which of the following is also required?

   (a) College education from an accredited college
   (b) Two years of experience in healthcare imaging or imaging informatics
   (c) IT or clinical credentials from an ABII-approved organization
   (d) Eighteen hours of continuing education credit in imaging informatics

Chapter 31
Availability and Notification

Jason Nagels

Contents

31.1 Introduction

Medical imaging encompasses a variety of systems and solutions. These systems will inevitably experience problems that result in service interruptions. An imaging informatics professional should be prepared to manage service interruptions across the healthcare environment. Properly managing service interruptions requires action plans that incorporate identification, management, and communications to users. Imaging informatics professionals can identify service interruptions proactively by using monitoring tools, or reactively when users place service tickets informing system administrators that there is an issue. In practice, service management models are used to streamline resolution processes and reduce risk when incidents and

J. Nagels (✉)
Department of Clinical Informatics, HDIRS, Markham, ON, Canada
e-mail: jnagels@shn.ca

© The Author(s), under exclusive license to Springer Science+Business Media, LLC, part of Springer Nature 2021
B. F. Branstetter IV (ed.), *Practical Imaging Informatics*,
https://doi.org/10.1007/978-1-0716-1756-4_31

problems occur. A key function of managing service interruptions is communicating with affected system users until a resolution is in place and normal operations resume.

31.2 Measuring Availability for Service Level Agreements

31.2.1 Key Services in Medical Imaging

- To accurately measure availability, you must have a comprehensive understanding of the services provided to your organization and have familiarity with the various Service Level Agreements (SLA) offered by each vendor.
- Some key services that your organization's imaging informatics team may rely on include:
  - Local Area Network (LAN)
  - Wide Area Network (WAN)
  - Virtual Private Network (VPN)
  - Hospital Information System (HIS)
  - Radiology Information System (RIS)
  - Picture Archive and Communication System (PACS)
  - Vendor Neutral Archive (VNA)
  - Enterprise Master Patient Index (EMPI)
  - Storage Platforms
  - Databases
  - Patient Portals
  - Cloud Services
- Each solution/service within your organization will have a unique SLA that defines the expected uptime and availability of service [1].

> **DEFINITION: Service Level Agreement (SLA)**
>
> A commitment between vendor and client that outlines aspects of the product or service related to quality, availability, and responsibilities of both parties. Service availability is a major component of the SLA.

> **FURTHER READING: Service Availability**
>
> Toeroe M, Tam F. Service availability: principles and practice. Hoboken: Wiley; 2012. https://doi.org/10.1002/9781119941378.

31.2.2 System Availability

- System Availability is the promise made by a vendor that their service or system will rarely malfunction. It is expressed as a percentage of time that the system is working.

> **DEFINITION: System Availability**
>
> A metric used to measure the percentage of time a service is operational and available to users.

- Percentages are described by their order of magnitude, referred to as "classes of nines" (e.g., 99.99% uptime is "four nines").
- Typically, downtime is measured across a calendar year, but service agreements may specify downtime measured monthly, weekly, or per downtime event.

- The following table shows the downtime that is allowed for a particular percentage of availability, assuming that the system is required to operate continuously 24 h a day, 365 days a year [2] (Table 31.1).

> **KEY CONCEPT: Automated Identification of Interruptions**
>
> Any SLA with an availability specification beyond "three nines" requires automated, proactive identification of service interruptions. It is impossible to meet higher levels of availability (e.g., 99.99% allows less than 5 min/month of downtime) through reactive processes.

Table 31.1 Uptime availability

Uptime availability represented in nines				
Availability (%)	Downtime per year	Downtime per month	Downtime per week	Downtime per day
90 ("one nine")	36 days, 12 h, 34 min, 55 s	3 days, 1 h, 2 min, 54 s	16 h, 48 min, 0 s	2 h, 24 min
99 ("two nines")	3 days, 15 h, 39 min, 29 s	7 h, 18 min, 17 s	1 h, 40 min, 48 s	14 min, 24 s
99.9 ("three nines")	8 h, 45 min, 56 s	43 min, 49 s	10 min, 4 s	1 min, 26 s
99.99 ("four nines")	52 min, 35 s	4 min, 22 s	1 min, 6 s	8.64 s
99.999 ("five nines")	5 min, 15 s	26.30 s	6.05 s	864.00 ms
99.9999 ("six nines")	31.56 s	2.63 s	604.80 ms	86.40 ms

Times calculated using www.uptime.is

> **HYPOTHETICAL SCENARIO: High Availability Thresholds**
>
> Service providers may agree to such a high level of availability on a system or service (e.g., 99.999% availability for their PACS uptime) that it cannot realistically be met or accurately measured. In this case, a violation of the SLA may be quite short and difficult to detect; for example, with five nines of availability, an SLA-violating interruption of 865 ms/day might easily go undetected.
>
> Despite a lack of user awareness of interruptions of availability, it is vital that your organization have the ability to detect and identify SLA violations to manage service provider performance effectively.

31.2.3 Defining Appropriate Service Level Agreements

- Prior to a service being implemented, the organization and service provider will work together to define appropriate, agreed-upon SLAs.
- Organizations must be confident that appropriate data collection methods are in place to **measure end-to-end system availability**, holding service providers accountable for any violation of system availability covenants defined in the SLA [3].

> **KEY CONCEPT: Establishing SLAs**
>
> For new infrastructure, applications, or services implemented at your organization, you must work collaboratively with the service provider and subject matter experts to develop mutually acceptable processes for support and well-defined availability and response times.

31.2.4 Identifying Service Level Agreement Breaches

- In order to identify service interruptions that affect system availability, automated monitoring tools are required.
- There are commercial and open-source monitoring tools that capture alerts when a service shows signs of degradation and/or when a downtime occurs.
- It is important to understand that service interruptions as defined in an SLA do not always directly impact end users. Yet any service interruption has the potential to affect users eventually and should be continuously monitored.

> **DEFINITION: Monitoring Tools**
>
> Monitoring tools provide the ability to keep track of a system or service, in order to have automated identification and notification of failures, degradations, or interruptions.

> **FURTHER READING: Monitoring Tools**
>
> Nagios (https://www.nagios.org/) is an open-source tool that monitors the entire infrastructure to ensure systems, applications, services, and business processes are functioning properly.

> **OUR EXPERIENCE: Monitoring Availability for a Health Information Exchange**
>
> A regional Health Information Exchange (HIE) located in Canada allows hospitals and clinics to publish images and reports to a central repository for exam sharing across the region. When measuring system availability, monitoring tools provide accurate stats. However, there are times when additional information is required, beyond what is captured by the monitoring tools. For example, monitoring tools can provide false positive uptime information when determining server uptime based on a ping response. Servers can respond positively to a network ping, but a service that affects the storage and retrieval of imaging studies may have stopped running.
>
> **KEY LESSONS LEARNED**
>
> - Beyond just server uptime, availability must relate to the specific services that the organization depends on – in the case of this HIE, the services related to publishing and consuming images/reports is essential.
> - It is important to look at all relevant indicators like inbound and outbound volumes per participating site, heat maps, and storage trends per time of day.
> - Using a blend of monitoring tools and other appropriate information provides insight into availability of the HIE services.

31.3 Identifying Service Interruptions

Identifying service interruptions is one of the first steps to properly manage disruptions. System interruptions can be identified by using both proactive and reactive identifications.

> **KEY CONCEPT: Proactive Versus Reactive Identification of Service Interruptions**
>
> Proactive Identification is using monitoring tools that detect when a service or system has become (or better yet, is at risk of becoming) unavailable prior to the awareness of an end user.
>
> Reactive Identification is when end users notify the Service Desk or system administrators about a disruption of availability.

31.3.1 Proactive Identification

- Organizations should strive toward proactive approaches when identifying interruptions for as many services and systems as possible.
- A proactive approach allows appropriate support resources to be aware of a system interruption and aims to resolve issues prior to end-user awareness [4].
- Monitoring tools are useful in detecting and measuring occurrences related to service interruptions and availability [4]. Organizations can leverage this data during SLA negotiations, especially when service providers violate SLA covenants.
- When planning and implementing monitoring tools, it is vital to have a comprehensive understanding of your enterprise topology and how each system and their services interact and exchange data.
- Awareness of the **data flows** for each system and identifying all potential **points of failure** is an important step when setting up and implementing monitoring tools.
- Service providers may provide monitoring tools built into their system.
  - For example, a PACS may come with tools that detect and report problems with image storage, such as detecting when a modality has stopped sending studies to the PACS or trends that demonstrate when study volumes, study sizes, or study object counts have dramatically increased or decreased.
  - These tools combined with third-party monitoring tools can provide a holistic view of potential service interruptions.

FURTHER READING: Proactively Monitoring Departmental Clinical IT Systems with an Open Source Availability System

Toland C, Meenan C, Warnock M, Nagy P. J Digit Imaging. 2007; 20:119–24. https://doi.org/10/1007/s10278-007-9063-2.

KEY CONCEPT: Root Cause Versus Cascading Interruptions

Within your medical imaging environment, many of the services and systems depend on each other. For example, if construction work cuts the fiber outside your building, this will affect network connectivity and may influence the internal local area network, the virtual private network, and other downstream services.

Another example is if the organization's VNA is unavailable, there may be an impact on the ability for the PACS to access prior imaging studies that are not stored on the local cache. Understanding how your organizational systems and services work together is essential when setting up error traps and monitoring tools.

The first thing to go wrong is the "root cause," which can then result in a cascade of service interruptions.

31.3.2 Reactive Identification

- Reactive Identification involves end users notifying the service desk about issues that they have experienced, before any monitoring tools were able to flag performance anomalies.
- End users will mostly report issues that are specific to their role. It will take further investigation by the imaging informatics professionals to determine if the reported issue is an isolated instance or an indication of an interruption that will affect many users.
- Reactive support, or **break/fix support** is correcting issues after they occur. This was the predominant support model used by early generation IT support.
- The reactive support model is undesirable for the following reasons:
  - Reactive support negatively impacts clinical operations.
  - The root cause of break/fix tickets can evolve to larger system issues that can be subsequently irreparable.
  - Slower responses lead to vulnerabilities to cyber and ransomware attacks.
  - Negative financial repercussions.
  - User frustration.
- Advanced analytic dashboards, system management tools, and emerging artificial intelligence-enhanced predictive models will lead to reductions in reactive support models as well as decreases in break/fix support tickets.

31.4 Service Interruption Management

- Imaging informatics professionals and other appropriate support resources troubleshoot issues reported via proactive and reactive methods to determine if they are isolated events or indicative of larger problems. The **service management model** tracks and monitors these responses (Fig. 31.1).

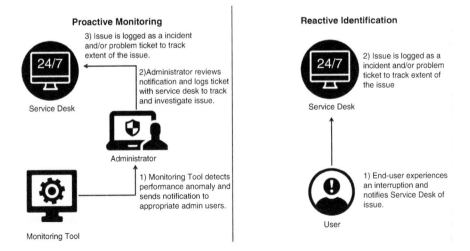

Fig. 31.1 The service management model

- **Information Technology Infrastructure Library (ITIL)** is a framework for managing IT service delivery in the business world and is a widely accepted approach when establishing service management protocols and systems.
- The purpose of the **ITIL 4 Service Level Management (SLM)** practice is to set clear business-based targets that aim to minimize the negative impacts of incidents.

FURTHER READING:
Transforming IT Service
Management – The ITIL Impact

Cater-Steel A, Toleman M, Tan W-G. Transforming IT service management – the ITIL impact. In: ACIS 2006: 17th Australasian Conference on Information Systems: Thought, Leadership in IS, 6–8 Dec 2006, Adelaide, South Australia.

31.4.1 Incidents

- Incidents are unplanned interruptions that have not yet affected service. Monitoring tools can provide insight regarding issues that reduce the quality of a service but have not yet directly affected users.

DEFINITION: Incident

An incident is an unplanned interruption to a service, or the failure of a component of a service that has not yet impacted service.

- The incident response plan should define what constitues the incident then identify who or what team is responsible for managing the situation.
- According to ITIL 4 the purpose of **Incident Management** is to minimize the negative impact of incidents by restoring normal service operation as quickly as possible [5].
- The incident management usually has five phases:
    - (i) Identification and logging
    - (ii) Classification and prioritization
    - (iii) Investigation, triage, and diagnosis
    - (iv) Resolution and recovery
    - (v) Incident closure

HYPOTHETICAL SCENARIO: Incidents and Monitoring Tools

A monitoring tool may indicate there are issues with the nightly database (DB) backup. The notification indicates that over the past week, the time to complete DB backup is taking much longer than usual. Although this may not immediately affect users, it is a reduction in service quality that can potentially lead to DB backup failures and could indicate other performance issues in the DB.

Tracking this as a service incident helps identify the right course of action, including who should handle the resolution.

STEP-BY-STEP: Incidents Managed Through a Service Desk

1. Identification and Logging:	Determine the right course of action, including who should handle the resolution, the extent of communication, and the speed of response. A major incident would be one that has significant impact and urgency, requiring an all-hands-on-deck approach.
2. Classification and Prioritization:	Incident classification identifies trends in the types of logged incidents. Incident prioritization assesses the urgency of an incident along with the impact.
3. Investigation and Diagnosis:	Involves initial diagnosis and determining if the service desk can solve the issue or if the incident requires escalation to a senior specialist team or the service provider. Escalation may be necessary to address the incident or if higher management levels need to communicate the details to stakeholders, approve emergency changes, or manage resource allocation.
4. Resolution and Recovery:	Focuses on finding a solution to the incident and communicating the solution.
5. Closure:	Involves talking with users to confirm they are satisfied that normal service has resumed.

31.4.2 Problem Management

- ITIL defines the purpose of Problem Management as the ability to reduce the likelihood and impact of incidents by identifying the actual and potential causes (aka root cause analysis) of incidents and known errors [6].
- Problem management is a support method that follows specific steps in the life cycle of a reported problem and seeks to deploy **workarounds** in order to minimize negative impacts and mitigate reoccurrences.
- Problem management can be proactive as well as reactive, although proactive is preferred.

DEFINITION: Problem

The underlying cause of one or more service incidents. Problems are tracked separately from incidents.

DEFINITION: Root Cause Analysis

A formal post-hoc analysis of a problem designed to identify the underlying systematic causes. Problems are often blamed on an individual or a vendor, but there may be productive ways that the entire system can change to prevent these errors (see **Chap. 25**).

STEP-BY-STEP: ITIL Problem Management

1. Problem identification:	Logging, categorization, and prioritization
2. Problem control:	Analyzing and documenting workarounds and known errors
3. Error control:	Fixing errors through change control and evaluating efficiency of workarounds

31.4.3 Managing Alerts

- Monitoring tools provide the ability to configure alerts according to specific organizational needs. Ideally, alert notifications are set to trigger on unique thresholds for each service.
- **Alert Fatigue** is when an overwhelming number of alerts desensitize the support team, such that legitimate alerts are missed or ignored.
  - A single alert is manageable and can be reviewed and responded to while managing daily operational duties or during afterhours on-call duties. However, managing a series of alerts is much more difficult. The more inbound alerts received the greater probability that a genuine interruption will be overlooked [7].

STEP-BY-STEP: How to Avoid Alert Fatigue

1. Establish intelligent thresholds:	Assign alerts according to urgency. Determine which alerts should be assigned to issues requiring an immediate response versus those that are less emergent and can be addressed later.
2. Define tiered alert priorities:	Not all alerts are equal. Set alert priorities and leverage visual indicators to highlight the priority of each report alert. (For example, Red = requires immediate attention, Yellow = non-urgent and can be reviewed later).
3. Specific actionable alerts:	Ambiguous alerts require more focus, attention, and time than specific, actionable alerts. If resources are already experiencing fatigue by an excessive number of alerts, ambiguous alerts are at risk of being disregarded.
4. Consolidate redundant alerts:	Consolidating redundant notifications and reducing reminders where possible can help keep the alert load more manageable, leading to better attention from resources.

31.5 Service Interruption Communication

31.5.1 Policies and Procedures

An organization must have well-defined **Downtime Policies and Procedures** to effectively manage and communicate all types of service interruptions. Interruptions in service can originate from internal and external forces, which is why business strategies, culture, regulatory compliance, available personnel, and financial resources drive policies and procedures. (For more about downtime procedures, see **Chap. 29**.)

- Composing clear and concise downtime policies and procedures requires fundamental knowledge of the roles and user workflows affected by the downtime.

- **Scheduled downtimes** are intentional service interruptions caused by maintenance or system enhancements. Although done

> **KEY CONCEPT: Policies and Procedures**
>
> A policy is a guiding principle used to set direction in an organization.
> A procedure is a series of steps to follow that produces a consistent approach to a specific task.

purposely, these types of downtimes are disruptive to clinical operations. Scheduled downtimes are necessary to keep systems operating smoothly.

- **Unscheduled downtimes** are service interruptions that occur unexpectedly and are the result of a system failure. Unscheduled downtimes can negatively affect patient care if not managed correctly.

- Organizations must have well-defined Downtime Policies and Procedures that include communicating the status of problem to the end users. This allows an organization's resources to understand:
  - **How** the communication will be delivered (e.g., email, in person, broadcast public address (PA) announcement).
  - **Who** the communication is intended for.
  - **What** verbiage and messaging will be contained in the communication. (This will depend on what service is unavailable and what users are affected.)
  - **Where** to find status updates. (Make sure your status page is available during the downtime – build redundancy.)

31.5.2 Notification Practices

Communication during and immediately after incidents or problems are reported provides assurances to users and stakeholders by reassuring users that the interruption is being managed and addressed with the level of seriousness it deserves.

- Scheduled downtime communications will be different from unscheduled downtime communications. Defining the content, verbiage, delivery methods, and frequency of downtime notifications should be contained in the organization's policies and procedures.
  - Notifying staff of the planned downtime ahead of time allows adequate preparations to ensure the continuity of patient care in a safe and effective manner.

- Advanced communication of the scheduled downtime must contain specific information including:

    The imaging system or application that will be down and the department/service areas that will be affected.

    The time that the downtime will begin and the expected

DEFINITION: Crisis Management Plan (CMP)

A CMP is a document that describes the processes that an organization should use to respond to a critical situation that could adversely affect its profitability, reputation, or ability to operate [8].

length of time the system or application will be unavailable.

The reason for the downtime and the expected changes once the planned downtime is completed.

In unscheduled downtimes, stakeholders should be immediately notified upon discovery of the interruption.

- Communicating updates throughout the duration of the downtime should be managed carefully to avoid inundating a user's email inbox.

    - **Regular and consistent communication** on the progress of the downtime, even if it is not good news, is more acceptable

DEFINITION: Disaster Recovery

A set of policies, procedures, processes, and systems put in place to enable the restoration and recovery of vital data and infrastructure following a natural or man-made catastrophic event.

to those affected by the downtime than no communication at all. When stakeholders and end users receive accurate and timely updates, frustration levels vastly decline.

- Throughout the business continuity and disaster recovery phases, communication is vital to ensure users are aware of any workaround procedures to access backup services during an interruption. The intention of communication during an outage include:

DEFINITION: Business Continuity

During a temporary downtime, business continuity provides access to the ePHI until the systems are fully restored to normal operating conditions (see **Chap. 29**).

- **Providing instruction**: Details about the interruption, the impact to care teams, workaround practices during the interruption, and notification of when the system interruption has been resolved.

KEY CONCEPT: Disaster Recovery Versus Business Continuity

Business Continuity is a backup system that gets used during brief planned or unplanned downtimes. You expect to use BC on a regular basis.

Disaster Recovery is a complete recovery of all data and infrastructure from the ground up, assuming everything got destroyed. You hope never to need DR.

- **Instill confidence**: Effective communication results in a better understanding of what is occurring in real-time and that the situation is actively being addressed.
- Depending on the type of downtime, communication may require a person-to-person communication or a telephone call. Consider using multiple communication tools and methods during planning.
- The ideal delivery method will depend on whether you are communicating to internal users, existing customers, or the public. Downtimes can be advertised using multiple communication channels.
  - Email is the primary method of communication; however, communication can be sent via social media, web pages, internal communication methods (e.g., organization's instant messaging platform), or on the application's sign-in page, if possible.
  - Online enterprise status page. It is important to ensure that the online status page consistently contains accurate and updated information. If possible, integrate the status notification updates on the ticketing tool virtual application page that users go to when creating tickets. This will inform users that the support team is already aware of the issue and provide them with real-time updates.
  - If the interrupted service runs on a mobile device, it may be possible to send in-app notification or push notifications containing details about the downtime.
  - A third-party online status website enables users to check the status of the system interruption.

> **DEFINITION: Online Status Website**
>
> Third-party website that reports the status of an interruption to end users. Subscriptions allow users to receive email or text updates regarding a specific interruption.

  - In some cases, it may be best to personally inform key stakeholders of the interruption and provide them workaround steps while the interruption persists.
- In addition to internal communication strategies, external communication strategies may be required as well.
  - When a PACS or VNA is experiencing a service interruption, this requires communication to all appropriate stakeholders within and outside your organization as this interruption could affect viewing images through the patient portal or other methods of external presentation.

CHECKLIST: Downtime Communication Best Practices

1. Acknowledge the problem.
2. Use communications to assure users that the situation is under control (if and when it is).
3. Include contact information or methods to receive additional information or updates.
4. Word things in a way that will resonate with the appropriate stakeholder (e.g., avoid technical language to nontechnical users, avoid jargon or acronyms).
5. Provide context to the stakeholder so they understand the impact.
6. Provide alternative options for working around the interruption.
7. Do not over promise – be as truthful and transparent as possible.
8. Provide a final communication related to the resolution, while providing users the opportunity to confirm that the service has resumed normal operation.
9. Include contact information to report issues that occur during or after the update.

HYPOTHETICAL SCENARIO: System Downtime Caused by External Factors

A service interruption is sometimes caused by an external variable and is not an organization's direct responsibility. For example, in 2017 a 4 hour outage related to Amazon's AWS cloud services caused service interruptions to hundreds of thousands of web services across the globe. If an organization's PACS or VNA relied on cloud storage for images during this outage, there would be a service interruption to the organization's end users.

Communications related to these types of interruptions should avoid blaming service provider, partners, or vendors. Depending on the user, they may require different levels of information – some users may find it useful to know what provider is responsible for the downtime, others may just want to know what is down, the workaround procedure, and when is will be resolved.

Even when the organization is not able to resolve the interruption or have a workaround, regular ongoing communication is essential!

PEARLS

- Service Level Agreements (SLAs) are predetermined system definitions and expectations mutually agreed upon between the system provider and the organization using the system.
- Service availability measures the percentage of time that a system is expected to be operational and available.
- Monitoring tools provide automated identifications and notifications of failures, degradations, or interruptions.
- Methods used to identify system interruptions are proactive or reactive.
- Incident management addresses unplanned interruptions that have not yet affected service.
- Problem management addresses underlying causes of one or more incidents.
- Policies and procedures are essential in documenting methodologies and approaches during downtime events.
- Communication is vital during system downtimes to assist care givers in providing business continuity.

References

1. Kearney KT, Torelli F. The SLA Model. In Wieder P, Butler JM, Theilmann W, Yahyapour R. (eds.). Service Level Agreements for Cloud Computing. Springer Science+Business Media, LLC. 2011; pp. 43–68. ISBN 9781461416142.
2. Singh VP, Swaminathan S. "Sample sizes for system availability," Annual Reliability and Maintainability Symposium. 2002 Proceedings (Cat. No.02CH37318), Seattle, WA, USA, 2002, pp. 51–55. https://doi.org/10.1109/RAMS.2002.981619.
3. Telecommunications: Glossary of Telecommunication Terms, Federal Standard 1037C. 1996. https://www.its.bldrdoc.gov/fs-1037/fs-1037c.htm.
4. Toland C, Meenan C, Warnock M. et al. Proactively Monitoring Departmental Clinical IT Systems with an Open Source Availability System. J Digit Imaging 20, 119–124 (2007). https://doi.org/10.1007/s10278-007-9063-2.
5. Cusick JJ, and Ma G. Creating an ITIL inspired Incident Management approach: Roots, response, and results, 2010 IEEE/IFIP Network Operations and Management Symposium Workshops, Osaka, 2010, pp. 142–148. https://doi.org/10.1109/NOMSW.2010.5486589.
6. Jäntti M, Miettinen A, Pylkkänen N, Kainulainen T. (2007) Improving the Problem Management Process from Knowledge Management Perspective. In: Münch J, Abrahamsson P. (eds) Product-Focused Software Process Improvement. PROFES 2007. Lecture Notes in Computer Science, vol 4589. Springer, Berlin, Heidelberg. https://doi.org/10.1007/978-3-540-73460-4_33.
7. Kelly M. Beware the danger of alarm fatigue in IT monitoring. InfoWorld [Internet]. 2018 [cited 12 September 2020]. Available from: https://www.infoworld.com/article/3268126/beware-the-danger-of-alarm-fatigue-in-it-monitoring.html.
8. Barton L. Crisis Management: Preparing for and Managing Disasters. Cornell Hotel and Restaurant Administration Quarterly. 1994;35(2):59–65. https://doi.org/10.1177/001088049403500219.

Self-Assessment Questions

1. What is the definition of "Service Availability":

   (a) A metric used to measure the percentage of time a service is operational and available to users.
   (b) A Service Level Agreement agreed upon by the customer and service provider.
   (c) Continuing business operations in spite of an interruption.
   (d) The ability to restore the data and services that run your business.

2. Which best describes the "Nines" concept of availability:

   (a) A commitment between a service provider and a client that outlines aspects of the service related to quality, availability, and responsibilities of both parties.
   (b) An organization is not able to accurately track availability for more than five-9's of services.
   (c) The ability to keep track of a system or service, in order to have automated identification and notification of failures, degradations, or interruptions.
   (d) Percentages of a particular order of magnitude are sometimes referred to by the number of nines or "classes of nines" in the digits as part of the service-level agreement.

3. From the list below, what is a step that can help avoid alert fatigue?

   (a) Responding after an overwhelming number of alerts desensitizes the resources assigned with reviewing and responding to alerts.
   (b) Establish intelligent thresholds. Determine which issues require an immediate alert and which can wait until normal working hours.
   (c) Avoid the use of monitoring tools and allow users to report issues as a means of identifying interruptions.
   (d) Ensure all administrators have a comprehensive understanding of the topology of the environment and how each system and service interact, exchange data, and depend on each other.

4. Describe the relationship between monitoring availability/uptime and the Service Management Model.

5. When a service interruption is caused by an external variable that is not your organization's direct responsibility, which one of the statements below is accurate:

   (a) Communication and updates regarding the interruption is not required as the organization is not responsible for the cause of the interruption.
   (b) Disable Monitoring tools throughout the period of the downtime.
   (c) Communication related to these types of interruptions should avoid blaming the service provider or vendor.
   (d) System Availability allows an individual to calculate the probability that a service/system is available.

6. Monitoring tools provide an organization the ability to:

   (a) Proactively identify potential service incidents before they have directly affected end users.
   (b) Receive updates on the holistic topology of the organization's network environment.
   (c) Log and track service incidents identified by the monitoring tools.
   (d) Identify scheduled and unscheduled downtimes.

7. What is the definition of Business Continuity:

   (a) The ability to restore the data and services that run your business.
   (b) Continuing business operations in spite of an interruption.
   (c) An unplanned interruption that has not impacted services yet.
   (d) An underlying cause of one or more incidents.

8. From the list below, select the items that would result in logging a service ticket with the service desk. Select all that apply:

   (a) Monitoring tools identify a potential issue with a service.
   (b) End-user reports an incident related to the inability to access the EMR.
   (c) Communication about a downtime is sent via email to affected users.
   (d) The online status webpage is updated to reflect a downtime.

9. From the list below, select the items that are defined in the Downtime Communication Policies and Procedures. Select all that apply:

   (a) Which delivery methods should be used to communicate the downtime.
   (b) Which services are affected when monitoring tools alert of a potential service issue.
   (c) How frequently to provide communication updates related to the downtime.
   (d) Which users should receive the communications about a specific downtime.

Part VII
Project Management

Chapter 32
PACS Readiness and PACS Migration

Steven C. Horii and Fred M. Behlen

Contents

32.1 Introduction

Since the previous edition of this book, most healthcare facilities have changed from film-based operation to full or partial PACS operation. Thus, this chapter will examine both initial PACS readiness and the more common scenario of switching to

S. C. Horii (✉)
Department of Radiology, University of Pennsylvania Medical Center, Philadelphia, PA, USA
e-mail: steve.horii@pennmedicine.upenn.edu, horiisc@email.chop.edu

F. M. Behlen
Medical Physics and Informatics, Laitek Inc. Homewood, IL, USA
e-mail: fbehlen@laitek.com

© The Author(s), under exclusive license to Springer Science+Business Media, LLC, part of Springer Nature 2021
B. F. Branstetter IV (ed.), *Practical Imaging Informatics*,
https://doi.org/10.1007/978-1-0716-1756-4_32

a new PACS. For any facility to make such a change, it is important first to ask a fundamental question, "Why do **we** want to make a change in our PACS?" If the radiology group has difficulty answering this question, either it is too early to make this decision or the group needs to do a more thorough study of the possible answers.

The migration of imaging data from one PACS to another forms the second half of this chapter. Because of the complexity of the decision to change systems or perform a data migration project, it is difficult in this short chapter to provide a comprehensive list of reasons for making the change. However, it may be useful to know some reasons that are *not* good ones.

Common but usually **improper reasons** for changing systems include:
- It's the trend.
- We have extra capital to spend.
- We expect to save a lot of money by making the change.
- Our imaging equipment vendor will give us a good deal on a PACS or long-term storage.
- A new PACS or long-term storage solution will solve our workflow problems.

32.2 Choosing to Change PACS

If your organization already operates with a PACS but there is an interest or need to change to a different system, some of the questions that were asked when you implemented your PACS the first time are bound to resurface. The usual reasons given for changing PACS vendors include:
- The existing system is not scalable and no longer meets our needs.
- Because of the merging or acquisition of healthcare systems, there is a need to have a single system.
- Your current PACS vendor is leaving the business.
- Teleradiology for expanded practice, reading from home, or off-hours coverage is nearly impossible with the current system.
- The existing PACS is integrated with a RIS, and your facility is changing to an electronic medical record (EMR) system that includes a RIS module.

The checklist of initial questions for PACS readiness also applies to the initial questions for changing a PACS.

CHECKLIST: Initial Questions for PACS Readiness

1. Why are we doing this?
2. What are our goals and expectations?
3. Do we have support for this change from the practice members and/or hospital administration?

32.3 Assessment

For changing from one PACS to another, the assessment process is similar to changing from a non-PACS to full-PACS operation. The overriding question is, "Why are we doing this now?" Answering this is not as simple as it may sound as it involves a thorough study of both the radiology department and its interaction with the rest of the healthcare facility [1]. A first step should be an assessment of the major interactions between radiology and the other departments. This can be useful in determining radiology report and image retrieval rates by the referring providers. The process of creating a detailed **functional diagram and specification** of the radiology department is performed after a PACS change readiness decision is made.

32.3.1 Assessing Workload

Workload assessments assess how much work is being done and where the specific work takes place. Is the work for a specific area urgent such as in emergency departments or surgical suites? What is the expected growth rate of the work?

If you are considering changing from one PACS vendor to a different one, or even replacing the existing system with a newer one from the current vendor, a major question regarding workload has to do with storage of studies. Workload data can be assembled from various sources and put into spreadsheets, which will make editing, analysis, comparison, and charting of data simpler. For facilities that already use PACS and are seeking to change systems, they can leverage the information already contained in the PACS database.

CHECKLIST: Workload Assessment

1. **Do you operate an electronic radiological information system (RIS)?**
   - If you do, this is a useful source of information to answer workload questions.
2. **How many studies of what kinds?**
   - These data elements are usually available from departmental logs, billing records, or the RIS.
3. **Of the number of imaging studies acquired, how many are acquired by each modality?**
   - Purchase records, examination orders, schedules, examination logs, and billing information are all potential sources of these data.
4. **How much radiology information is stored in your PACS database?**
   - How much data is added per time (day, week, month, etc.)?
5. **Estimate of growth rate:**
   - Extrapolate or project from existing data, trends, and any known expansion of services or facilities.
   - Radiology business managers usually do this analysis regularly.
6. **Are imaging studies read where they are acquired or are imaging studies read remotely?**
   - Is this expected to change with the new PACS? If so, how?
   - This is important in assessing where images are read so network capacity can be estimated.
7. **Where and how are images viewed by clinicians?**
   - This may require surveys of the clinicians both on-site and those practicing in outside offices.
   - Is important to determine the number and types of workstations needed.
   - If you are changing PACS, then this should be reassessed due to probable changes since acquiring your existing PACS.
8. **What other systems do you have that interface with the PACS?**
   - RIS
   - Reporting systems (e.g., digital dictation, speech recognition)
   - Medical records (if separate from the RIS)
   - A hospital information system (if different from the medical record system)
   - Accounting and billing
9. **Do you have a dedicated PACS storage system or are you operating a single archive for all your healthcare information (an "enterprise" archive)?**
   - The imaging informatics professionals that support clinical operations and the information services team should know this information.

32.3.2 *Workflow*

There are two very important workflow questions when preparing for a new PACS:

1. How do we do what we do?
2. How is the new PACS going to do those things? Determining how to perform the various tasks needed from the onset of when an imaging study is requested to the when the imaging report made available to the referring practitioner (final product) is a difficult process. If you do a count of the number of

> **KEY CONCEPT: Workload vs. Workflow**
>
> Workload assessment examines how much volume of work is being performed and how it is being divided among the members of the group.
>
> Workflow assessment examines how each person performs their job with the goal of increasing efficiency. See **Chap. 25** for more information on workflow assessment.

tasks and who performs them, you are likely to discover that there are numerous steps and people involved. Even if you already have a PACS in place and are seeking to change to a different one, you will still need to analyze your present workflow as it most likely changed when you deployed your existing PACS [2]. A simple way to think of workflow steps – each step has:

- Some sort of **input**
- A **task** performed on or with the input
- Some sort of **output** based on the task performed

A workflow assessment involves determining the various tasks performed by your organization – remembering that some of the tasks are performed outside your organization, even the steps within those tasks.

For some PACS-based operations, each task would be performed by different people. However, to accomplish each of the tasks, there are several steps. In PACS-based operations, information moves electronically but still involves the same type

> **KEY CONCEPT: Interface Engine**
>
> Handles messages between systems such as RIS and PACS. The interfaces may be unidirectional (one way) or bidirectional (two way).

of information that would have been moved in a film-based practice using paper forms, logbooks, and printed pages. Even in a PACS-based operation, printing of paper documents may still be required (e.g., printing a report for the requesting practitioner who does not have a connection to your electronic healthcare information system). Also required for electronic systems are the **interfaces** between a person and a system or between different systems.

There are several methods used to perform the workflow assessment process. These are typically based on a more detailed examination of what the practice does currently. Typical methods include:

- **Follow something** – In this method, you follow various things to see what happens to them and where they go. You could simulate a typical imaging workflow by pretending to be a patient (or follow an actual patient if they give their permission) and record all the places they go:
  - Observe what happens to them at each place.
  - Identify who is involved at each location from when the patient comes in to when they leave.
  - Follow other personnel (technologists, radiologists, file room clerks, referring physicians, etc.)
  - And follow "things" (films, reports, mobile equipment, information systems, etc.) using a similar process

TROUBLESHOOTING: "Follow the Film"

We had done a workflow analysis process of following our films to determine the locations where imaging studies were being viewed by our clinical colleagues. At the time, we discovered that films were being sent to the medical ICU (MICU) as expected. But we did not initially realize that a radiologist would go to the MICU each morning to review the imaging studies *with* the MICU clinicians. As a result, we located a PACS workstation in the MICU. When preparing for the replacement of our PACS, we repeated our "follow the images" analysis and found that since the original PACS was installed, the increased number of operating rooms and emergency department treatment areas meant that the number of workstations outside of radiology had to be increased considerably. This led to discussions between the radiology department and hospital administration about budgeting for the additional equipment and hospital network expansion.

- **Brainstorm** – This requires less manual labor but does require that you meet with the people involved. You gather those who work in your practice and ask them to describe in detail what they do. This method has the disadvantage of potentially missing steps; you can minimize this by having several people who do the same task describe their workflow. Keep in mind that this option requires that your personnel be given the time to attend these brainstorming sessions. You want to know:
  - What they do
  - What systems or information they have or need
  - When they do it
  - Who is involved
  - Where the person or thing they work with came from
  - Where the person or thing is going
- **Perform a gap analysis** – After identifying current workflows, have several working sessions with your personnel to demonstrate how these tasks will be accomplished in the new PACS and to determine if you have uncovered any gaps in the workflow processes.

- **Hire someone** – This is certainly a viable option, but keep in mind two things: (1) the cost and (2) that you want to be sure that all the information you want collected is included in the description of what your expert will do.

These efforts result in what can be thought of as a workflow "catalog" – a comprehensive list of tasks and performance steps involved. The objective of developing a workflow catalog is to determine how the PACS will accomplish existing tasks done in the legacy system. The importance of analyzing workflow is to be sure no tasks or steps are inadvertently overlooked.

A more complete discussion of workflow analysis is available in **Chap. 25**.

OUR EXPERIENCE: A Short Workflow Story

In preparing to implement PACS in our ultrasound section, we did some time-and-motion studies of our sonographers. We found that the time they spent interacting with the RIS was between 3 and 5 minutes per patient. For our daily volume, that amount of time could mean at least an additional examination done per sonographer per day. Even after PACS, though the RIS interaction time has been reduced, a follow-up study showed that the time had decreased to just under a minute per patient. The main reason for this is that the sonographers still must interact with the RIS to complete examinations. The reduction in time resulted from DICOM Modality Worklist which automated loading of patient information into the ultrasound machines. We still do not have DICOM-performed procedure step, which when the examination is completed on the ultrasound modality would allow for the status update information flow back to the RIS.

32.3.3 Personnel

A radiology practice is labor-intensive. You are certain to discover that most tasks are accomplished by people. While some automation is now common, the performance of imaging procedures is still done by technologists and radiologists. The goal of personnel assessment is to ensure that the new PACS will be able to perform and support the different roles in your department and permit each role to have access to all needed functionality.

KEY CONCEPT: Personnel Assessment

Assessment of personnel and their roles is essential for planning for a PACS. Determining personnel roles should be done at the end user level as well as supervisors and administrators.

HYPOTHETICAL SCENARIO: Using Job Descriptions

Do not be tempted to use job descriptions alone to determine tasks and steps performed by personnel. People often find "shortcuts" to improve the speed or reduce the number of steps involved in their tasks. When developing the lists of tasks that our various personnel would be "allowed" to do in our electronic medical record (EMR) system, the surveyors from the vendor often relied on information from managers and administrators about "who did what." We discovered one problem with this approach; when some exams were performed at the end of the day, the technologist did not track these exams to "complete" status in the system. This meant that the radiologist could not dictate these studies because they did not appear on their worklist. The radiologist had tried to complete the studies herself, as she had been able to do in the legacy RIS, but it was not a task that showed up for *any* radiologist in the new EMR. Subsequently, the radiologist located a technologist who was still in-house to complete the studies. Later, when she asked the EMR support person about this, she was told, "Administration said that radiologists do not complete exams; only technologists do that."

32.3.4 Interfaces

Information, whether it is analog or digital, must move between equipment and personnel to accomplish workflow tasks. This requires equipment-to-equipment, people-to-equipment, or people-to-people interfaces. As described in the Assessment section, the various interfaces within your organization need to be cataloged and coupled with the workflow evaluation. The various tasks you discover in building your workflow assessment will all likely require some type of interface. An example is order entry and scheduling (this scenario assumes a separate EMR and RIS):

- A provider requests a radiology examination: This can be a person-to-person interface or, more commonly, a person-to-EMR workstation or EMR application interface.
- The EMR sending this information to the radiological information system (RIS), a system-to-system interface.
- The request information is picked up from the RIS and entered in the scheduling module within the RIS, a person-to-system interface.
- The RIS scheduling module returning the schedule confirmation to the EMR, a system-to-system interface.
- The EMR notifying the requesting provider and usually the patient that the examination has been scheduled, a system-to-person interface.

This example is much simplified. If you examine your organization's workflow, it is likely that you will determine that there are other steps and interfaces required. Also, some of these interfaces may move information between systems without a person working between them.

> **OUR EXPERIENCE: An Interface Story**
>
> In the process of changing from a radiology department RIS to an EMR that had an integrated RIS, we developed a catalog of RIS interfaces. We were quite surprised by the number – it was over 100 interfaces.

When you build your catalog of interfaces and what information moves between them, it is likely you will find a large number of interfaces that need to be considered, either when planning for a first PACS installation or when replacing an existing PACS.

CHECKLIST: Interface Catalog

- Interface type: Person-to-person, person-to-system, and system-to-system.
- What personnel (by role or task) are connecting for a person-to-person interface?
- What personnel (by role or task) are connecting to what system?
- What system is connecting to what other system or systems?
- What initiates the information movement across the interface?
- What information is moved or exchanged – including the information type and format or encoding?
- Is there an acknowledgment system as part of the interface operation?
- How are errors on the interface handled (e.g., a failure to connect; a failure to send the information; incomplete information sent or exchanged; an unexpected termination of the information movement or exchange)?
- Is there a way to detect data corruption as it is moved or exchanged across the interface?
- What would happen if a particular interface fails?
- Remedies or workarounds if the interface does fail.

OUR EXPERIENCE: Interface "Lockup"

One problem in designing an interface is how to handle an error. Some poor designs are unable to skip a process running on an interface if the task fails. One suboptimal response is to report the failure and stop. Another method is to retry the task, which is not a bad method so long as the number of retries has a limit. An interface that can manage itself could retry the task a fixed number of times, and if the problem repeats each time, log the problem for troubleshooting and proceed to the next task in the queue. A log of the interface failures would allow troubleshooting personnel to determine what task caused the problem.

We had a problem with a machine that failed on sending a study to the PACS. It kept retrying to send the same study, which meant other studies that were queued to be sent to the PACS were held up. The only error message displayed to the technologist was "Something wrong on the DICOM protocol" (not a very helpful message). It turned out to be an error with a DICOM mandatory element being omitted from the DICOM metadata. We suspected that the problem was corruption due to a "bit flip" as the metadata in the other images was correct and examination of the error image showed that the value in the element tag was wrong. The workaround was to tell the machine to start sending the next studies in the queue.

32.3.5 What Kind of PACS?

This section is not to recommend a particular PACS for initial acquisition or change but rather to examine a fundamental question for what the overall design of your PACS will be. With subspecialties such as breast imaging, ultrasound, nuclear medicine, and imaging subspecialties that use advanced visualization (3D and 4D imaging, virtual or augmented reality), it may be difficult to find a single PACS vendor that supports all these subspecialties with the functionality they need. Most of these particular requirements have resulted in the development and evolution of systems to support them. In some cases, these are processing systems that carry out necessary functions for clinical operation:

- Breast imaging typically uses very high-resolution displays and workstation controls suited for the rapid display and comparison of studies with a minimum of menu item selections and mouse movements.
- Nuclear medicine/molecular imaging often needs mathematical operations performed on the images.
- Ultrasound may have to display multiple **cine loops** simultaneously and support the ability to control them (playback speed, playback direction, freeze, and even select a frame to copy as a separate image) plus some obstetrical measurements not typically done with usual PACS measurement tools (e.g., measuring a fetal heart rate or **Doppler waveform**).
- Virtual and augmented reality displays may be used in an operating room but will require that image update rates and manipulation of the images by the surgeon happen in real time.

Because these requirements may exceed PACS functionality, some of these sub-specialties use **mini-PACS** developed for their area of expertise. The question for those seeking a first PACS or a replacement one is whether the PACS can perform all the functions needed by the subspecialties or will the mini-PACS continue to be used. If a candidate PACS can truly meet all subspecialty needs, then a single PACS should do (provided it also meets other requirements you have specified). Otherwise, the solution is to implement a "federated PACS." In this scenario, essential mini-PACS (those with functions the main PACS cannot perform) are retained and integrated (ideally) or interfaced to the main PACS. The concern with a federated PACS design is that there can be maintenance problems. If the studies on a mini-PACS fail to display on the main PACS, which system (interface concerns in this situation) has caused the problem? This assumes that the role of the main PACS is that the workstations would be used for the display of all (or almost all) the studies for reading whether captured directly by the main PACS or sent from one of the mini-PACS.

The subspecialty systems may not be a mini-PACS but a separate processing system designed to handle particular imaging. An example is the advanced visualization system that accepts images from various imaging equipment and generates the needed 3D or 4D images. These systems may need separate workstations or, in some cases, launch their application in a window on the main PACS workstation. Federated systems will require additional analysis of how the studies generated or processed by a mini-PACS or processing system are to be viewed for interpretation.

32.4 Change Management

A change from one PACS to another is a major change for any medical imaging practice. A part of readiness assessment is to examine the problems that will drive change management [3]. Unfortunately, change management is often not fully considered, or is assumed to be so obvious it is deemed trivial. A failure to consider change management principles is an invitation to a much more difficult process than would otherwise be the case.

There is a significant amount of literature on change management, but the principles applied to PACS readiness analysis include:

- From the very inception of the idea, all the way to making the change to a different PACS vendor, communicate the idea, the goals, and the processes involved as widely as possible. Keep communication frequent, regular, and informative.
- Involve those affected.
- Be realistic about expectations and goals; do not oversell the project.

For a complete discussion of change management, please see **Chap. 26**.

32.4.1 Training Issues

A useful aspect of going through the process of analyzing workflow and personnel roles is that these processes will provide insight into which areas will need the most training when a new system is considered. Because of the common implementation of PACS, training for the "changing PACS" scenario is more likely. However, both have the following elements in common:

- Training is labor- and time-intensive.
- If you have previous experience with introduction training for new systems (EMR, RIS, HIS, etc.), it is useful to use the successful aspects of that training curriculum and address the deficiencies you found.
- Finding the time for training due to the busy schedules of your personnel will be one of the most difficult challenges.
- Consider a "train the trainers" approach – have vendor training experts train your personnel who would like to be trainers themselves. They have the advantage of knowing both their colleagues and the operations of your facility.
- It is very helpful to have a "test system" or "playground" that those being trained can use. This fosters a safe training environment without fear of causing problems with the "live" system or taking up clinical resources. It should be possible for your personnel to use the training system whenever they have the time, even potentially by remote access.
- The training system should provide ample hints for users, and if errors are being made at the same step of operation repeatedly, it is useful to log these so the vendor can use that information to mitigate the cause of the errors.
- If the vendor is willing (or is required in your purchase or lease agreement) to have training personnel on-site, it is better to set an agreed-upon endpoint. The trainers should remain on-site until that endpoint is reached. This is a more suitable option for system training rather than training for a fixed amount of time. An endpoint can be as simple as the percentage of your personnel trained and who then can pass a "test" of using the system functions relevant to their role.
- Make sure that training plans will train "all materially affected users." If you have per diem, remote, research, or part-time users, they must be included in training plans.
- Don't forget to train referring providers. Many of them are strong PACS users!

Many problems with training on new systems arise because the training occurs way ahead of go live or the amount of time estimated for training is too short. Vendors may estimate training time simply on a count of users, though the types of users should also be considered. Some users will require training on more modules or functions than others and will take longer to train. Other groups of users, particularly radiologists and other physicians, are likely to find it difficult to fit training into their schedules. Administration should consider this and provide for dedicated training time that is not counted against vacation or other time off, and if metrics such as work relative value units (RVUs) are used to compute incentive or bonus payments, adjustments for training time should be made.

> **OUR EXPERIENCE: Training for a Replacement PACS**
>
> During a recent enterprise PACS replacement project, we were juggling numerous tasks and had a significant amount of personnel to train. In an effort to be efficient, we started scheduling our technologist training 3 months ahead of the go-live date. During the training sessions, we found that most of the technologists were disengaged because they felt they still had time to learn the system. When go-live day approached, many technologists were mildly panicking because they had forgotten what they learned 3 months earlier.
>
> **LESSONS LEARNED**
>
> Schedule training 1–3 weeks before go live. Personnel will most likely remember training points while it is still fresh in their memory and because go-live day is quickly approaching.

How a vendor approaches training for their systems should be a major consideration in the vendor selection process. They should provide a complete and comprehensive plan for training your personnel and, if possible, provide some reference sites where such plans have been used successfully. Ideally, a reference site should have similarities to your own in terms of the type of facility, examination volume, numbers of personnel, and how much experience the personnel have with information systems.

32.4.2 IT Historians and Their Roles and Importance

A forgotten aspect of implementing systems is to maintain a historical record. For many critical systems within healthcare, hardware and operational histories are the norm. The importance of establishing a catalog of equipment and historical interfaces integrated to the equipment cannot be understated. While it sounds simple, healthcare equipment is often replaced, software is updated, new equipment is added, and storage capacities of machines and servers are expanded. The difficulty is that different people perform updates to equipment and software at different times. These updates can be performed by support teams within your organization or by the vendor.

When considering changing to PACS or replacing/updating an existing PACS, there can be difficulties if the historical information is not readily available. Those responsible for making decisions about PACS requirements, those who build interfaces and equipment catalogs, and those who assess workflow processes need historical data. A PACS vendor is very likely not just to ask what equipment you have but what software version is running on it is and when it was last updated.

OUR EXPERIENCE: Software Updates and Loss of Function

A story heard from several IT managers is the sudden change in behavior of a piece of imaging equipment. As an example, at the beginning of the workday, the CT modality would not send images to the PACS. The machine itself was operating properly; it could scan patients and images were being stored on the local storage and displayed on the operator's console. However, the images could not be found on the PACS reading worklists. IT troubleshooting finds that the studies are not moving across the DICOM interface to the PACS. Low-level network testing shows that the network itself is fine – the IT folks can "ping" the PACS from the CT machine and vice versa. The DICOM interface is not working. After many telephone calls, the team learned that the CT modality's vendor performed a software update overnight. That software update changed the DICOM AE Title of the machine. The PACS no longer recognized the machine as a valid device so it would not establish a connection with it.

CHECKLIST: Equipment Database (IT Historian)

- Device, interface, or system type.
- Change flag: A change in one of the fields has been made.
- Importance category:
  - Critical
  - Failure tolerant (you can operate without it or there is a backup immediately available)
  - Needed on demand (surge application)
  - Descriptions of changes; planned or already accomplished
- Date of acquisition
- Acquisition cost (or periodic lease fee)
- Source of acquisition funding
- Start date of vendor warranty
- End date of vendor warranty
- Performance specification details
- Downtime (scheduled or unscheduled) with date, time, and duration
- Current hardware, firmware, and software versions
- Updates and changes of hardware, firmware, or software
- Descriptions of changes; planned or already accomplished
- Links to interfaced devices or systems
- Responsible personnel (system owners or those who manage the device)

Establishing the role of an IT historian could help prevent a number of problems. Establishing a database indexing imaging equipment, interfaces, and systems is a very useful tool. However, the goal of such a database is to use it to log information about all of the items important for the facility.

In a large medical facility, the maintenance of an imaging equipment inventory database could be a full-time job. Even then, one person might have difficulty tracking all of the things that change within the scope of items being followed. It may be useful to have the supervisors and managers of the various divisions or sections within a department take responsibility for updating the applicable portions. Another alternative is having personnel from the various divisions or sections within a department take responsibility for updating the applicable portions of the database with the "IT historian" overseeing these responsibilities.

When there is an anticipated or unanticipated change, the inventory database would be able to quickly provide information about the various equipment and software used in the facility. The records documented by the IT historian would include what interfaces were affected by software updates or if the system stopped working when software update was deployed. Without the IT historian, system administrators would be required to search numerous files for answers. Ideally, such a database would provide useful information:

- **Notification system**: If changes occur, a notification of the change and for which equipment should be automatically sent. The ability to send notifications via e-mail or text messages can simplify this. Some filtering could be done so that the messages would be sent to those affected by the change.
- **Dashboard**: A second possibility is for the database to drive a "dashboard," which is a graphical display of systems and their status. This allows all personnel to quickly view the overall status of systems. Dashboard displays are common in other industries as well: power plant control rooms, aircraft pilot displays, military "situational awareness" displays, chemical plant process controls, etc.

Long term, a history database could be used for research purposes (e.g., technology assessment) and quality assurance (e.g., performance meeting specifications). The cost of an IT historian is likely justifiable and is likely to be allocated as an operating expense. The potential cost savings of employing an IT historian can be gained from avoiding litigation with vendors over matters of system performance or uptime, improving the response time for fixing problems, and setting budgetary goals (e.g., when to purchase a replacement piece of equipment).

HYPOTHETICAL SCENARIO: The Value of an IT Historian

The warranty: You purchase and install a new piece of imaging equipment. In the contract, the vendor warrants that the system will have a guaranteed uptime of 99.99%, based on the agreed-upon decision of how that uptime is calculated. The equipment unexpectedly fails. The vendor's service department tells you that the failure does not mean the uptime guarantee was not been met, so you are expected to pay for the service. If you do not have access to the detail of the uptime agreement terms and how long the equipment is down before repair, you may have to accept the vendor's claim.

PACS performance: You have changed from film-based operation to a PACS. The vendor agreed to the condition that until the PACS could replace film use for specified applications, they would deduct the cost of the film from your lease payments for the PACS. Although the radiologists are reading the chest images on the PACS after the first month of operation, the MICU physicians find that either they do not have PACS workstations installed yet or the performance is too slow. As such the clinicians continue to ask for printed film for rounds. Chest imaging was included in the applications that were supposed to be completely PACS-based. The vendor says you are required to document the missing workstations and how the PACS performance speed is suboptimal. Unless you can prove your assertions and the vendor is wrong, they will not pay for the film you are still using.

32.4.3 Getting Help

The decision to change an existing PACS to another is an expensive one. Both over- and underspecifying a system can increase the cost. As this chapter has shown, there is much work involved in deciding whether to change to a different PACS involves much work and expertise.

Because the costs of PACS acquisition and change are high and the risk of making the wrong decisions would add to the costs, it may be worth considering getting outside help. There are consultants who are experts and do the sort of work described in this chapter. Consultants gather the information needed about existing equipment, personnel responsibilities, workflows, and training needs. A consultant would be required to learn about your systems and operations. If you rely on your own personnel instead of an outside consultant, they may unconsciously perform some of the tasks needed for documentation and fail to consider them during the information-gathering phase of the project. There are usually workarounds or shortcuts team members created because of workflow deficiencies or bottlenecks. A consultant should know to ask if the person performing a task uses shortcuts, and if so, why If this phase is not done, the answer to the main question of "How is the new PACS going to do those things?" may not be properly addressed.

32.5 Data Migration

When you install a new PACS, you will have to be able to access historical image data for comparison studies. You will have to choose between keeping the old archive running (and interfacing to it from the new system) and migrating the data out of it. The migration is usually directed to the new PACS, but many hospitals

> **DEFINITION: VNA**
>
> A vendor-neutral archive is a large storage system that maintains image data and can interface with any PACS. This enables multiple PACS interfaces to all access the same data. It permits "best of breed" systems.

are installing vendor-neutral archives (VNAs) at a separate enterprise facility. Either way, it is a data migration, and when you have completed the project, you will want to decommission the legacy PACS. There are four basic approaches to data migration (see Fig. 32.1).

- **Retain access to the legacy system**:
  - Keep the old system running.
  - When required, the new system queries the legacy archive for DICOM studies.

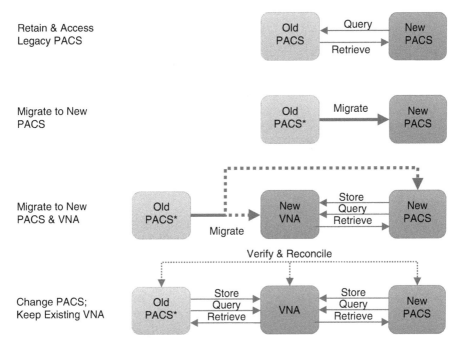

*Decommission system at completion

Fig. 32.1 Means of providing legacy data

- Some facilities even continue to use the legacy PACS workstations for viewing historical images, though at significant inconvenience for radiologists.
- **Migrate to new PACS**:
  - Transfer all historical data to the new system.
  - Decommission the old PACS.
- **Migrate to VNA**:
  - When transferring the historical data to a new vendor-neutral archive (VNA), the existing PACS will retrieve historical images when needed.
  - Often this migration is to a new PACS, which subsequently archives the data to the VNA. Thereafter, the legacy PACS is decommissioned.
- **Change PACS using existing VNA**:
  - If an institution already has a VNA that is used by the PACS, the need for data migration to the new PACS may be reduced. Special attention may still be required before the legacy PACS is decommissioned.
  - There may be differences between the PACS data and VNA data that do not appear when images are viewed from the PACS that wrote them, in particular:

    Data in PACS storage that for any reason is not yet archived. For example, waiting for the report to be finalized before archiving.

    Changes in PACS not propagated to the archive. Patient demographic changes in the PACS may not have been propagated to the VNA. The PACS may automatically update the demographics when the study is displayed on the PACS, thus hiding the inconsistency.

    Data stored in private attributes. The legacy PACS may archive annotation or measurement data in private attributes in the DICOM data. As a result, those annotations are visible only when the data is displayed in the legacy vendor's PACS.

    Data that is in the PACS database only and is not archived to the VNA.

> **KEY CONCEPT: Migration vs. Decommissioning**
>
> *Migration* is the process of getting enough data transferred to the new system to enable its full clinical use.
>
> *Decommissioning* is the process of shutting down the legacy system, requiring that all needed data in the old system has been extracted and secured.

> **OUR EXPERIENCE: Retiring the Legacy PACS**
>
> Practical factors of complexity, maintenance and operating costs, and reliability usually favor solutions in which the legacy system is retired and decommissioned.

The need for PACS data migration is not new [4]. But unsurprisingly, the designers of existing PACS did not pay much attention to how the data would be exported to a new system. In fact, the earliest PAC systems had no provisions whatsoever for the export of data, but nearly all systems in use today have DICOM Query/Retrieve interfaces allowing other systems to find and retrieve stored studies. These were originally designed for use in clinical workflows. For the purposes of migration, those interfaces are limited in a number of respects:

- **Speed.** Your existing PACS was provisioned to handle the data traffic from normal clinical operations, not for data migration at many times that rate.
- **Robustness.** Migration traffic from the Query/Retrieve port may compromise the clinical performance of the existing system, or even destabilize it.
- **Completeness**:
  - It takes a fair amount of art just to get a complete inventory using a DICOM Query/Retrieve interface. Every PACS has a limit to the number of records that are returned in a query response. This limit is usually in the hundreds or thousands. For some systems, that limit is not a fixed number of records, and no explicit notice is given that the response has been truncated. Migrators usually query by ranges of study date and study time, but even so, some additional tricks are required to get a complete inventory.

    > **KEY CONCEPT: Migration Limitations**
    >
    > Overcoming migration limitations requires going inside the source PACS to extract data.

  - The Query/Retrieve interface may not export data from special features in the existing system, as we will discuss below.

32.5.1 Migration Methods

Conventional migration retrieves studies by DICOM Query/Retrieve and sends them, either directly (third-party MOVE) or by store-and-forward method to the new PACS. Rapid migration (sometimes called media migration) extracts data directly from source system storage and database, transforms it into current DICOM form, and stores it in the new PACS (Fig. 32.2).

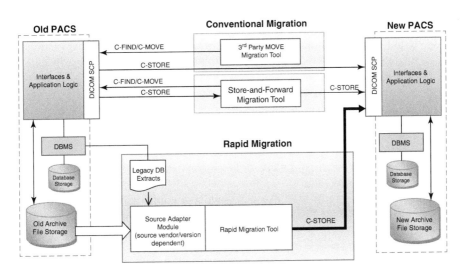

Fig. 32.2 Basic methods of data migration

Both new and old PACS have the basic architecture that you input and output data through a DICOM standard interface. That interface is part of the archive software, the "Interfaces and Application Logic." The archive software stores image data on a data storage system, and stores information about the images in a database. The format of the image files and the format of the database are totally up to the implementer, or it could be proprietary, so long as the DICOM interface behaves consistently as specified in the system's DICOM Conformance Statement.

- **Conventional migration** tools just interact with the DICOM interface of the source archive:
  - It has the advantage that one migration tool design can work for any legacy DICOM archive.
  - It has the disadvantage that it can only migrate data as fast as the old archive can deliver it, and migration projects can stretch out to years.
- **Third-party migration** tools invoke the transfer directly from the source to the destination PACS:
  - Store-and-forward tools have the ability to modify the DICOM data before transfer to the new system.
- **Smart features**: Some migration tools have smart features to make clinical life easier during the period of migration, such as things that watch HL7 message feeds to give priority to migrating currently active patients.
- **Rapid migration** takes a more brute-force approach of:
  - Directly extracting information from the PACS database.
  - Directly reading the image storage media.
  - Assembling the information into multiple DICOM output streams.
  - Sending the data into the new archive, often as fast as the new archive can take it.
  - Transfer rates measured in terabytes/day are achievable.
  - The disadvantage of this method is that the rapid migration appliance needs custom engineering for each make, model, and version of source archive, and it is not available for all types of source archives.
  - Rapid migration projects usually have greater setup times than conventional migration, a fact that can favor conventional migration in smaller projects.

32.5.2 What to Migrate

Your assessment needs to take stock of the content of your existing system, and you will need to decide which, if not all, of the patient data needs to be migrated. Your existing PACS may contain:

- **Images** in a variety of SOP classes, single and multi-frame, including photographic images. Note that the display of an image may be modified by other objects in the study.
- **Presentation states** that define how images are displayed, including grayscale window/level/lookup table, flip/rotate, and masking. Presentation information

may be stored as DICOM Grayscale Softcopy Presentation State ("GSPS") objects, in which case they will automatically come along with images in a DICOM study retrieval. Yet some systems store this information in their database and do not export it as DICOM format. Annotations (described below) may be encoded in GSPS objects.

- **Key Object Selection** (KO) objects are coded "post-it notes" tagging images, series or studies, used for a host of purposes, including:
  - "Best in Set" or "For Referring Provider" to note images of interest to clinicians
  - Critical information such as "Rejected for Quality Reasons" or "Rejected for Patient Safety Reasons"
- **DICOM Structured Reporting (SR)** objects contain:
  - Measurements and findings acquired in the imaging exam, such as in cardiology or ultrasound.
  - Results from computer-aided diagnosis (CAD) and similar post-processing.
  - Radiology reports. Note that there may be some reports in SR form, such as those that came in with imported image sets, even if regular reporting did not produce SR results.
- **Orders** are usually adequately represented in study and report data, and not needing to be explicitly migrated. However, paper orders and hard-copy documentation are frequently present as scanned documents encoded as DICOM Secondary Capture objects.

DEFINITION: Secondary Capture

The Secondary Capture (SC) Image Information Object Definition (IOD) specifies images that are converted from a non-DICOM format to a modality-independent DICOM format.

Examples of types of equipment that create Secondary Capture Images include:

- Video interfaces that convert an analog video signal into a digital image
- Digital interfaces that are commonly used to transfer non-DICOM digital images from an imaging device to a laser printer
- Film digitizers that convert an analog film image to digital data
- Workstations that construct images that are sent out as a screen dump
- Scanned documents and other bitmap images including hand-drawings
- Synthesized images that are not modality-specific, such as cine loops of 3D reconstructions

Source: dicom.nema.org

- **Tech notes** are stored in some systems. These free-text notations associated with a study are not encoded in DICOM data, and may or may not be clinically relevant, depending on your facility's history of using these features.
- **Reports** in a PACS are usually copies of documents that officially reside in other systems such as the RIS or the EHR, but may include reports received with outside studies or other sources. Still, it is usually necessary to populate the new PACS with reports, from the EHR, the PACS, or both.
- **Teaching files** are collections of images or studies maintained by attending radiologists in residency programs. Various PACS have different ways of supporting these types of user needs. Some are met using standard workflows such as making a second copy in a teaching library, which is easily migrated. Others offer special features, which are supported in the PACS database and require custom extraction.
- Waveforms, radiotherapy data, DICOM raw data objects, and a host of other DICOM SOP classes may be present, and will be migrated if the new PACS is configured to receive them.
- **Annotations and measurements.** Radiologists may wish to add a circle or arrow pointing out a finding for the convenience of the referring provider. More significantly, measurement tools may create annotations; when the area or major diameter of an irregular-shaped lesion is in the report, it is

> **DEFINITION: Annotations**
>
> Your PACS contains not only DICOM data received from modality devices or specialty workstations but also information created in the course of image management, viewing, and interpretation in the PACS.

useful to show where that measurement was made on the image. This is also of value to radiologists in subsequent examinations, so migrating these annotations is important. The expendable "grease pencil" markings of the past are no longer the standard of practice.
- **Laterality corrections.** Pay special attention to how laterality corrections are made in your present and historical workflows, and how they are represented in your archived data. These occur primarily in radiography, where a misplaced lead marker is on the image, or in ultrasound, where an image was acquired with a wrong laterality setting. Such errors may be present in the image or the DICOM laterality metadata (or both). Best practice is to fully correct these errors using a QA workstation, but common practice is to use annotation tools to overlay the laterality corrections. If this has been, or may have been, present in your workflow, then the migration of annotations is a patient safety requirement.
- **Annotations may be represented as**:
  - Overlay planes embedded in the DICOM images
  - Overlay planes in DICOM Standalone Overlay objects
  - Vector graphics in DICOM Grayscale Softcopy Presentation State (GSPS) objects
  - Pixel overlays in DICOM Grayscale Softcopy Presentation State (GSPS) objects

- Regions of interest in DICOM Structured Reporting (SR) objects
- Proprietary data in the legacy PACS database

In the installed base of systems today, we find overlay data mostly embedded in the images, in GSPS objects, or in proprietary data. The other forms are rare. However you do it, the migration process will need to convert the data you have to a form displayed by your new system. All PACS can display embedded overlays, but sometimes configuration settings need to be modified to enable their display. The most popular standard representation is vector graphics in Grayscale Softcopy Presentation State (GSPS).

32.5.3 Data Enhancement in Migration

Integral to any PACS operation is the presentation of prior exam data for comparison with new data. The task of data migration is to assemble historical data in the new system to support that operation. Ideally, the result is seamless, i.e., data from the old system looks just like it had been acquired in the new. That usually requires some enhancement to data from the old system. For example:

> **OUR EXPERIENCE: Overcoming PACS Syntactic Peccadillos**
>
> Some imaging equipment emit data with minor violations of the DICOM standard. A good PACS will tolerate minor violations that do not interfere with patient care, yet different vendors have different levels of tolerance. Historical data may need to be fixed during the migration process.

- **Changed clinical context.** Patient IDs, accession numbers, or procedure codes may need to be mapped when facilities are consolidated in a merger or acquisition.
- **Updated codes.** Even within the same organization, a system change may a good opportunity to update or consolidate exam descriptions or other codes.
- **New productivity features** in the new system, such as hanging protocols, may be sensitive to study or series descriptions. Technologist training and workflows will address this in going-forward data, but priors should be made consistent with new practice.
- **Violations of the DICOM standard.** These are things like overlength fields, malformed UIDs, hierarchical inconsistencies, and so forth.
- **Proprietary tags**: In addition, proprietary features of the legacy system may create historical data. You need to decide which of the historical features need to be supported in the new system.

32.5.4 Data Cleansing and Reconciliation

Data cleansing usually refers to a reconciliation. That is, we have an authoritative list of exams or patients from the RIS or other information system, and we match the attributes in the image data with a record in this "gold-standard" list of patients or exams:

- **Patient-level reconciliation**: Matches the basic patient attributes, patient ID, patient name, administrative gender, and birthdate.
- **Exam-level reconciliations**: When you do exam-level reconciliation, you have more to work with. In addition to the basic four patient attributes, you have an accession number, modality, and timestamps that you can match to corresponding attributes in orders from the RIS. This is the kind of reconciliation that is usually done (see Fig. 32.3).

The methods used to do this matching can be either deterministic rule-based methods or heuristic/probabilistic methods based on proprietary algorithms or maximum likelihood classification schemes. Often the latter

> **KEY CONCEPT: Dirty vs. Junk Data**
>
> When people talk about "dirty" PACS data, it is usually valid medical images from a real patient. We refer to it as dirty because we don't know who that patient is, because the patient name, ID, sex, birthdate, accession, or some combination thereof is wrong. This may be because of error when the data was acquired, or because for any reason the system did not receive the HL7 ADT update messages when the patient demographics changed.
>
> There may also be true "junk data." These are test images made by service engineers or QA personnel, or images discarded for one reason or another, research images accidentally stored in the PACS (we once found an MRI of a rat in a patient folder), or other stuff that might have been imported from a CD. They're pretty easy for a person to spot, because they have goofy names, etc., but they can be nontrivial for a computer to detect.

Fig. 32.3 Study-level reconciliation

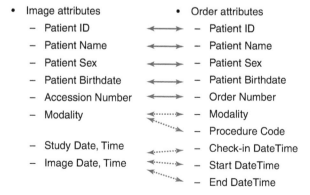

methods get a little higher matching results, at the expense of not knowing exactly how they work.

A certain amount of fuzzy matching is required to accommodate varying representations and meanings of data. For example, what is the exam time? In DICOM data, study date: time could be the timestamp of the first image in the study, or it could be an order timestamp that was imported from the modality worklist or an HL7 Order feed. Which of the various timestamps in the RIS (order entered, exam started, exam finished) it best matches depends on the RIS and on the operating practices of the imaging technologists. These are definitions that need to be clarified at the start of your project.

Doing some form of RIS-PACS reconciliation in the migration process can be particularly valuable. This introduces a task dependency that can have a major impact on project schedules. More often, the following processes overlap, with reconciliation, review, acceptance, and transmission processes occurring in a processing pipeline.

- Matching and cleanup operations can be performed:
  - Before images are moved. Working only with the inventory lists, which is nice because they are less bulky than images
  - While migration is in progress
  - Remediation as part of exception handling, as when an image or study is rejected by the target archive
- The value of the RIS-PACS reconciliation:
  - Today's PACS are likely to have a higher degree of RIS-PACS integration than older systems you have in place now.
  - Many current PACS expect an HL7 Order and/or ADT registration message to be received **before** the patient exam. When the PACS receives an image, it will try to link it to an order that it has already received through an HL7 interface.

  > **OUR EXPERIENCE: HL7 Interfaces**
  >
  > Start your HL7 interfaces running early in the migration process, because otherwise they are going to hold up data migration, which can hold up your go-live.

  - If a matching order is not found for the image, it creates an exception condition.
  - You need to migrate the orders and/or results **before** migrating images.

32.5.5 Do-It-Yourself Migration

In certain situations, it is feasible to do the migration yourself. For example, suppose you have a mammography operation with its own mini-PACS, or you have an imaging center with a small archive, and you want to fold this data into the main PACS archive. These can be cases where:

1. You don't have too many studies.
2. You're happy with the DICOM data you get out if it, so the complications we discussed previously are of tolerable scale.
3. You like doing this and have the time.

There may be a "send" utility on your legacy PACS you can use, an "import" utility on your new PACS, or one simple way to do it yourself is you go to your favorite general-purpose DICOM workstation, read in a batch of studies from the old PACS, and then push them out to the new PACS. All these methods are pretty arduous, and you'll exhaust yourself if you have to do a lot of it, but it is possible.

For small and simple migration jobs, DIY may be the best way to go if you have a pretty good PACS and someone with a decent IT skillset in-house. But it gets old fast when you've got a lot of data to move or when you're facing the kind of complications mentioned earlier.

> **OUR EXPERIENCE: Do-It-Yourselfers**
>
> Do-it-yourselfers may want to download some free utilities and write some command files to transfer the whole lot. For example, the OFFIS toolkit (Google for OFFIS DICOM to find it) has a DICOM C-MOVE client program called **movescu**. You can use this program to tell the old PACS archive to send a study directly to the new PACS archive. A little simple scripting can do this for a number of studies, but it is important to check the destination system to confirm that everything you sent is there. There are some commercial and freeware tools that do these basic inventorying, traffic management, and verification functions.

32.5.6 Commercial Migration

Migration can be done as a part of the new system procurement contract, or you can engage a migration contractor directly. The former provides simpler contractual lines of responsibility – "one throat to choke" is the charming phrase in the industry – whereas the latter gives you more control of the project and your data. All PACS and VNA vendors offer data migration services, usually subcontracting large and complex projects to migration specialists.

Start by considering what you need:

> **DEFINITION: One Throat to Choke**
>
> This colloquialism describes the advantage of purchasing goods or integrated services from a single vendor. That way, when things do not work as they should, there is only "one throat to choke." It contrasts with "best of breed."

- Decide what you need and write it down.
- Take stock of your current state: How much data you have, where your data is stored, where/if/how it is backed up, and how old it is.
- Decide what data you need moved. These are policy decisions about what to keep and what to discard.

- Consider what kind of options you want: data matching/data cleansing, presentation states, annotations, and so forth.

32.5.7 Specifying a Migration Project

Start with understanding your data and operational history. If you have the good fortune of having an IT historian, you are already there. This is good information to have at hand when you start talking to vendors. For your legacy PACS, you should have:
- The make/model and software version number
- The version history including the dates of major upgrades
- An inventory of the number of studies, series, and images
- A reading of the number of terabytes you have stored

A clear specification of the target system configuration will help the migration contractor understand what kind of resources will be at the receiving end of the migration streams. For your new PACS, it is important to know:
- The configuration of the hardware
- What kind of storage system the new PACS has on its back end
- The sustained total input rate, which is often expressed in terms of maximum numbers of images per second and total data terabytes per day

If you are planning to include any data matching or cleansing operations, it is especially important to know:
- The history of RIS/PACS integration in your setting
- What fraction of your studies were acquired using modality worklist on the input devices
- The mapping of ordered imaging procedure to a study

You need to decide what data you want moved. If you want reports moved, that is usually done by an HL7 feed directly from the RIS to the new PACS, but keep in mind that data may need to be migrated from the PACS as well. Some PACS contain reports that are not in the EHR, requiring migration from the PACS, or it can be included in the migration specification. You probably will want to move all of your data, but some institutions may choose to cull the data back to legal retention requirements.

OUR EXPERIENCE: Mapping Orders to DICOM Studies

There are a couple of different approaches out there, and the differences are laid bare in the handling of grouped procedures. For example, when you have a chest-abdomen-pelvis CT, which of the three accession numbers from your ordering system goes in the DICOM accession number? That whole area is a big mess, with well-entrenched camps espousing different approaches. (The mapping in IHE Scheduled Workflow, by the way, represents only one of those camps.)

Some systems have nice features that allow radiologists to flag key images for referring physicians. Radiologist-generated annotations, as cautioned above, may also be present in the old data:

- Some systems store these selections and annotations as derived images copied into a separate series, and when they do, they will come right across in the image migration.
- Others use some of the Standalone Overlay features of DICOM that never caught on and may not be supported in your destination PACS.
- The annotations may be completely proprietary in the old system. If you want to move this data, you will need to learn what form your new PACS wants it in.
- The preferred DICOM encodings today are as Key Object Selection (KO) objects or Grayscale Softcopy Presentation State (GSPS) Object that include annotation.
- Also, take note that annotations in GSPS may be in either vector or bitmap form, and if the new PACS does not display both forms, make sure the migrated data is in the form supported by the new PACS.

Data matching and "cleansing" options may be important in terms of their value to your organization and workflow. It is common to hear that older data is "dirty," and it is natural to want to put only "clean" data in your new PACS, but the real value of consistent and reconciled data is its facilitation of smooth workflow.

Different vendors offer different

> **OUR EXPERIENCE: Optional Features**
>
> If you want optional features, you may wish to request them as separately priced options in your bid solicitations. They can be expensive, and you will want to be able to reconsider their value in relation to their cost.

kinds of business approaches. Some will do the whole job per a statement of work (SOW). Some offer migration software for you or other service providers to use. Whatever path you take, the basic practices of protecting your interests apply:

- Find the right amount of flexibility in your requirements: Too loose and you do not get what you need; too strict and you pay too much.
- You might want to have penalties or incentives on meeting schedules, but remember that if you ask for penalties, they usually cut both ways, and you could end up paying if the project is extended at no fault of the contractor.
- And of course, the usual nondisclosure, Information Security, and HIPAA Business Associate agreements must be in place before any data is exposed to outside persons or organizations.

References

1. Berkowitz SJ, Wei JL, Halabi S. Migrating to the modern PACS: challenges and opportunities. Radiographics. 2018;38(6):1761–72.
2. Bramson RT, Bramson RA. Overcoming obstacles to work-changing technology such as PACS and voice recognition. Am J Roentgenol. 2005;184(6):1727–30.
3. Warburton RN. Evaluation of PACS-induced organizational change. Int J Bio-Med Computing. 1992;30(3–4):243–8.
4. Behlen FM, Sayre RE, Weldy JB, Michael JS. "Permanent" records: experience with data migration in radiology information system and picture archiving and communication system replacement. J Digit Imaging. 2000;13(2 Suppl 1):171–4.

Self-Assessment Questions

1. A good reason for considering implementing a PACS or changing to a new one is:

   (a) A PACS or a new PACS will significantly reduce our expenses.
   (b) Our major equipment vendor has offered to add or change a PACS for us at a lower cost than other vendors if we purchase their PACS.
   (c) Most of the area practices have made the switch to particular PACS vendor; we want to stay with this trend.
   (d) We have requirements from radiologists and other physicians for near real-time imaging and cannot meet these requirements with film or our existing PACS.

2. Reasonable questions to ask when considering changing PACS include:

   (a) Why are we considering changing to PACS or changing our PACS?
   (b) What are the goals and expectations we have for such a change?
   (c) Do we have support for this change from the practice members and/or hospital administration?
   (d) We are merging with a larger health system; do we need to change to their PACS?
   (e) All of the above.

3. Usual assessment categories include the following *except*:

   (a) Workload
   (b) Workflow
   (c) Personnel
   (d) PACS RFP
   (e) Interfaces

4. When assessing personnel requirements and tasks, we should:

   (a) Use only the job descriptions of personnel, as they are the most specific description of what personnel do.
   (b) Interview and observe end users and ask about what they do in addition to what their job descriptions indicate they do.
   (c) Ask radiologists what job duties the technologists who work with them perform, as they will have the best assessments.
   (d) If personnel are observed taking shortcuts and using workarounds, these should be reported to supervisors and administrators so the personnel who use these should be educated in the proper procedures and tasks.
   (e) Make it known that a PACS or new PACS may result in changes in personnel schedules, job descriptions, and staff reductions so that change management is incorporated into personnel requirement assessment.

5. A list or catalog of interfaces should be created and maintained because:

   (a) Interfaces between people and equipment are more reliable than electronic ones.
   (b) The speed of interfaces is always high so operation of them is of primary importance.
   (c) The interfaces between people and equipment and equipment to equipment are key to the operation of systems.
   (d) Error handling in interfaces is always automatic, and the list or catalog of them is important in establishing maintenance requirements.
   (e) Listing or cataloging is the best way to determine the importance of interfaces.

6. True or false: Replacing an existing PACS should be to a single system that can perform the functions of existing subspecialty systems, even if some of the functions are not fully implemented in the single existing system.

   (a) True
   (b) False

7. Which of the following are you most likely to accept as a training plan from your PACS vendor:

   (a) The vendor should be willing to establish a training program based on local needs and an agreed-upon endpoint such as percentage of your employees trained, demonstrated success of trained employees to use the system, and concentrated training for tasks in which your employees make errors.
   (b) On-site personnel for training all your employees for a fixed time, which is determined by comparison with the vendor's successful training experience at facilities similar to yours.
   (c) Establishing training sessions with fixed schedules and session times based on the vendor's study of typical employee level of experience.
   (d) The vendor should establish in-person training during operating hours and host all other training times with online educational resources.
   (e) Because a "train the trainers" approach can take your personnel away from their usual duties, the vendor should offer to have their trainers on-site. The number of trainers and the length of time they will be present will be subject to contract, and any additional training required will be at a negotiated cost.

8. Considering data migration, which of the following is true:

   (a) If you have a vendor-neutral archive (VNA), you will not have to migrate data if you change PACS vendors.
   (b) Data migration has the potential to impact clinical operations.
   (c) If all the information in your existing PACS archive is stored as DICOM objects, migration would be as straightforward as copying the DICOM objects from the existing PACS to the new PACS storage system.
   (d) The standard way in which vendors store annotations and measurements means that these can be migrated easily along with the images.
   (e) It is likely you will overestimate the time it will take to migrate your data.

9. "Junk data" in your PACS storage system may be the result of:

   (a) Test images created by service personnel.
   (b) Images from research studies.
   (c) Images that were "deleted" on a workstation, but the deletion did not delete the image in storage.
   (d) Images and other information imported from CDs created at another facility.
   (e) All of the above.

10. True or false: Data migration is likely to be the most time-consuming aspect of changing PACS even if you don't have a petabyte archive and even if you already have a VNA.

    (a) True
    (b) False

Chapter 33
Procurement

Keith J. Dreyer, Tom Schultz, and Karen J. Roberts

Contents

K. J. Dreyer
Mass General Brigham, Boston, MA, USA

Informatics Massachusetts General Hospital and Brigham and Women's Hospital, Boston, MA, USA

Harvard Medical School, Boston, MA, USA

ACR Data Science Institute, Boston, MA, USA
e-mail: kdreyer@partners.org

T. Schultz
Enterprise Medical Imaging and Clinical Data Science Office, Mass General Brigham, Boston, MA, USA
e-mail: tschultz@partners.org

K. J. Roberts (✉)
Enterprise Medical Imaging, MGB Mass General Brigham, Boston, MA, USA
e-mail: kroberts3@partners.org

© The Author(s), under exclusive license to Springer Science+Business Media, LLC, part of Springer Nature 2021
B. F. Branstetter IV (ed.), *Practical Imaging Informatics*,
https://doi.org/10.1007/978-1-0716-1756-4_33

33.1 Introduction

A well-planned strategy for procurement of products and services is vital to the success of any organization. Choosing the type of PACS solution based on the institution's demands, workflows, and infrastructure requires extensive investigation and considerable analysis. Over a decade ago, imaging departments were transitioning from analog to digital workflows and had the growing pains associated with moving to a PACS platform. Due to technological advancements in the medical imaging industry, many organizations are once again looking at PACS solutions to replace their legacy PACS. Imaging stakeholders recognize that their requirements have vastly changed since their first PACS purchase.

> **DEFINITION: Procurement**
>
> The act of researching market solutions and engaging with industry vendors to evaluate and purchase products that keep your organization running optimally.

Vendor agnostic enterprise imaging (EI) platforms as well as emerging technologies in advanced visualization, image sharing solutions, and artificial intelligence (AI) offer many options. Procurement is the act of researching market solutions and engaging with industry vendors to evaluate and purchase products that keep organizations running optimally. Finding a suitable vendor that can satisfy all organizational requirements is challenging as technologies in diagnostic imaging are rapidly evolving. Formulating a smart implementation strategy can mitigate excessive costs, risk, and downtimes in the short and long term, as well as provide leverage during the contract negotiation process.

33.2 Standard Practices for Acquisition of Technology

Innovations in Radiology Information Systems (RIS), the DICOM standard, and Picture Archive and Communication Systems (PACS) have revolutionized medicine in a very short time and the momentum does not appear to be slowing down. Medical imaging stakeholders fundamentally understand that delaying a PACS replacement solution can significantly influence patient care. Keeping up with the rapid change in medical imaging technology, effectively controlling operational and capital spending, and providing quality patient care begins with a solid procurement strategy.

33.2.1 Developing an Appropriate Business Plan

- Create a PACS Procurement Committee to define the organizational needs and ensure that the procurement of a new PACS solution is in alignment with the organization's strategic plan.

- **Strategic Planning** involves the creation of objectives and goal setting for near-term and long-term periods. Strategic planning approaches include:
  - Competitive analysis
  - Environmental scanning and forecasting
  - Internal organization analysis
  - Determining long- and short-term objectives
  - Identifying strategic alternatives
  - Strategy evaluation and selection
  - Strategic control systems
- Consider the requirements of all stakeholders:
  - Radiologists
  - Technologists
  - Radiology administrators
  - Clinician specialists – surgeons, orthopedics, emergency medicine, referring providers
  - Information Technology (IT) Department
- Assess existing practice in detail and develop a **needs assessment** that includes:
  - Operational analysis (workflow)
  - Technical analysis (existing infrastructure, storage and network requirements, and HIS/RIS integrations)
- Create a business plan and perform a **cost-benefit** analysis
- Incorporate return on investment (ROI) analysis. Include estimated costs for initial and ongoing expenses versus expected cost savings.
- Factors to consider:
  - Cost of data storage
  - Potential liabilities
  - Improvements in workflows
  - Decreased workload
  - Improvements in patient care

> **CHECKLIST: Members of the PACS Procurement Committee**
>
> - Radiology Chairman
> - Chief Medical Information Officer
> - Hospital Management
> - Imaging Department Director
> - Biomedical Engineering Director
> - Imaging Informatics Professional
> - Finance Director
> - Lead technologists
> - Clinicians

> **FURTHER READING: Procurement Readiness**
>
> Oosterwijk H, Hardin N. Health imaging and informatics (CIIP) study guide. OTEch Inc.; 2009. www.otechimg.com.

> **DEFINITION: Return on Investment**
>
> Most purchases require an initial capital investment but (hopefully) reduce operational costs in the long term. ROI is a measure of how long it will take for the operational savings to make up for the initial investment.

33.2.2 Request for Information

- A Request for Information (RFI) is considered a preliminary step in the procurement process that is designed to obtain general information from potential vendors that have been identified for a pending project.
- The RFI document describes attributes necessary to be included in a Request for Proposal. These attributes can vary, but typically included:
  - Information about the company
  - Product portfolio
  - Experience in the relevant field
- Based on the results, a customer will decide whether to include the vendor in the product selection process.

> **KEY CONCEPT: Request for Information Versus Request for Proposal**
>
> **Request for Information (RFI)**: A document delivered to vendors early in the product selection process. It provides general information about the problem and invites descriptions of potential solutions.
>
> **Request for Proposal (RFP)**: A document distributed to vendors late in the product selection process, after the type of product is known, to solicit specific information about the vendor's solution. Responses are compared between vendors to select the optimal solution.

33.2.3 Request for Proposal

- A Request for Proposal (RFP) is a lengthier document submitted to vendors that indicates specific costs, offering of service, and their ability to meet the requirements of the project.
- This well-documented process is a standard practice for obtaining vendor bids, avoiding conflicts of interest, and maintaining public records for business relationships and transparency.
- The main objectives of an RFP are:
  - To provide the vendor with an overview of the organization.
  - To provide a detailed description of the specifications with the intent of including the vendor's response in the final contract.
  - To obligate the vendor to deliver per the requirements specified.
  - To solicit responses that facilitate comparison among the vendors particularly with respect to the issues identified as the selection criteria.
- Vendors respond to an RFP with a Proposal that includes:
  - Information related to the company
  - Product
  - Service offering
  - Pricing for the product of interest
  - Solution details specific to the organization

33.2.4 Technology Acquisition Components

Many organizations are bound to follow guidelines of the RFI and RFP processes for all purchases. However, if you have some flexibility in choosing vendors, the following criteria could be used to evaluate possible candidates. This does not mean that a formal RFP process still cannot be used, but there can be more value and risk mitigation in using a more creative approach. When acquiring a technology solution where the standards of functionality and performance are uncertain because it is cutting edge, the following flow chart provides guidance for each purchase and what approach to take. Narrowing the PACS purchase from among the five core approaches can provide organizations with a strategic path to success (Fig. 33.1). The five core approaches are:

1. Commodity-based purchase
2. Functionally differentiated
3. Best of Breed
4. Monolithic
5. Collaborative/Co-development

- **A1: Commodity-based purchase**
  - Often times these are generic technology services driven by hospital institutional standards.
  - Personal computers are an example of a commodity-based purchase since they are more straightforward in nature.
- **A2: Functionally Differentiated**
  - If the market is less mature, an RFP can aid decision making.
  - This should include a detailed checklist of desired functionalities from all aspects of the project (e.g., PACS system purchases from 10 years ago and upcoming Artificial Intelligence applications of today).
  - It is important to get timelines for version releases and future functionality defined while in the procurement process.
- You may need to make technical decisions that encompass multiple solutions. When the technology procurement comprises multiple solutions, you must choose between monolithic and best of breed strategies.
  - **Monolithic**: Selecting one single vendor to solve all solutions. If there is a clear vendor path that will solve all aspects of the project, a monolithic approach is best. If a single vendor has the best solution for each component of the project, you could have a single source for all issues. Monolithic purchases are ideal, but unfortunately, not always realistic.

> **HYPOTHETICAL SCENARIO: Commodity-Based Purchase**
>
> Your IT department may be standardized on a particular PC brand. Typically, the purchase is dependent on availability of product, reliability, cost, and longevity. If there is no big differentiator in functionality between vendors, then it is a commodity purchase. These are fully mature products without major unknowns.

TECHNOLOGY ACQUISITION FLOWCHART

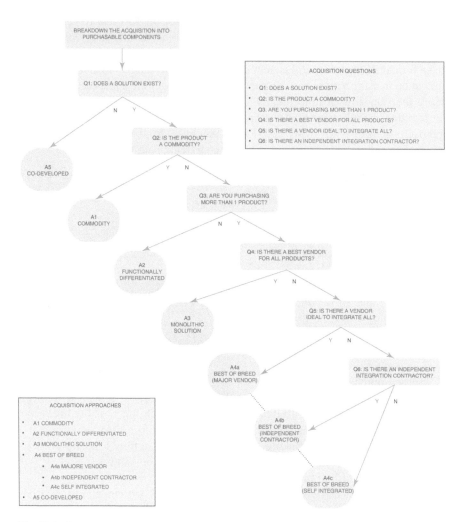

Fig. 33.1 Choosing an acquisition approach

- **Best of Breed**: Alternatively, a best of breed approach could provide you with an opportunity to select the best component for each problem. However, this strategy introduces challenges with integration and coordination of

DEFINITION: Best of Breed Strategy

A process of selecting the best products or systems that will meet your business requirements. This often requires different vendors for different components of the project.

disparate solutions working together. In that best of breed approach someone in your organization needs to be the general contractor. Most likely that is one of three choices:

Major Vendor: One of the vendors that you chose for the components acting as a coordinator for the other vendors.

Independent Contractor: An external consultant hired to coordinate and manage the project.

Your Organization: If careful consideration is toward using a major vendor or contractor, the responsibility of coordination will be up to your organization to manage.

- **A5: Collaborative/Co-development**: If no product exists to meet your needs, you may be able to develop your own. Many organizations work independently or collaborate with vendors to co-develop an in-house solution to a technology need.

33.3 Requirements

Transparency between purchaser and vendor is essential. Historically, the procurement process was held at a distance from healthcare workers. However, involvement of key players in the procurement process helps build close and collaborative relationships, fostering discussions and solutions instead of pursuing legal recourse when issues arise. Being mindful of potential conflicts of interest, the value of transparency between both sides is key to a strong relationship.

33.3.1 Vendor Management Strategies

- The goals, objectives, and expectations of the imaging department and the healthcare enterprise should be explicit:
  - Extent and time for the project
  - The expected improvements in departmental and enterprise productivity
- General information about the healthcare enterprise:
  - Single site or multiple sites across a larger healthcare enterprise
  - Number of sites
  - Types and number of specialties
  - Locations of the key departments
  - Patient populations
  - Inpatient and outpatient imaging volumes at each site
  - Number of inpatient beds at each site
  - Plans for future expansion projects
  - Business strategies of the enterprise as a whole

- Operational and workflow information about the imaging department and other departments with access to PACS.
  - Workflows
      Patient registration to exam scheduling
      Ordering and performance of studies
      Interpretation of the examination by the radiologists
      Report generation
  - Specific workflows
      For individual sites in a multisite organization
      For each imaging modality at each site
- Workload for professional staffing and exam volume information
  - Number of location of imaging sites
  - Number of imaging modalities at each site
  - Exam volume by modality at each site
  - Inpatient versus outpatient mix
  - Number and location of interpretation sites
  - Subspecialties at each site
  - Number of radiologists, including number of staff members, fellows, and residents
  - Number of examinations reported per day
  - Number of radiologists reading simultaneously
  - Division of work within the department
  - Departments such as emergency medicine and intensive care units may require high-resolution, primary grade monitors similar to those deployed at diagnostic workstations.
  - Other consumers of medical imaging such as referring physicians, radiotherapy, surgeons, orthopedists, and remote sites requiring images for their medical practices
  - Teleradiology operations
  - Volume change projections
- Carefully documenting internal clinical workflows and expected outcomes/ changes based on the acquisition of technology is paramount to ensuring that vendors understand the goals. Vendors can then effectively propose solutions that match the clinical and technical workflows of the institution.
- Choosing a vendor that best aligns with the goals of the project will help establish practices of transparency from the start.
- An important aspect of the decision-making process comes down to mutual amicability and motivation between the customer and the vendor throughout the RFP negotiation process.
  - Do the vendors possess the communication skillset the customer requires?
  - Just evaluating a vendor on cost and functionality alone can leave organizations vulnerable if their team is not up to the task.
  - Make sure the vendor can offer a committed team that works well with your internal delegates for the project.

- Relationship Management during the project is also crucial to transparency. To avoid delays and unexpected issues:
  - It is important for organizations to set expectations with the vendor for performance metrics and timelines critical to roll outs and "go live" dates.
  - In turn, the vendor should be completely transparent regarding their ability to meet those needs and provide proper staff and resources.

OUR EXPERIENCE: What We Wished the Vendor Knew/What the Vendor Wished We Knew

Procurement Team Challenges
- Gathering accurate organizational requirements for prospective vendors
- Documenting clear expectations and what success of the project means to the organization
- Providing consistent evaluation criteria that facilitate comparable elements
- Composing an RFP that provides context and asks the right questions
- Providing adequate transparency to all vendor participants
- Creating sufficient scoring guidelines
- Allowing sufficient time for vendor response
- Availability of procurement committee members in order to carefully examine vendors' proposals
- Facilitate a follow-up process
- Avoiding procurement committee member conflict of interest

Vendor Challenges
- Interpreting unclear RFP objectives
- Uncertainty of the product's intended use
- Obtaining a firm understanding of customer's expectation (avoiding assumptions)
- Transparency to organization of what the vendor can do and what it cannot do
- Tracking down answers to ambiguous questions
- Subject matter expert collaboration
- Meeting target dates when completing lengthy RFPs
- Providing quantitative and qualitative responses
- Mistakenly responding to lose-lose RFPs

- Defining Success:
  - What a successful PACS acquisition looks like from the organizational perspective should be transparent in the early stages, and well documented in detail.
  - Depending upon the type of application or system being implemented, uptime guarantees, performance metrics, daily use, and the interaction with other applications will vary in urgency and importance.
  - The vendor should fully understand the intended use of the product or service and its level of criticality in order to determine if their product is a good solution for the organization.

33.3.2 Technical and Hardware Requirements

- **Modality inventory**: List the imaging modalities including vendors with model numbers, dates of purchase, software versions, and DICOM Compliance for each modality.
- **Archiving and storage of images**:
  - Estimate and explicitly specify requirements for online cache storage capacity as well as long-term persistent storage.
  - Preferred method of imaging study storage:

    Lossy compression in online storage versus uncompressed or lossless compressed images in long-term storage.

    Specify if long-term storage will be online or will act as near line storage from which the images are prefetched.

    Presence of priors versus no priors contained within online storage.

    Specify timeframe during which images must be immediately available online.

    Requirements for backup and disaster recovery storage.

    Confirm integration requirements with preferred storage vendor (if different from the PACS vendor).

- Requirements for image retrieval and interpretation:
  - Workstation requirements:

    Number of workstations

    Diagnostic monitor requirements (resolution, singe/dual/quad configuration)
  - Software functionality—determine user interface:

    Worklists

    Queries

    Report displays

    Image displays

> **KEY CONCEPT: Supply Chain Asset Management**
>
> Supply chain asset management is the task of deciding when new purchases are needed and when equipment has passed its useful life. Asset management databases store pertinent imaging modality data and provide the essential information needed in making cost-effective decisions about procurement and decommissions. Supply chain software companies use artificial intelligence (AI) algorithms to identify and recognize modality usage patterns and provide the information needed for purchase, redundancy, and decommission planning.

> **KEY CONCEPT: PACS Functional Requirements**
>
> System functionality for the end user is a critical aspect for PACS. Therefore, this section in the RFP should be extremely detailed.

Paging

Stack mode

Hanging protocols

Prior report display

Image manipulation (e.g., window/level, zoom, pan/scroll, measurements, annotations)

– Advanced visualization imaging workflow options from the PACS vendor or the need for integration with third-party software and hardware:

MIP

MPR

Volume rendering

PET/CT fusion

Cinematic Rendering (CR)

Artificial Intelligence (AI)

Quantitative treatment planning software

Digital Breast Tomosynthesis software

> **KEY CONCEPT: RFP Construction**
>
> • Provide detailed specifications of the institution's software functionality and hardware performance requirements for both primary interpretation and clinical review.
> • Request that vendors specify whether they can provide these features and describe any available alternatives.

• Determine **web distribution** requirements:

– Allows for distribution of images for clinical review across the healthcare enterprise.

– Specification for areas with access to PACS images:

Technologists

Referring providers

Film librarians

• Integration requirements:

– Specify the integration requirements for existing systems (Electronic Medical Record (EMR), Radiology Information System (RIS), voice recognition, advanced visualization platforms, etc.).

– Request vendor specifications, prior experience, and pricing for interface builds.

• Data management requirements

– Specify the requirements for patient demographic and image data management, which is typically done with commercially available database management systems (e.g., Oracle, MS/SQL, Sybase).

– Request the specification of data management systems and provide a detailed description of any redundancy features of this system component.

Could expose a single point of failure (SPOF)

– Request a description of image reconciliation tools (moving images, merging or separating imaging studies, etc.)

- Image management requirements
  - Image importing software
  - Image sharing platforms
  - Image compression rules (what images can be compressed and what images cannot)
  - Image Lifecycle Management
  - Routing rules (sending to third-party applications or other destinations)
  - DICOM functions (query/retrieve, DICOM copy, etc.)
- Networking infrastructure
  - Description of the existing enterprise networking infrastructure.
  - Assessment of suitability of the existing infrastructure.
  - Define the minimum acceptable performance requirements for several measurable scenarios based upon various representative image sets.
    The vendor should specify the maximum time taken by the PACS to fully display various imaging study types at the radiologist workstation.
  - Demand in writing that the network is adequate for proposed system.

> **KEY CONCEPT: Breast Imaging Compression**
>
> Digital Breast Tomosynthesis and 3D breast imaging technology have high image storage demands. The FDA requires that facilities store breast imaging studies in original or lossless compressed formats.

33.3.3 Additional RFP Information

- **Timeline for Installation and Implementation Responsibilities**
  - PACS implementation typically requires a multiphase approach. The timeline for each phase should be clearly defined.
  - Outline the customer's expectations priorities and objectives within the implementation timeline
  - Request details on the implementation responsibilities and personnel:
    Time to spent at the site
    Costs associated with implementation
    Personnel minimum qualifications
- **Training requirements**
  - Request details for various user classes:
    Technologists
    Radiologists
    Referring providers

> **KEY CONCEPT: Legality of RFP**
>
> An RFP is a legal document and should be signed by appropriate representatives of the institution and the vendor. The vendors are thereby obligated to meet the requirements they have specified in the RFP even if not specified in the final contract.

Imaging Informatics Professionals

System owners

Training venue

Hours

Number of sessions

Reference materials

- **Financial terms**
  - Provide an itemized (line item) pricing form to facilitate comparison of the bids among the vendors solicited.
  - Include details on all components of the system and services offered:
    Software
    Hardware
    Technical costs
    Labor costs
    Upgrades
    System integration
    Installation
    Training
    Extended maintenance services
- Warranties:
  - Describe expected warranty coverage and duration along with upgrades included during this period.
  - Request detailed description of what the warranty includes.
  - Demand the vendor the same uptime guarantees and service response times as the support committed to in the maintenance and support section.
  - Demand that the PACS offered must remain compliant with all applicable laws and regulations, including those regulated by the Food and Drug Administration (FDA).
- Maintenance and Support
  - Request expected vendor commitments during the implementation and planning including:
    Vendor support strategy
    Staffing
    Nearest sales and service office
    Expected uptime
    Service response times for remote and onsite support
    Software release schedule
    Installation procedures for software updates
- System Security:
  - Request a description for security and authentication supported by the system and compliance with HIPAA standards and regulations.
  - Request details on backup and disaster recovery techniques.
  - Involve your security division of your IT department

OUR EXPERIENCE: Establishing DICOM Security at the Onset

If you are implementing a DICOM-based system, try to establish DICOM security requirements at the onset of the project. There are many attack vectors via DICOM that can be leveraged by hackers. Many DICOM devices are not very secure and are susceptible to impersonation, insecure communication, and in some cases cannot easily prevent unauthorized access. We strongly urge you to consult with potential vendors early in the process to understand their strategies in combatting security vulnerabilities.

33.3.4 Defining Expected Performance and Product Stability

Measuring performance and reliability of the products used at your organization is crucial to assuring system stability. The most import aspect in guaranteeing uptimes is approaching a product decision with known uptime requirements and **Uptime Guarantees**. It can be possible to increase your degree of certainty in their reliability by addressing the following criteria in the RFP:

* Reviewing the Service Level Agreements (SLAs) or building guarantees and remedies into the vendor contract.

KEY CONCEPTS: Business Continuity Versus Disaster Recovery

   Business Continuity (BC): The ability to maintain essential business functions during routine system disruptions.
   Disaster Recovery (DR): Processes and systems that put into production to prepare for adverse events associated with catastrophic system failures such as natural disasters (fires, floods, earthquakes) or human-made disasters (ransomware attacks).

* Clarification on what the vendor is promising and determining that the vendor meets organizational expectations.
* Scheduled downtimes/maintenance.
* Hardware, Services, Applications—establish an approach for each area.
* Determine how application responsiveness will be continuously measured.
* Architecting a solution early in the vendor selection process to address the above will define the capabilities as well as expose shortcomings of a given product and the vendor's technical team.
  - Try to design a solution that enables multiple independent instances of the system to be implemented.

- Work with the vendor to enable an Active-Active design where both instances are clinically operational. Advantages of an Active-Active design include:
  - Multi Datacenter instances
  - If only one location is available, then consider two independent environments within the single site.
  - Cloud Implementation.
  - Provides significant geographic redundancy.
  - One instance can be on-site and one can be maintained by a cloud provider.
- Accepting a solution that provides passive standby components rarely work due to the inactive nature of the passive system.
  - During normal operations, passive systems are not in service and it is not until the primary system fails when you will learn if the passive system is truly operational and properly configured/maintained.
  - To test the passive system it will require a scheduled downtime of the primary system. Often there is more downtime due to passive system testing then there are real issues.

FURTHER READING: RFP

Oosterwijk H. All you need to know about a PACS RFP, you learned in kindergarten. Radiol Manage. 1998;20(5):39–43.

Orenstein BW. On the right path – preparing an RFP for a successful PACS purchase. Radiol Today. 1998;6(13):14.

Schweitzer AL, Smith G. Creating the PACS request for proposal and selecting the PACs vendor. In: Dreyer KJ, Hirschorn DS, Thrall JH, Mehta A, editors. PACS: a guide to the digital revolution. 2nd ed. New York: Springer-Verlag; 2002.

Williams J, Riggs A. Mastering the PACS RFP. Radiol Manage. 2005;27(4):46–8, 50.

33.4 RFP Review

33.4.1 Review Responses to RFP

Written responses can help the buyer compare the merits of each system and make the appropriate selections of the solutions most suitable for their facility. The PACS procurement committee should set aside ample time to review each of the RFP responses. Using a predefined scoring system, where each of the RFP elements can be ranked according to the degree of actionable components.

STEP-BY-STEP: Reviewing Responses to the RFP

1. The PACS procurement committee should short list the vendors to a manageable number (about 4–6 vendors); selecting those who appear to be most suitable for their requirements.
2. The RFP should be sent out to these vendors giving them a firm response date (generally less than 8 weeks to respond).
3. The responses to the RFP should be summarized and tabulated for evaluation. All discrepancies or ambiguities should be clarified with the vendor.
4. For evaluation of the responses, each criterion being judged should be first weighted by importance using consensus of the PACS procurement committee.
5. Each vendor should be scored for each criterion and these scores weighted based on the importance of the category being analyzed.
6. The scoring should be based on the responses to the RFP as well as prior knowledge of the vendors.
7. The totals of the weighted scores should then be calculated for each vendor.
8. Based on the evaluation, the vendors should be narrowed down to 2–3 preferred and alternative vendors for manageable contract negotiations.

33.4.2 Site Visits

- The PACS procurement committee should schedule one or more site visits at locations where the PACS under consideration is already in use.
- Schedule site visits close to each other in time to ensure better comparison.
- The buyer does not necessarily have to go to the sites chosen by the vendor. Buyers can choose to visit other sites with the system version that their institution is intending to purchase, and who emulate similar workflows, business requirements, and IT infrastructure (e.g., EMR, RIS, voice recognition).
- The review team should attend the site visits in order to identify technical and operational issues. The review team could include:
  - Radiologists
  - Technologists
  - Imaging Informatics Professionals
  - IT staff
  - radiology administrators
  - Clinicians

KEY CONCEPT: Site Visits

Visits to other healthcare institutions that are already using the product permit feedback from experienced users. By observing the system in action, a comprehensive site visit can help the team discover and anticipate many potential issues that may undermine a successful implementation.

FURTHER READING: Site Visits

Archer LH, Pliner N. PACS site visits: when where, who, and how. Radiol Manage. 2006;28(5):48–53.

CHECKLIST: Site Visit Sample Questions

- Radiologists should evaluate the workstation and observe different users to assess the time taken and the steps involved for actions such as:
  - Opening a new imaging study
  - Viewing images
  - Manipulating images, annotating, saving
  - Accessing prior reports and images
  - Retrieving prior exams for comparison
- Technologists should evaluate the networking and steps involved in sending completed studies to PACS.
- Imaging Informatics Professionals (IIPs) should ask for a demonstration of a merge, name change, and other elements associated with data management.
- Administration should assess workflow impact of PACS.

- For an enterprise-level PACS, the clinicians' opinion is important. However, since site visit teams are limited (6–8 people), only the key players should be included in the site visits. Often a Chief Medical Information Officer (CMIO) will represent the clinician perspective in the absence of local expertise amongst the clinicians.
- Site visit planning includes:
  - A specific site agenda
  - A list of questions and evaluation criteria should be provided to the target site prior to site visit. This practice optimizes the time spent during the site visit.
  - The individual members of the review team should focus on their own area of expertise and schedule time to talk to their peers during the site visit.
  - The team should engage the key stakeholders at the site without the vendor being present.

33.4.3 Proof of Concept (POC)

- Before commencing to the overall contract review process, it is strongly suggested to perform a POC (Proof of Concept) that "tests" the system against expectations.
- Even if the vendor requires some funding for resources, this is the only opportunity to vet the system and reject the product before being shackled to a bad deal that cannot be undone.
- If the provider pushes back, move on to your next best choice.

DEFINITION: Proof of Concept

A small-scale test environment that runs proposed software solutions inside your hospital system. Enables the buyer to see how the system integrates with existing solutions and test functionality before a purchase is finalized.

- Factor in additional non-expiring professional service (PS) hours beyond implementation that can be applied to any vendor resource.
- This up-front negotiation will give you leverage for possible reduced rate hours or additional hours at no charge.
- A POC will enable project owners to address items missed during the original scoping or add additional scope to the project without having to secure new/additional funding.
- A POC enables both parties to address items in a timely fashion without bureaucratic delays.

33.4.4 Deconstructed PACS

Deconstructed or Best of Breed can deliver awesome capabilities to the clinical users but can also create significant integration issues. There are bound to be issues when there are two or more systems that depend on the information from one or more systems in order for its data/state to be clinically accurate.

OUR EXPERIENCE: Best of Breed "Beware"

Spend significant effort capturing all workflow events and working with the selected vendors to ensure detailed requirements for functionality and integration are documented before commencing a deal.

- Standards only go so far.
- There are many workflow conditions that are not properly captured leading to inconsistence between systems that interact for clinical state.

33.5 Contracts

An important part of procuring products for your institution is risk mitigation. There is no greater opportunity to protect your purchases then with standard practices for Vendor Contract negotiations that cover three main areas: business, technical, and legal terms.

33.5.1 Business Terms

- Have a designated **Contract Manager** take the lead internally on vendor contract negotiations and review.
  - Having a designated point person to coordinate discussions reduces project delays.
  - This delegate should have full knowledge of the organization's standard business terms to ensure the organization is properly represented in the contract.

- Some aspects to consider with each contract:
  - Nonnegotiable terms, such as payment terms, tax exempt status, and other business-related standards enforced by your organization.
  - A full understanding of the corporate expectations for submitting invoices, getting vendors set up in the organization's active directory, contacts for accounts payable, etc.
  - Contract term—most vendors have a specific term built into their SLA and maintenance agreements.
    - Committing to a 3-year term initially, and each year after the contract renews.
    - Negotiate the actual start and end date of the contract.
    - Define automatic renewals.
    - Establish product and environment testing requirements before the actual start date.
- **Payment milestones** mitigate risk of recovering funds if goals are not being met. Payment milestones should be coordinated with the technical team to keep the vendor on the hook for:
  - Completing the implementation in stages
  - Proper testing
  - Providing financial incentives for meeting goals
- A contract manager can tie a proof of concept stage to the contract process, working with the technical team to establish a baseline test before going too far down the contract process.

> **OUR EXPERIENCE: Sometimes There Is No Guarantee**
>
> Building safeguards into contracts and SLA's is definitely the recommended approach. Establishing a remedy for falling outside the promised guarantees with applied penalties or credits should be negotiated and included in the contract language. However, in our 25 years of experience we have never once received a payment or credit back from a vendor. The best you can do is follow protocol to mitigate risk and put your organization in the best possible position, but ultimately there are no guarantees the penalties will stick.

33.5.2 Technical Terms

- There should be a point person or technical team in place to answer any contract questions relating to the technical aspects of the project.
- These team members should read the actual contract to understand the terms of the contract.
- The following areas of the contract should comport with the organization's expectations:
  - Hardware requirements.
  - Determine if the software needs to communicate with any other products already in place.

- Determine how the license fee is calculated.
- Stages of implementation with proper testing milestones (this will relate to the payment milestones mentioned above).
- Maintenance requirements:
  Determine if the organization needs additional maintenance outside of what the contract stipulates.
  Decide if an annual auto renew option is beneficial.
  Requirements for scheduled maintenance downtimes.

33.5.3 Legal Terms

Internal discussions with your legal department at the onset of the contract negotiations will lead to a more effective and advantageous negotiations with the vendor. Simply sending a vendor contract to your legal department asking them to review the terms can cause a series of issues and delays. Advantages of including a **designated attorney** include:

- Your organization will be protected legally.
- All relevant concerns can be addressed.
- Internal discussions of the issues will lead to more effective and advantageous negotiations with the vendor.
- When sending your legal department a vendor contract that has been reviewed and red-lined with proposed business and technical edits ahead of time, your legal counsel will become an integral team member involved in any purchase to be sure you are protected.
- Every boilerplate vendor contract has legal terms that should be familiar to your attorney and can be negotiated to properly protect your organization.
- You will have the most leverage with contract terms if you have your attorney take the lead on negotiation discussions with the vendor.
- Relevant members of the technical team, as well as your contract manager, should be present during negotiations.
- It can take several rounds of negotiations to get a sound contract that meets the needs of the organization.

33.5.4 Negotiating the Contract

- To obtain the best possible contract terms, it is generally helpful to simultaneously negotiate with two or more vendors regarding:
  - Price
  - System options

- Hardware
- Software upgrades
- Software licensing
- Service contracts

33.5.5 Payment Terms and Budgeting

- Cost negotiations should be discussed internally and ahead of time.
  - Determine how fees are calculated.
  - Review the options and determine which will work best for the organization.
- Be mindful of price caps as it may weaken the incentive for lower prices.
  - Many vendors will offer a great up-front price, but if a cap on fees is not nego-tiated for the years to follow, your budget may take an unexpected hit.
- Include associated costs such as:
  - Implementation
  - Maintenance
  - Software licenses
  - Interface customization fees
  - Other factors such as loss of time and productivity during implementation
- Consider several options such as traditional capital purchase, lease applica-tion service providers, where pricing is typically based on the annual exam volume.
- The decision between the different options usually depends on the financial resources at the given institution.
- At the time of negotiation, it is important to factor in:
  - Initial costs
  - Maintenance:
      Maintenance costs
      Version changing costs
      Replacement costs
  - Operational costs:
      Cost per exam (user must carefully define an exam to offset any confusion and surcharges)
      Costs with fluctuation of exams per year
      Fluctuations with training of staff due to changes in the version of software or hardware.

KEY CONCEPT: Payment Options

1. Traditional capital purchase: needs substantial up-front capital investment, which may negatively impact cash flow. Ownership of equipment bears the risk of technological obsolescence but allows complete ownership and flexibility.
2. Capital or operational lease: needs less initial investments on software or hardware and has steady predictable costs.
3. Software only option: needs less initial costs as the vendor markup on hardware may be more expensive when compared to other sources. However, institution needs to have the expertise and resources to buy, support, and maintain the hardware.
4. Combined options like capital purchase of equipment with leasing the software.

PEARLS

- Assemble a PACS procurement committee.
- Develop a strategic business plan.
- Determine software, hardware, and workflow requirements.
- A Request for Information is a preliminary step in the procurement process.
- A Request for Proposal (RFP) is a document with explicit objectives, and goals. General information about the enterprise and departments utilizing PACS, and a detailed list of requirements and specifications.
- Review the responses to the RFP by weighing each category and *scoring* the responses to narrow the field to two or three preferred and alternative vendors.
- Transparency is mutually beneficial to both the customer and the vendor.
- Perform comprehensive site visits.
- Negotiate service contracts, payment terms, and budgeting.

Self-Assessment Questions

1. What is the first step when selecting a vendor?

    (a) Developing a strategic business plan
    (b) Writing an RFP
    (c) Negotiating the contract
    (d) Site visits
    (e) Deciding payment options

2. When sending out the RFPs, how many vendors should be selected by the imaging informatics team?

    (a) 1–3
    (b) 2–4
    (c) 4–6
    (d) 8–10
    (e) 10–15

3. Which is the correct order of operations?

    (a) RFP, RFI, site visits
    (b) Site visits, RFI, RFP
    (c) RFI, site visits, RFP
    (d) RFI, RFP, site visits
    (e) RFP, site visits, RFI

4. For an enterprise-level PACS, generally clinicians are a part of the site visit team:

    (a) Always true—clinicians must always attend
    (b) True to a certain extent—experts in different divisions may attend within group site constraints
    (c) False—consultants replace the clinicians in all visits as the number of people visiting sites is limited
    (d) Vendor decides if clinicians must attend

5. What is *not* true about site visits?

    (a) Location should be decided by the vendor.
    (b) The review team can include radiologists and clinicians.
    (c) One or more site visits should be made.
    (d) Different visits should be close to each other.
    (e) A specific site visit agenda should be established.

6. What is the correct order for the following steps?
    1. The responses to the RFP should be summarized and tabulated for evaluation.
    2. The RFP should be sent out to the vendors giving them a firm response date.
    3. Each vendor should be scored for each criterion and these scores weighted based on the importance of the category being analyzed.
    4. The PACS selection team should short list 4–6 vendors selecting those who appear to be most suitable for their requirements.
    (a) 4,2,1,3
    (b) 1,2,3,4
    (c) 2,1,3,4
    (d) 2,4,1,3
    (e) 2,3,1,4

7. How much time should be given to the vendors to respond to the RFP?

    (a) Less than 16 weeks

    (b) Less than 8 weeks

    (c) Less than 2 weeks

    (d) They can take as much time, as long as they address all the questions in the RFP.

    (e) Less than 4 weeks

Chapter 34
Imaging Program Management

Kevin W. McEnery

Contents

34.1 Introduction

While implementations of PACS have revolutionized the healthcare delivery, imaging project portfolios now extend well beyond PACS. The scope of imaging program management includes image storage architectures, post-processing

K. W. McEnery (✉)
UT M.D. Anderson Cancer Center, Houston, TX, USA

© The Author(s), under exclusive license to Springer Science+Business Media, LLC, part of Springer Nature 2021
B. F. Branstetter IV (ed.), *Practical Imaging Informatics*,
https://doi.org/10.1007/978-1-0716-1756-4_34

applications, clinical decision support, and, more recently, the implementation of artificial intelligence and machine learning-based applications. Regardless of the application under consideration for installation, a consistent method for project management is essential for successful imaging program management.

34.2 Imaging Program Oversight

The oversight of the imaging informatics portfolio involves ensuring ongoing successful operations of existing systems along with managing their implementations and upgrades. One essential responsibility is maintenance of the current imaging infrastructure for day-to-day reliability. However, a necessary component of reliability is to maintain a program of perpetual software version upgrades as well as the implementation of an entirely new imaging software and hardware infrastructure when needed. Maintaining uptime during system upgrades and large-scale rollouts is particularly challenging.

CHECKLIST: Imaging Program Committee Members

Radiology Representation
- Chief Radiologist – Department Chair. This person presumably has the authority oversight for many aspects of the clinical practice.
- Radiology department manager/administrator.
- Radiology operations manager.
- Radiology information system manager.
- Chief technologist(s) – the number of technologists necessary on the committee will vary depending upon the size of the practice and the organization structure.
- Chief of service for group responsible for imaging equipment – in some practices this will be imaging physics or biomedical system engineers.
- Radiologists – modality or subspecialty section leaders.
- Radiologist champion – this person will be expected to assist in encouraging and coordinating radiologist participation – may be one of the above radiologists.
- Radiology nursing representative (or institutional nursing).
- Imaging informatics professional (PACS administrator) – when organization already has PACS installed and project needs an upgrade from existing system.
- Contracts and purchasing officer (local or from institution).
- Project manager (PM).

Institutional Representation
- Information system representative (CIO or a direct report)
- Electronic medical record and/or health information management (HIM) department representative

34.2.1 Imaging Program Committee Membership

A core leadership group is usually instantiated as a committee focused on the maintenance of the existing imaging systems as well as strategic and tactical planning for future implementations and installations. Imaging informatics project committee representations include key stakeholders; some within the imaging department and others from the healthcare enterprise. Over time, this operations workgroup should function at a high level of efficiency, continually resolving problems and updating open issues.

34.2.2 Strategy and Tactics

The imaging informatics committee creates strategies aimed at improving organizational, departmental, patient, and provider satisfaction:

- Strategic plans are developed in 3–5-year cycles. It is essential for informatics to be involved in the development of these plans.
- Tactics represent selected projects and initiate proposed actions to address the outcomes identified in the strategic plan.
- Strategic and tactical examples:
  - Strategy: Improve the value of radiology reporting.
  - Tactics: Implement structured reporting templates.
  - Tactics: Implement common data elements in reporting for improved data mining.
- Imaging informatics projects can serve as cornerstones to the strategic plan or in support of other mission areas such as clinical care, research, and education.
- Strategic plan development:
  - A key component of strategic and tactical planning is having the knowledge of current and emerging technologies that will be available during the period of the proposal.

> **DEFINITION: Strategic Plan**
>
> General plan of action to achieve an overarching goal or outcome in a specific time period (usually 3–5 years).

> **DEFINITION: Tactical Plan**
>
> Specific projects and process improvements designed to meet the goals of a strategic plan.

> **OUR EXPERIENCE: Strategic Planning**
>
> Diagnostic imaging strategic planning occurs in parallel with institutional strategic planning in 5-year cycles. Following establishment of the institution's major strategic focus areas, the imaging strategic plan aligns to the institution's plan with imaging strategy and tactics proposed to support the major focus strategies.

- A "best of breed" strategy entails selecting different systems or parts from different vendors. It may be a good option for organizations but total cost of ownership may exceed single vendor option.

> **DEFINITION: Best of Breed Strategy**
>
> A process of selecting the best products or systems that will meet your business requirements. This often requires different vendors for different components of the project.

- Communication with imaging vendors regarding product upgrade plans or features of upcoming releases can also assist with creation of forward-looking tactics.
- Alignment of proposed potential projects with the organization's (or imaging department's) strategic plan enables a greater probability of funding for large investment projects.

34.2.3 Imaging Operations Workgroup

While imaging informatics committees can establish the "big picture," many imaging informatics professionals find it useful to form a specific team of individuals to oversee a given project. The size and diversity of roles in the project group must align with the goals and outcomes of the project under consideration. The purpose of this workgroup is to discuss and collaborate on resolutions to issues (even unexpected ones), which the project plan requires.

CHECKLIST: Imaging Operations Workgroup Members

- Imaging program administrator
- Imaging program support personnel
- Project manager(s)
- Electronic medical record (EMR) team
- Radiological information system (RIS) leadership
- Imaging physics representatives
- Vendor representative
- Desktop IT support
- Network administrators

- The workgroup membership should include membership from those groups who are actively participating in the project implementation.
- Meeting agenda should continually track open issues and their resolution:
  - The meeting minutes can be saved on a shared hard drive for reference during the week by team members.

34.3 Identify Goal, Scope, and Risks

34.3.1 Imaging Project Goals

- An initial focus of the project committee must be to create a **project charter**, which defines the overriding goals for the entire project. Although each constituent group will bring their own perspective on how the project will affect their area, it is important to keep the focus on the project goals. The success of the project depends on the alignment of individual goals.
- A good place to start when initiating alignment is in the context of the institution's **mission statement**, and then polling individual stakeholders to obtain perspective of how the proposed imaging project would allow them to achieve their mission specific goals:
  - End-user surveys are a valuable tool to validate or guide the project committee in regard to assumptions and priorities.
- Alignment of imaging projects with the imaging department's goals as well as **institution mission and goals** provides a higher level of visibility for the project in prioritization for funding and access to necessary implementation resources such as educational opportunities for stakeholders both inside and outside of the imaging department.
- Project goals serve to provide clear statements of purpose required by a project committee to meet the proposed outcome.

34.3.2 Imaging Project Scope

- A project scope statement is the description of the project, major deliverables, assumptions, and constraints.
- Once the project goals are established, **specific project deliverables** must be defined, which enable the objectives of the project goals. Specific project deliverables directly affect the project plan and resource allocation.
- The project **statement of work** (SOW) should explicitly define which areas of diagnostic imaging operations are included and which areas are excluded from the project.
- A **change management process** should be agreed upon by the committee in advance to deal with those instances where the PACS project chose not to address a specific area or a new area of work presents itself. A formal change management process allows the appropriate allocation of existing resources or the request for additional resources.

> **DEFINITION: Statement of Work**
>
> Defines fulfillment of contractual requirements for scope of work, location, period of contract, schedule for project deliverables, and acceptance criteria for work performed.

- Controlling the project scope is managed through a **change control** process. The uncontrolled expansion of the project is "scope creep," which includes:
  - Trading one functionality for alternative functionality
  - Adding functionality that can be accomplished within the contingency

DEFINITION: Scope Creep

Incremental changes to the project, or the addition of features that were not identified in the original project charter. Scope creep delays the timetable and can prevent a project from ever being completed.

  - Adding a subsequent phase for addressing the needs of other facilities
  - Adopting a new information model that better meets the plan
- The scope should also define whether the proposed project represents the installation of an existing application or represents the development of a new application.

34.3.3 Project Milestones

- The project plan defines a series of steps that must be accomplished for project success.
- Expected delivery dates for project components assist in defining those steps.
- Milestones are selected from the tasks defined in the project plan.

DEFINITION: Project Milestones

Key events and deliverables in the project timeline. Milestones are attached to specific tasks' start and end dates.

- Milestones should include critical path completion steps.
- Milestones assist the project team in the coordination of resources
- Project deployment or go live typically occurs late in the project life cycle. The go-live phase is the timeframe between project completion and handover.
- Delay in completing critical path milestones will most likely delay the completion of the project

OUR EXPERIENCE: Team Building

Ongoing collaborations on short-term operational projects with colleagues both within the imaging department and across the enterprise enable effective collaboration in the allocation and coordination of organizational informatics resources.

34.3.4 Project Team Membership

- Membership of the project team reflects the resources that need to be coordinated.
- Projects which impact the enterprise beyond diagnostic imaging will require alignment of institutional resources.
- Leveraging resources both within and outside of the imaging department is especially important in large-scale projects such as PACS deployments, system upgrades, as well as pre- and post-integration implementation and support into the electronic medical record.
- The resources of the responsible development groups should be involved at the outset of the project of responsibilities and milestone timelines.

34.3.5 Common Risks for Imaging Informatics Projects

Imaging informatics projects are subject to failure for the same reasons other IT projects fail. First-generation PACS projects were subject to a high degree of risk because of the diversity of stakeholders involved by the process. Today, these are less risky because PACS projects are no longer novel. There are many instances of proven successful PACS implementations in a variety of medical practice settings. Although PACS projects are no longer new and uncertain, there are still reasons why imaging informatics projects could fail:

- Project leadership committee member represents their own personal interests and opinions and not those of the group they were selected to represent.
- Inadequate communication from informatics project leadership to end users subsequently leading to disengagement in the project.
- Lack of training opportunities or training in a test environment, which did not simulate the **local work environment**.
- A generic system workflow in the test environment that vastly differs from the existing workflow with no expectation or plan to change workflows.
- Failure to understand the **culture of the institution** with regard to IT-enabled change. Generally, there will be resistance to change, especially in organizations that have difficulty in adoption with other electronic clinical systems (EMR, order entry, electronic results review, etc.). (See **Chap. 26**.)
- An aggressive deployment schedule with no accommodation for unexpected events.
- Failure to provide a **small-scale pilot project** to validate project assumptions. This is especially important in the adoption of internally developed systems, which have not otherwise been tested or deployed at other sites.
- Lack of a **back-out plan** in the event that system "go live" demonstrates unexpected critical project defects.
- Implementing two unproven IT systems on the same "go-live" event – for example, implementing voice recognition software along with PACS.

- Lack of detail in project plan with minimal detail in the contract's statement of work.
- Unrealistic deadlines, which subsequently lead to project delays and cost overruns for non-budgeted system change requests.
- Failure to provide necessary network infrastructure or anticipate the requirements of the new system's interface to the institution's existing interface engine or within the electronic medical record.

DEFINITION: Back-Out Plan

Steps needed to return the system to the state prior to the upgrade or deployment. It gets triggered if there are unforeseen consequences to other hospital systems. Also it is referred to as "roll-back" plan.

34.3.6 Risk Mitigation Strategies

- Clearly define the communication and training strategy in the project plan.
- Prospective vendors should provide examples of successful project implementation plans in similar size institutions.
- **Limited system deployment** with parallel workflows.
- When transition to a new PACS vendor, continue to utilize existing PACS during pilot in parallel with new system.
- When transitioning to a new vendor-neutral archive (VNA), maintain the availability of the existing archive solution until transition is successfully completed.
- Vendor should submit a detailed **environmental survey** that outlines all anticipated integration interfaces and integration responsibilities.
- Acceptance of detailed project plan should be part of the contract negotiation with selected vendor including specific remediation steps agreed upon prior to implementation.

34.4 Evaluation of Project Feasibility

In the early days of PACS, opposing viewpoints of whether images could be efficiently and effectively digitally captured, interpreted, and distributed were often open to debate. The perseverance of early adopters has matured into readily available vendor systems that are fully capable of meeting the promise of comprehensive digital medical imaging systems. Forecasting project costs and viability for first-generation imaging systems was undoubtedly met with a certain amount of trepidation. However, using feasibility analysis benefits these types of projects by affirming why the project should move forward or exposing the potential unforeseen costs or risks that could derail the project. The evaluation of a project's feasibility considers various aspects such as infrastructure, technical, and financial resources.

34.4.1 Local Environment Assessment

- Available resources for project management should be identified:
  - Existing infrastructure needs to be fully assessed.
  - Identify those projects that will facilitate the replacement of or upgrade to existing applications vs. projects, which bring net new functionality to an organization.
  - Determine the infrastructure needed to support the project and assess adequacy of existing infrastructure.

34.4.2 Physical Plant Assessment

- Imaging IT project planning must account for infrastructure requirements, which must be available for the success of the project.
- While organizations will likely have an existing IT infrastructure for **current** operations, the impact of the proposed project on the IT infrastructure once deployed must be taken into consideration (e.g., resource allocation).
- Assessment consideration:
  - **Storage availability** – does the project increase imaging storage requirements?
  - **Network availability** – impact of application on capacity.
  - **Security infrastructure** – does the project require changes or updates?
  - **Server room infrastructure** – what are the physical space and power requirements of the proposed project?
  - **Image workstation** – do the existing installed base of imaging workstations have the local memory and storage needed for the proposed application **and** existing applications?
  - **Image display** – are updates needed to existing diagnostic monitors (e.g., new video cards)?
  - **Remote access** – vendor requirements to support remote application server access.

34.4.3 Financial Feasibility

- Regardless of size, organizations have a defined process for capital project approval for which larger IT projects must navigate. Imaging informatics professionals must learn the project funding guidelines specific to their institution.
- Project spending thresholds are likely already in place to help determine what level of organizational approval is needed for the proposed imaging project. In turn, the imaging project committee must understand this approval process and determine the likelihood of successful funding. Imaging project plans and fund-

ing requests must be submitted into the applicable approval framework to enable the highest likelihood of project approval.

- Project timelines must include estimation of approved for funding timelines, as delays in funding will almost certainly delay project completion.
- From the outset, involvement of appropriate stakeholders from outside of diagnostic imaging will provide the appropriate context that an imaging project such as a PACS not only benefit the diagnostic imaging department but the efficiency and effectiveness of the entire institution.
- Implementation of traditional PACS typically entails a large capital investment to purchase necessary workstations and storage modalities.
- There are **alternative PACS funding models** available today including both traditional capital purchase systems and operational cost models where a fee is paid for the storage of individual examinations. It is also possible to purchase PACS software from one vendor and the storage archive from another vendor.

> **KEY CONCEPT: Operating Expenses vs. Capital Expenses**
>
> **Operating expenses (OPEX)** are funds allocated for the day-to-day functioning of running a business.
>
> **Capital expenses (CAPEX)** are funds allocated for future benefits, projects, or investments that are expected to add long-term value to the business.

- The project committee must fully understand the procedure volume, average study size, and **anticipated procedure volume growth** to provide an accurate model of overall system cost. Many institutions also require return on investment calculation, which compares the proposed system implementation cost to the benefits received in either tangible terms (e.g., improved productivity, increases in procedure volumes) or intangible terms (e.g., patient satisfaction).
- Imaging project implementations must also include accounting for costs to the organization outside of the imaging department.

34.4.4 Project Prioritization

Standardization of project prioritization is essential for management of the overall project portfolio. Objective assessment tools such as **benefits vs. complexity decision matrix** can assist in project prioritization:

- Project complexity is not specific to the application being installed but rather the environment in which the application is intended to be installed.
- Project implementation experience at "early adopter" sites can provide insight into relative weight of complexity scoring for other organizations.
- Projects scored in the "high benefit/low complexity" quadrant are preferred (Fig. 34.1)
- Projects in the "low benefit/high complexity" quadrant in general should be avoided.

Fig. 34.1 Benefit vs. complexity decision matrix

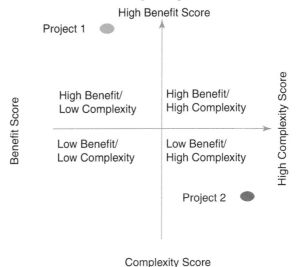

Benefit vs. Complexity Decision Matrix

CHECKLIST: Benefits vs. complexity matrix calculations

Example benefit score components	Example complexity components
Strategic alignment	Resource impact – project and operationally
Patient safety	IT resource coordination
Patient experience	Anticipated design needs/internal knowledge
Improved productivity	Organizational complexity
Regulatory/compliance	Vendor requirements
Finance	Scope clarity
Operational continuity	Number and complexity of integrations/interfaces
	Anticipated end-user training support
	Application customization needed
	Analytical reporting impacts
	Operational deadline

34.4.5 Project Management Methodology

Informatics project management varies across organizations. The medical imaging IT team (MIIT) must determine the organization's existing processes that are involved in project approval.

CHECKLIST: Imaging IT Project Responsibilities

- Set clinical and operational goals for the project.
- Establish project scope and ensure project remains within the scope.
- Allocate necessary resources to implement project plan.
- Ensure that all roles and responsibilities are defined in the project plan.
- Develop and approve a detailed project plan.
- Provide project oversight.
- Serve as a communication resource for all the constituent groups represented on the committee.
- Schedule regular meetings to review project milestones. At a minimum, monthly during project implementation, consider biweekly during initiation and vendor selection phases.

34.5 Common Project Management Tools

- The principles of project management can be applied to any project requiring the coordination of numerous resources over an extended period.

  > **DEFINITION: Project Management**
  >
  > The discipline of planning, organizing, and managing resources to provide optimal project outcome

- A project management framework also allows all those involved in project execution to make specific decisions regarding the project scope, quality, time, and budget.
- These **project constraints** provide the context for which the imaging project will be judged as well as empower rational decision-making regarding project timelines and project budget:
  - For example, reducing the scope of a project will usually shorten timelines and decrease the project budget.
- Allowing the scope of a project to widen without appropriate oversight during its execution will invariably lead to missed project deadlines, delayed project milestones, and budget overruns.

In most institutions, the project management framework is well established, and one needs to be aware of the project management framework utilized in a given institution. The framework usually follows a traditional project management process designed to provide a consistent process for all project management within an institution.

STEP-BY-STEP: Traditional project management process

1. Initiation	Identification of the business needs
2. Assessment	Involvement of stakeholders to define project charter and scope as well as risks
3. Planning	Create detailed project plan including communication and training strategy. Also includes vendor selection
4. Execution	Project implementation as well as change management process
5. Monitoring	Observation and verification of project deliverables to ensure project completed on time, within scope and on budget
6. Completion	Performance reports, benefits analysis, and lessons learned

34.5.1 Project Development Stages

Regardless of the methodology used, the project development processes share similar stages. At some institutions, these phases are combined, and at other institutions, the phases are divided into subphases. A typical project management life cycle consists of four major phases.

1. **Initiation phase**
   - **Define** the project objectives, scope, purpose, and deliverables.
   - **Business needs** that project is targeting are identified.
   - **Feasibility** study is conducted with expected financial return on investment (ROI).
   - **Project sponsor and stakeholders** are identified and participate in group oversight.

   > **DEFINITION: Project Sponsor**
   >
   > The fiscal or administrative entity that has overarching responsibility for the project.

   - **Project charter** is a document that formally authorizes approval and existence of a project and includes:
     - Project objectives
     - Project scope
     - Stakeholders
     - Project constraints
   - **Project team** is created.
2. **Assessment**
   - Review existing workflow operations.
   - Determine existing IT environment including necessary IT system and imaging modality interfaces.
   - Determine end-user requirements:
     - (i)   Radiologists
     - (ii) Technologists
     - (iii) Nurses

    (iv) Management

    (v) Customers (e.g., referring providers)

- Develop **project specification documentation**:
  - Final project documentation, including budget, tasks, deliverables, and anticipated project schedule
- In this phase it is very important for the committee to understand those requirements that are unique to their institution and to establish these as internal "discriminator criteria." These criteria should also have higher weight during vendor selection scoring.

3. **Planning phase**
   - **Procurement** planning; vendor selection process
   - **Vendor site visits**
   - **Request for information (RFI)** delivered to prospective vendors. The responses from prospective vendors explore how they might resolve the business needs. Attributes that prospective vendors may include in the RFI:
     - Information about the company
     - Product portfolio
     - Experience in the industry
   - **Request for proposal review (RFP)** usually follows the RFI. The RFP is a type of procurement document distributed to prospective vendors which requests information related to the vendor's capabilities.
   - **Contract negotiations** of selected vendor:
     - Must include development and approval of a project plan
   - **Budget planning** specifies the budgeted costs that will be incurred upon the completion of the project.
   - **Project plan** is created outlining:
     - Schedule
     - Activities
     - Tasks
     - Dependencies
     - Milestones
     - Timeframes
   - **Change management** process specification.
   - **Scope management**: identify the resources and strategies.
   - **Acceptance criteria** for system or application.

> **DEFINITION: Request for Information**
>
> A document delivered to vendors early in the product selection process. It provides general information about the problem and invites descriptions of potential solutions.

> **DEFINITION: Request for Proposal**
>
> A document distributed to vendors late in the product selection process, after the type of product is known, to solicit specific information about the vendor's solution. Responses are compared between vendors to select the optimal solution.

- **System performance criteria** as well as agreed-upon definitions for system downtime and remedies.
- **Communication plan** for application deployment:
  - Enterprise-wide deployments should leverage existing communication channels.
- **Application training** requirements for end users.

4. **Implementation (execution) phase**
   - **Implementation** of system based upon project plan
   - **Coordination** of vendor and customer resources
   - **Oversight** from imaging informatics committee implementation
   - **Decision** to have system activated (go live)

> **OUR EXPERIENCE: Project Stages**
>
> At MD Anderson Cancer Center, project execution and initial analysis of project completion are combined into a single step appropriately entitled "Execution and Control."

5. **Monitoring**
   - Observation and verification of project deliverables
   - Observation of project milestones
   - Update project sponsors and stakeholders on project status
   - Report project milestone completion to project stakeholders and sponsor
   - Review of budget reports and initial ROI estimates
   - Confirm project is within scope, on-time, and in-budget

6. **Completion phase – project closeout**
   - Final deliverables are released.
   - Communication of project closure to stakeholders.
   - Compilation of **lessons learned** from the project (review of what worked and what didn't).
   - Assessment of actual project milestone deliveries.
   - Transition capital expenses to operational expenses (if applicable).
   - Release of project resources (personnel); if salary support from project, it must be transitioned to another project.

34.5.2 Project Management Methodologies

Traditional project management is well suited for the use of commercially available project management software. Imaging informatics professionals (IIPs) are likely to be involved in projects that involve the development, installation, and deployment of novel or innovative applications. If these applications were developed within the organization, project timelines and milestones from prior installation projects can be emulated and established.

Project management methodology involves principles, practices, techniques, and procedures used in project delivery and require well-defined process throughout the project's life cycle. There are various project approaches used by project managers; two widely held project management methodologies are waterfall and agile:

- **Waterfall methodology** is the traditional method for managing a project. It uses sequential and linear phases and is well suited for projects with software requirements. Waterfall "plans ahead" by developing a project plan and review that focuses on meeting deliverables. This approach is well suited for projects that seek to automate an existing, well-functioning process and is well suited for scope development projects. The phases of the waterfall model are:
  - Requirements
  - Design
  - Implementation
  - Testing
  - Deployment
  - Maintenance
- **Agile methodology** is a process of continuous iteration that values adaptability and involvement. The agile approach has different development methodologies. The scrum methodology breaks the project into individual deliverable time-boxed pieces called **sprints**. This approach is well suited for projects that seek to improve an existing poorly functioning workflow and/or process. The core principles in the agile model are:

> **DEFINITION: Scrum**
>
> A type of agile project management that is executed in discrete iterations called sprints. A sprint typically lasts for a few weeks. Requirements for each iteration are defined at the start of the sprint, and the incremental outcome is assessed at the conclusion of each sprint. The process repeats until the final project is delivered.

  - Adaptability
  - Customer involvement
  - Lean development
  - Teamwork
  - Time
  - Sustainability
  - Testing

34.5.3 Project Management Forms and Tools

It is common for imaging informatics projects to compete against other institutional clinical informatics projects for funding prioritization. Imaging informatics professionals (IIPs) and/or the project managers must effectively complete the required documentation in order to have the best opportunity for project funding.

Successful projects mean working smart by using the right tools. In most institutions, oversight groups that practice formal project methodologies use **project templates, spreadsheets, and tools** that assist with setting goals, assigning tasks, and keeping the project on schedule. There are many useful project management templates and tools commercially available.

1. **Project charters and project plans**
   - Contains project justification and expected outcomes including anticipated return on investment (ROI)
   - Explicitly defines the project scope and serves as a reference to evaluate project change request
   - Provides summary information to assist upper management in project approval and prioritization
2. **Monthly reports for project tracking and budget management**
   - Provides ongoing summary of project progress.
   - Uses Gantt charts.
   - This document is shared directly with oversight committee primarily responsible for the project.
   - This document is usually forwarded to the institutional IT oversight committee.
3. **Task checklists**
   - Monitors the progress of deliverables
   - Used to set priorities
   - Aids in holding project team members accountable
4. **Timesheet**
   - Optimizes time management
5. **KPI monitoring**
   - Key performance indicator (KPI) monitoring is essential throughout a project.
   - KPI metrics allow accurate assessment of the project's overall health.
6. **Communication plans**
   - The institution could also have a process to provide project status updates to leadership and committees outside of the imaging department.
7. **Risk identification and mitigation plan**
   - Risk identifications facilitate risk mitigation.
8. **Team management**
   - **Stakeholder involvement** by identifying key personnel they would like to see participate in the project and confirm personnel that are already identified in the project.
   - **Personnel resource allocation** provides listing of personnel currently assigned to project and their level/percentage of participation.
9. **Gantt charts**
   - Invented by Henry Gantt (1861–1919)
   - Provides a sequenced view illustrating project tasks and timelines

   > **DEFINITION: Gantt Chart**
   >
   > A graphing model for project management that shows tasks as horizontal bars indicating start and end dates.

   - Provide overview of tasks with expected initiation and completion (usually represented in terms of weeks)
   - Can define who is responsible for specific task completion
   - Open-source and commercially available project management

- Well-suited method where project tasks and resources are well established from prior implementations (Fig. 34.2)
10. **PERT charts**
    - Acronym for Project Evaluation and Review Technique.
    - Initially developed by Booz Allen Hamilton with the US Navy Special projects office to support the Polaris nuclear submarine.
    - Designed for complex projects especially those in research and design where time to complete specific tasks can be difficult to estimate.
    - Project task steps are organized in a flowchart methodology.
    - Project tasks are defined as flowchart nodes.
    - Nodes are connected by arrows, which serve to define the dependencies across project steps.
    - PERT is intended for very large-scale, one-time, complex, nonroutine projects.
    - Regardless of project scale, PERT can be valuable in planning for projects which have not been previously implemented.
    - Helpful to gain appreciation of codependencies for project implementation (Fig. 34.3).

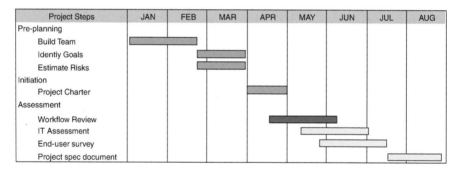

Fig. 34.2 Sample Gantt chart

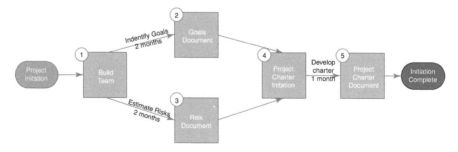

Fig. 34.3 PERT chart

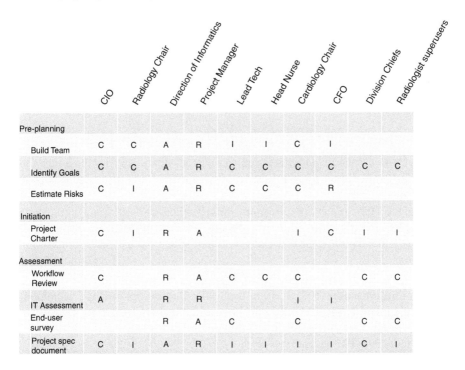

	CIO	Radiology Chair	Direction of Informatics	Project Manager	Lead Tech	Head Nurse	Cardiology Chair	CFO	Division Chiefs	Radiologist superusers
Pre-planning										
Build Team	C	C	A	R	I	I	C	I		
Identify Goals	C	C	A	R	C	C	C	C	C	C
Estimate Risks	C	I	A	R	C	C	C	R		
Initiation										
Project Charter	C	I	R	A			I	C	I	I
Assessment										
Workflow Review	C		R	A	C	C	C		C	C
IT Assessment	A		R	R			I	I		
End-user survey			R	A	C		C		C	C
Project spec document	C	I	A	R	I	I	I	I	C	I

Fig. 34.4 Sample RACI chart

11. **RACI diagram**
    - Is an acronym that stands for responsible, accountable, consulted, and informed.
    - Also referred to as the **responsibility matrix** diagram.
    - Designed to **mitigate ambiguous task assignments** between project participants.
    - Defines the reporting relationships for primary stakeholders and project managers or participants.
    - In a spreadsheet matrix, task descriptions are defined on rows and the involved roles are defined in columns.
    - For each task, a designation of "R," "A," "C," or "I" is entered which explicitly defines person's role concerning specific tasks (Fig. 34.4).

34.5.4 The Role of the Imaging Informatics Professional

In many organizations, a professional project manager is involved in the implementation of large-scale informatics projects and then steps aside once the project is closed out. Imaging informatics professionals (IIPs) participate in complex system implementations such as PACS upgrades or PACS replacements, as well as relatively noncomplex projects such as software installations on existing infrastructure for a small number of users. During the implementation of a PACS upgrade, a project manager is instrumental in project plan oversight, and the IIP will likely be fully engaged in implementing the tasks outlined in the project plan, leaving little time for the project oversight. For smaller projects like software installations, a project manager is not required, and the IIP may be asked to lead the project.

KEY CONCEPT: PMI Certifications in Project Management

Certified Associate in Project Management (CAPM): Ideal for those beginning their project management careers but do not yet have project management experience.

Project Management Professional (PMP): The gold standard of project management certification. Those who earn the PMP certification are recognized as having the experience, skill, and competency required to lead and manage projects.

- The project manager (PM) oversees the available resources from the institution, including the IIP. The PM will collaborate with the designated system owner on administrative activities specific to the site.
- If an outside PM consultant is commissioned for the imaging project, they should be hired at the initiation of the project in order to contribute to its specific requirements such as project plan development and implementation.
- The IIP will assist in all aspects of implementation including acceptance testing, system configuration, workflow reengineering, and user training.

OUR EXPERIENCE: Project Managers

Assignment of a dedicated project manager to large-scale informatics projects provides a dedicated personnel resource to supplement existing operational resources.

- As part of their contractual obligation, imaging informatics vendors should be required to provide the PM all vendor activities as it relates to the project plan to facilitate project coordination and planning. The IIP will work alongside the vendors for system configurations and as needed.
- Upon completion of the imaging project implementation, the IIP should assume responsibility for daily system maintenance and local oversight.
- After system go live, the system owner should continue to employ aspects of project management in the ongoing system maintenance including formal change management processes.
- As organizations increase local experience in project management, they could likely assume more responsibility in project implementation management and reduce the need for outside consultant expertise.

Further Reading

1. Project management. http://en.wikipedia.org/wiki/Project_management. Accessed 1 Oct 2020.
2. A Guide to the Project Management Body of Knowledge (PMBOK Guide), Sixth Edition, Project Management Institute. 2017. ISBN-10: 9781628251845.
3. Fournier C. The manager's path: a guide for tech leaders navigating growth and change paperback. O'Reilly Media; 2017. ISBN-10: 1491973897.
4. Houston SM, Kennedy RD. Effective lifecycle management of healthcare applications. CRC Productivity Press; 2020. ISBN-10: 9780367373894.

Self-Assessment Questions

1. In the project management process, selection of the project management team occurs in phase:

   (a) Assessment
   (b) Budget planning
   (c) Planning
   (d) Monitoring
   (e) Project closure

2. The earliest step in developing the plan among those listed below should be:

   (a) Defining the detailed functionality requirements
   (b) Selecting the hardware and software to be used
   (c) Defining the project team
   (d) Setting project milestones
   (e) Successful completion of contract

3. Roles of the imaging project committee include all *except*:

   (a) Ensure that any request for changes in the project plan align with initial project scope.
   (b) Review project plan to ensure it represents the clinical and technical requirements.
   (c) Ensure the current dominant imaging vendor receives the imaging project contract.
   (d) Serve as a project advocacy group in requesting of institutional funding.
   (e) Serve as an oversight group for project milestones and proper budget spending.

4. For large-scale imaging products with impact across the enterprise, committee membership should include in the stakeholder group:

   (a) Hospital IT representative
   (b) Cardiologists
   (c) Imaging physicist
   (d) Medical records representative
   (e) All of the above

5. The RACI matrix in project management is an acronym for:

   (a) Representative and actionable contact information
   (b) Responsible, accountable, consulted, and informed
   (c) Reasonable action for consultant integrity
   (d) Responsible activity for continual improvement
   (e) None of the above

6. Good project management should include all *except*:

    (a) Frequent team meetings
    (b) Project management software
    (c) Frequent adjustment of schedules to match achievements
    (d) Communications with oversight groups/individuals
    (e) Occasional external reviews

7. Scope creep includes all of the following *except*:

    (a) Trading some functionality for other functionality
    (b) Adding functionality that can be accomplished within the contingency
    (c) Adding a subsequent phase for addressing the needs of other facilities
    (d) Adopting a new information model that better meets the plan
    (e) Changing the standard video display card for PACS workstations

Answer Key

Chapter 1

1 – (d); **2** – (b); **3** – (c); **4** – (e); **5** – (d); **6** – (b)

Chapter 2

1 – (b); **2** – (c); **3** – (c); **4** – (a); **5** – (c); **6** – Axial (transverse), coronal (frontal), sagittal (lateral), or median (midsagittal); **7** – The body is upright facing the observer with feet placed flat on the ground directed forward with arms positioned at the body's sides with palms of hands facing forward; **8** – Anterior (A), posterior (P), right (R), left (L), head (H), and foot (F)

Chapter 3

1 – (d); **2** – (b); **3** – (b); **4** – (d); **5** – (a)

Chapter 4

1 – (b); **2** – (c); **3** – (a); **4** – (d); **5** – (c); **6** – (b); **7** – (b)

Chapter 5

1 – (d); **2** – (a); **3** – (c); **4** – (b)

© The Editor(s) (if applicable) and The Author(s), under exclusive license to
Springer Nature Switzerland AG 2021
B. F. Branstetter IV (ed.), *Practical Imaging Informatics*,
https://doi.org/10.1007/978-1-0716-1756-4

Chapter 6

1 – (d); **2** – (c); **3** – (b); **4** – (b); **5** – (c); **6** – (c); **7** – (b); **8** – (e); **9** – (c); **10** – (d); **11** – (b); **12** – (c); **13** – (c)

Chapter 7

1 – (d); **2** – (c); **3** – (a); **4** – (b); **5** – (d); **6** – (a); **7** – (e); **8** – (d)

Chapter 8

1 – (e); **2** – (d); **3** – (c); **4** – (e); **5** – (b)

Chapter 9

1 – (b); **2** – (c); **3** – (d); **4** – (c); **5** – (c); **6** – (a–c); **7** – (b); **8** – (a); **9** – (d); **10** – (b)

Chapter 10

1 – (b); **2** – (d); **3** – (a); **4** – (c); **5** – (b); **6** – (a); **7** – (b); **8** – (c); **9** – (d); **10** – (c)

Chapter 11

1 – (b); **2** – (b); **3** – (b); **4** – (a)

Chapter 12

1 – DICOM conformance statement; **2** – Each study may contain many series; **3** – IHE integration statement; **4** – HL7; **5** – DICOM

Chapter 13

1 – Medical record number. According to the security elements in the Health Insurance Portability and Accessibility Act, Social Security number can no longer be used as an MRN; **2** – CPT codes tell WHAT was done to a patient; ICD-10 codes tell WHY it was done; **3** – To ensure the appropriateness of diagnostic imaging services provided for Medicare beneficiaries; **4** – To assist referring providers in optimizing their choice of imaging procedure; **5** – Five alphanumeric characters; 6 – Seven alphanumeric characters; **7** – Name, DOB, facility, DOS, Dept, Adm date, Dis date

Chapter 14

1 – (a); **2** – (b); **3** – (e); **4** – (e); **5** – (c); **6** – (a)

Chapter 15

1 – (d); **2** – (c); **3** – (a); **4** – (a); **5** – (b)

Chapter 16

1 – (a); **2** – (d); **3** – (b); **4** – (d); **5** – (a)

Chapter 17

1 – (c) Slows down transmission of image data over networks. One of the main uses of compression of any kind (lossy or lossless) is to speed up transmission of data; **2** – (d) Spatial resolution, contrast resolution, and color vision. Spatial resolution is needed to discern fine details, contrast resolution is needed for visual acuity, and color vision is required in medical image areas that use color images (i.e., pathology); **3** – (c) 200 microns. Visual acuity and contrast sensitivity indicate that 2.5 cycles/mm or *200-micron pixel size is best*; **4** – (a) DICOM grayscale standard display function. HDTV is a broadcasting standard for television. The SPMTE was also developed for television and was used in radiology before the development of DICOM but is no longer recommended; **5** – (c) 20–40 lux. A moderate amount of light is recommended for viewing rather than too dark or too bright; **6** – (b) Digital mammography. The inherent resolution of digital mammography images is high and exceeds the display resolution of small matrix displays. To avoid extended use of zooming to access the high-resolution data and to view the entire image as close to full resolution as possible, a large matrix display should be used for mammography; **7** – (a) Distinguishing between objects and background in an image. Contrast perception is important for discriminating subtle shades of gray between lesions and background; **8** – (b) 50. Psychophysical studies have shown that a ratio of 50 is best; **9** – (c) 20–30 minutes. Dark adaption starts as soon as ambient lighting changes, but full dark adaptation typically takes 20–30 minutes; **10** – (d) Medical-grade (MG) displays are most appropriate. COTS displays are more appropriate for technologist viewing for quality assurance. VR and AR displays are more appropriate for simulation and training applications; **11** – (b) See Reference [31]. A Lmax of at least 420 cd/m^2 is recommended; **12** – (d) The MQSA establishes no specific *requirements* for resolution, color vs. monochrome, or FDA approval; **13** – (a) Response rate applies to LCD. Refresh rate was for CRT displays; **14** – (c) See Reference [40]. Digital mammography performed better than screen-film in younger women and those with dense breast tissue

Chapter 18

1 – (c); **2** – (b); **3** – (b); **4** – (c); **5** – (a); **6** – (c); **7** – (d)

Chapter 19

1 – (e); 2 – (a); 3 – (d); 4 – (b); 5 – (e)

Chapter 20

1 – (c); 2 – (a); 3 – (b); 4 – (c); 5 – (a); 6 – (b); 7 – (a); 8 – (d); 9 – (b)

Chapter 21

1 – (c); 2 – (d); 3 – (a); 4 – (d); 5 – (b); 6 – (d); 7 – (d); 8 – (d); 9 – (a); 10 – (b)

Chapter 22

1 – (d); 2 – (d); 3 – (b); 4 – (b); 5 – (a); 6 – (a); 7 – (b); 8 – (c); 9 – (b)

Chapter 23

1 – (e); 2 – (b); 3 – (b); 4 – (c); 5 – FAQs, knowledge bases, tutorials, and step-by-step troubleshooting instructions; 6 – Ability to write a report, present complex data, and practice active listening; 7 – The IIP can recognize problems before users even notice there is a problem; 8 – Proactive monitoring of entire system; 9 – Automatic ways for email reminders for forgotten passwords or a 24/7 help desk; 10 – Visit community medical association meetings as a guest speaker, attend staff meetings for other practices or departments, and publish newsletters and blogs with tips for better viewing and access to images

Chapter 24

1 – (c); 2 – (a); 3 – (b); 4 – (c); 5 – (d); 6 – (d); 7 – Reaction, learning, behavior, results; 8 – Defines elements of what the trainee will be able to do following the program; 9 – (b); 10 – (c)

Chapter 25

1 – (a); 2 – (b); 3 – (d); 4 – (c); 5 – (d)

Chapter 26

1 – (b); 2 – (c); 3 – (c); 4 – (d); 5 – (e); 6 – (e); 7 – (d)

Chapter 27

1 – (d); **2** – (a); **3** – (e); **4** – (a); **5** – (e); **6** – Any of the following: (1) Inappropriate lookup tables (LUTs), (2) Media failures, network failures, (3) Database failures, (4) Software bugs, (5) Improper association of exam and image information, (6) Image retrieval and distribution failures; **7** – (1) QC data, (2) Turnaround times (TATs) of exam, (3) Receipt and viewing of images; **8** – (1) How the display is calibrated? (2) How equipment is maintained? (3) How the equipment is operated? (4) Use digital test patterns; **9** – (1) Verify patient ID and exam info, (2) Verify patient positioning, (3) Verify image quality, (4) Reconcile patient data/image counts in PACS, (5) Report substandard images, (6) Erase cassette-based image receptors, (7) Compile and review reject analysis data, (8) Verify display calibrations, (9) Review QC indicators, (10) Verify receptor calibrations, (11) Verify X-ray generator functions; **10** – (1) Contrast, (2) Resolution, (3) Noise

Chapter 28

1 – (b); **2** – (a); **3** – (c); **4** – (b); **5** – (a); **6** – (a); **7** – (d); **8** – (d); **9** – (b); **10** – (d)

Chapter 29

1 – (c); **2** – (b); **3** – (e); **4** – (d); **5** – (e); **6** – (c); **7** – (c); **8** – (b); **9** – (b); **10** – verbal, email, dashboard, application splash screen

Chapter 30

1 – (b); **2** – (c); **3** – (d); **4** – (a); **5** – (b); **6** – (c); **7** – (d); **8** – (c); **9** – (d); **10** – (d); **11** – (a); **12** – (b)

Chapter 31

1 – (a); **2** – (d); **3** – (b); **4** – Proactively monitoring systems allows system administrators to identify issues even before the end users realize there are issues. This enables support teams to proactively correct issues, hence reducing break/fix tickets. If the monitoring tools fail to identify issues and customers do open service tickets, service management models streamline resolution processes and reduce risk when incidents and problems present; **5** – (c); **6** – (a); **7** – (b); **8** – (a & b); **9** – (a & d)

Chapter 32

1 – (d); **2** – (e); **3** – (d); **4** – (b); **5** – (c); **6** – (b); **7** – (a); **8** – (b); **9** – (e); **10** – (a)

Chapter 33

1 – (a); **2** – (c); **3** – (d); **4** – (b); **5** – (a); **6** – (a); **7** – (b)

Chapter 34

1 – (a); **2** – (c); **3** – (d); **4** – (e); **5** – (b); **6** – (c); **7** – (e)

Glossary

Acceptance Tests Tests that determine whether predefined specifications and requirements have been met before deploying a new system. This includes operational and user acceptance tests.

Accession Number A unique identifier for a single billable examination. From an accession number, your PACS database can determine which patient, what date, and what type of exam was performed. Sometimes, a single examination is coded with multiple accession numbers, only some of which have associated images.

Actionable Finding Any imaging finding that requires nonroutine communication to the ordering physician or patient. This includes urgent findings that might immediately affect patient care and also nonurgent findings that might slip through the cracks. Personal phone conversation is the preferred mode of communication. This task must be documented in the report.

Addendum (*Plural*: Addenda) Once the radiologist has finalized a radiology report, it cannot be modified, as it is a permanent part of the medical record. Any changes and/or clarifications must be appended to the end of the report as a separate section without modifying the original report.

Advanced Practice Providers APPs (also called physician extenders) are healthcare providers with degrees such as physician assistant or registered nurse practitioner who can provide independent care to patients with indirect physician supervision.

Annotations Your PACS contains not only DICOM data received from modality devices or specialty workstations but also information created in the course of image management, viewing, and interpretation in the PACS.

API An application programming interface allows software engineers from your institution to create customized software that uses functions from the vendor's software.

Artifact Any component of the image that is extraneous to the representation of tissue structures; can be caused by a technique, technology, hardware, or software error.

B. F. Branstetter IV (ed.), *Practical Imaging Informatics*, https://doi.org/10.1007/978-1-0716-1756-4

Artificial Intelligence A field of computer science focused on creating programs that perform tasks normally assigned to human intelligence, thus simulating human intelligence.

Assigning Authority The HL7 assigning authority value is a unique identifier generated by the system that created the patient's medical record number. The HL7 assigning authority maps to the DICOM Issuer of Patient ID (IPID).

Asynchronous Communication Two workers communicate asynchronously when they do not need to be simultaneously available. Thus, each worker can integrate the data into their workflow more efficiently. Email is the most familiar example of asynchronous communication.

Audit Trail A record of all the changes made to a database, usually with timestamps and user logs.

Authentic Assessment Using real work tasks in the actual work environment to evaluate the success of training.

Back-Out Plan Steps needed to return the system to the state prior to the upgrade or deployment. It gets triggered if there are unforeseen consequences to other hospital systems. Also it is referred to as "roll-back" plan.

Bandwidth The maximum amount of data that can be transmitted over a medium, usually measured in bits per second.

Base Case The base case is the most frequent task that is performed. Workflow design should address the base case first and foremost, even if less frequently utilized workflows are made less efficient. For example, radiologists often use distance measurements – this function should be easily available, even if it would make more logical sense to have it in the same place as all the other PACS tools.

Batch Mode A radiologist may sign each report as it is dictated or dictate several reports and sign them all in a batch.

Best of Breed Strategy A process of selecting the best products or systems that will meet your business requirements. This often requires different vendors for different components of the project.

Big Data Extremely large datasets that are analyzed computationally to reveal unexpected patterns, trends, and associations. Data may be structured, semi-structured, or unstructured. Data may grow exponentially with time.

BI-RADS Breast Imaging-Reporting and Data System is a reporting and QA tool owned by the ACR and used for mammography reporting. After the success of BI-RADS, similar systems have been developed for other anatomic regions, such as NI-RADS (neck), PI-RADS (prostate), etc.

Business Associate Agreement (BAA) Any individual or entity that performs functions or activities on behalf of a HIPAA-covered entity and has access to PHI is considered a business associate, according to Health and Human Services (HHS). Examples include a consultant who does hospital utilization reviews or an attorney who has PHI access while providing legal services to a healthcare provider. Business associates must have a documented BAA that ensures HIPAA Privacy Rules are followed and that PHI is protected.

Business Continuity During a temporary downtime, business continuity provides access to the ePHI until the systems are fully restored to normal operating conditions.

Classification The assignment of a meaningful name like "lung" to a group of pixels or voxels.

Clinical Decision Support CDS systems are software add-ons to the EMR that assist referrers who are ordering imaging exams, in the hope that this will reduce inappropriate utilization of imaging. Many of these systems are based on guidelines such as the ACR Appropriateness Criteria or the ESR iGuide. They calculate appropriateness scores for the requested test, and if the test is inappropriate, the referring physician is advised (but not required) to modify the selection.

Codec Short for coder-decoder. Devices or computer programs that compress data so that it can use less storage space or transmit more quickly. The coder compresses the data; the decoder is needed to reconstitute the original.

Commoditization A commodity is a service or product that is interchangeable between vendors. Crude oil is a typical example, since it doesn't matter which well it is pumped from. Services like radiology interpretation can be treated like commodities if there is no discernable difference in the quality of the interpretations and no added value (such as consultations or patient interactions) from an in-house radiologist.

Common Data Element A CDE is a fragment of a dictation with heavily structured content, including data types and allowable values. CDEs are designed to be reused and recombined in different dictation templates.

Compression Compression reduces the volume of data to reduce image processing, transmission times, bandwidth requirements, and storage needs. *Lossless compression* allows for reconstruction of exact original data before compression without loss of information. *Lossy compression* uses methods that lose data once the image has been compressed and uncompressed, but provides a greater degree of compression.

Computer Vision Syndrome Long periods in front of a computer can cause "myopization," which is temporary nearsightedness that results in eyestrain and irritation.

Convolution The multiplication of a neighborhood of pixels by a "kernel." Each value in the kernel is the number by which the corresponding neighborhood pixel is multiplied. If all the values in the kernel are "1," the result is the mean.

Covered Entity Any organization to which the HIPAA Privacy Rule applies, namely, health plans, healthcare clearinghouses, healthcare providers, and business associates of those entities.

CPT Current procedural terminology codes are used to precisely classify medical, surgical, and diagnostic services and procedures.

CPT Code Current Procedural Terminology codes indicate which procedure was done to a patient by a physician. These can be physical examinations, operations, or interpreting radiologic tests. CPT codes should not be confused with ICD codes, which are used by hospitals (and other facilities) to indicate patient diagnosis.

Crisis Management Plan (CMP) A CMP is a document that describes the processes that an organization should use to respond to a critical situation that could adversely affect its profitability, reputation, or ability to operate.

Critical Result According to the National Patient Safety Goals set forth by the Joint Commission, a critical result represents a finding that could threaten a patient's life.

Critical Test Results Management Software and processes to ensure that important radiologic results are properly communicated and do not slip through the cracks.

C-suite Short for "corporate suite," C-suite colloquially refers to the roles on the business side of healthcare.

Dashboard Display A graphical interface that summarizes input from many sources into a small visual area that can be quickly understood. More detailed information is available by expanding individual elements of the dashboard.

Data Analytics Collecting information, looking for patterns, and managing the information.

Data Governance Governance includes monitoring data quality to ensure that the organization successfully realizes its desired outcomes and receives business value from data management activities.

Data Use Agreement A data use agreement (DUA) is a specific type of agreement that is required under the HIPAA Privacy Rule and must be entered into before there is any use or disclosure of data from the medical record to an outside institution or party usually for one of the three purposes: (1) research, (2) public health, or (3) healthcare operations.

Data Warehouse A database that collects a large amount of clinical or imaging data without a defined research question or purpose. Subsets of the data can later be mined to answer newly framed questions.

Database A structured collection of data. Data which is housed in a database is more amenable to analysis and organization. Databases are ubiquitous and are the essential component of nearly every computer application that manages information.

Decision Support An interactive software tool that assists providers in making care decisions. In the context of radiology, clinical decision support is software that guides referring physicians to choose the optimal imaging technique for a given clinical situation.

DICOM An industry standard for the format of digital medical images and the communication of images from one software system to another.

DICOM Conformance Statement This document, provided by a system manufacturer, describes the DICOM services and structures that the system supports. Be sure to read this to gain key insights into your systems when integrating.

Digital Test Patterns Standardized images with numerous shades of gray that can be used to test whether displays are performing optimally.

Disaster Recovery A set of policies, procedures, processes, and systems put in place to enable the restoration and recovery of vital data and infrastructure following a natural or man-made catastrophic event.

Dose Index Monitoring The process of monitoring radiation dose used in diagnostic imaging procedures that use ionizing radiation, such as computed tomography (CT), interventional radiography (IR), projection radiography, and mammography.

Downtime A period of time when a digital information system, an application server, or the network are unavailable or fails to provide its primary function, resulting in data communication interruptions.

Encounters-Based Imaging Encounters-based imaging is defined as being performed during a clinic visit or procedure when image content acquisition is not considered the purpose of the visit. There is usually no indication preceding the visit that imaging will be performed and imaging is at the sole discretion of the provider, as with dermatology photographs.

Enterprise An entire system of healthcare delivery that encompasses hospitals, outpatient services, and business administration.

Ergonomics The study of human efficiency in the work environment. It encompasses physical (human responses to physical and physiological loads), cognitive (mental processes such as perception, attention, and cognition), and organizational (organizational structures, policies, and processes) elements.

Escalation Process Defines who to contact next when the first point of contact does not respond in a timely manner. The sequence of individuals is an escalation policy.

Exception An image whose patient demographic and exam information disagree with the RIS. These images are usually quarantined until the discrepancy can be reconciled.

Fat-Finger Error Manual typing is inherently error-prone, especially when the data is numerical. Fat-finger errors are typographical errors that could be avoided by pre-populating data fields.

Fault Tolerance The ability of a given system to continue functioning even if one of its components fails.

Filter A processing method that enhances or removes a specific component in a signal or image. The name could reflect what is removed, what is enhanced, or the calculation that is used.

Flag Reminder or indicator that new data is available. Usually it is an auditory or visual cue within a software program. For example, "You've got mail!"

Food and Drug Administration Responsible for protecting the public health by ensuring the safety, efficacy, and security of human and veterinary drugs, biological products, and medical devices and by ensuring the safety of the US food supply, cosmetics, and products that emit radiation.

Fourier Transform A Fourier transform converts an image from a familiar Cartesian matrix (the usual X-Y-Z coordinate space) to the frequency domain, where the image is represented by the summation of numerous sinusoidal patterns. Fourier space is hard to conceptualize.

Gantt Chart A graphing model for project management that shows tasks as horizontal bars indicating start and end dates.

GSDF The grayscale display function is a DICOM method that defines the relationship between the pixel value of an image and the luminance of the display. It is designed to optimize human perception and is a necessary part of display calibration in radiology.

Hanging Protocol By default, a PACS will display images in the order that they were produced on the scanner, using default windows from the scanner. But this may not be the most convenient way to interpret the images. A hanging protocol is a reproducible way of organizing images when they are displayed on the PACS. Hanging protocols are based on DICOM tags.

Health Literacy The degree to which individuals have the capacity to obtain, process, and understand basic health information and services needed to make appropriate health decisions.

Histogram A graph that reflects how many pixels of each brightness are on the image. The horizontal axis is brightness, and the vertical axis is number of pixels.

HL7 An industry standard for the format of messages sent from one medical software system to another.

Hounsfield Unit CT number representing absorption values of tissues; expressed on a scale of −1000 units for the least absorbent (air) to the maximum X-ray beam absorption of bone (+3000 for dense bone). Water is used as a reference material for determining CT numbers and is, by definition, equal to 0. Set ranges of CT numbers can designate tissue type, and differences in tissue Hounsfield units can indicate abnormal findings and/or pathology.

ICD-10 ICD-10 codes are used to classify medical diseases and a wide variety of signs, symptoms, abnormal findings, complaints, social circumstances, and external causes of injury or disease.

IHE Integrating the Healthcare Enterprise is an initiative that has created a framework for medical workflow in which different electronic systems can exchange information.

Imaging Biobank Organized database of medical images and associated imaging biomarkers (radiologic and clinical) shared among multiple researchers and linked to other biorepositories.

Incident An incident is an unplanned interruption to a service, or the failure of a component of a service that has not yet impacted service.

Incident Report Post-downtime report provided by the vendor that explains the cause of any unscheduled downtime.

Incidental Finding A finding that is unexpected and unrelated to the reason the imaging examination was ordered, but still requires downstream follow-up.

Integrated Change Control An element of project management in which *ALL* system changes undergo a formal process of request, approval, management, and documentation. ICC is typically coordinated at an enterprise level.

In-the-Wild Threats Exploits propagating in real-world computers and not just in test labs.

Ionizing Radiation Radiation capable of producing energetically charged particles that move through space from one object to another where the energy is absorbed. These tests are potentially hazardous to patients.

Isotropic Having the same size in each dimension.

IT Governance The structure around how organizations assign roles and make IT decisions.

Just Culture An adverse event reporting/debriefing system in which individual blame is de-emphasized and underlying systematic reasons for failure are addressed.

Just Noticeable Difference The minimum amount that the luminance can be changed for the human eye to perceive a difference. The JND varies with the current display luminance; a JND Index Curve is an element of diagnostic monitor evaluations.

Leadership Force Multipliers These individuals, when placed in the right roles, and given the right levels of empowerment, can dramatically increase the effectiveness of a group – creating a team and a series of outcomes that is more than the sum of its parts.

Learning Management System System that supports the delivery, tracing, and management of training resources and user evaluations.

Lexicon A lexicon is a common vocabulary to standardize and enhance communication and potentially reduce healthcare-related communication errors.

Limited Data Sets LDS are a HIPAA exception. They include partially de-identified data that excludes most (but not all) protected health information. Things like geographic divisions smaller than a state and dates can be included. LDS is permitted for research, public health, and healthcare operations if specific criteria are met.

Load Balancing Ensuring that work is distributed optimally to avoid having some workers (or IT components) idle while others are overworked.

Lookup Table for Display A lookup table converts the pixel values of an image into brightness values for the display. Lookup tables are defined for each display monitor individually, so they can be used to ensure that an image looks exactly the same on every display.

Lossless Compression Digital data compression in which all the original data information is preserved and can be completely reconstituted.

Lossy Compression Methods of digital compression in which the original information cannot be completely reconstituted.

Machine Learning A field of study in which a machine learns by itself and elaborates a model from a training database.

Macro In the setting of speech recognition, a macro is a short phrase that represents a more complex set of keystrokes, text, or actions. The dictator speaks the macro and the report automatically populates with a large amount of text. This text may have blanks built in that need to be filled.

Man in the Middle A cyberattack in which the attacker places a device on the network within an institution and is able to intercept or modify the traffic from a sending system to a receiving system.

Medical Coding Accurate and efficient completion of patient paperwork so that it can be submitted to the insurance carrier for reimbursement.

Medical Imaging Several different technologies that are used to visualize the human body in order to diagnose, monitor, or treat medical conditions.

Medical Physicist A medical physicist is a professional who applies the principles and methods of both physics and medicine for the prevention, diagnosis, and treatment of human diseases, with a specific goal of ensuring quality services and safety to the patients exposed to radiation. The medical physics field can be divided into three main categories: radiation therapy, diagnostic imaging, and nuclear medicine.

Megapixels MP is the number of pixels contained in the display, measured in millions of pixels.

Microsleep A brief period of sleep in which the person is not even aware of dozing off.

Mission Critical Application A mission critical application is software or a suite of related programs that must function continuously in order for a business to operate.

Mission Statement Versus Vision Statement A mission statement defines the purpose of a company, institution, or working group. Mission statements include current objectives and the approach to those objectives.A vision statement, on the other hand, is aspirational – what do we want to become?In other words, mission statements focus on today, while vision statements focus on tomorrow.

Modality The word "modality" may refer to a technology used to create images (e.g., CT) or to a specific machine that is producing images (e.g., CT scanner #3 in the emergency department).

Monitoring Tools Monitoring tools provide the ability to keep track of a system or service, in order to have automated identification and notification of failures, degradations, or interruptions.

MQSA The Mammography Quality Standards Act and Program of the US Food and Drug Administration define numerous standards by which institutions become accredited to perform mammography.

Nighthawk Preliminary interpretations provided for studies performed overnight and on weekends. A nighthawk radiologist or reading service is tasked with interpreting studies within a few minutes of receipt, and then sending back preliminary reports. This is a service used by many healthcare organizations, particularly those that do not have radiologists available to provide 24x7 onsite support.

Noise Random fluctuations in the image information that can obscure the true elements in the image. Noise reduction is synonymous with improving the signal-to-noise ratio (SNR) or contrast-to-noise ratio (CNR).

On-Axis Viewing The viewer should be directly in front of the display, with line of sight perpendicular to the surface of the display.

One Throat to Choke This expression describes the advantage of purchasing goods or integrated services from a single vendor. That way, when things do not work as they should, there is only "one throat to choke." It contrasts with "best of breed."

Online Status Website Third-party website that reports the status of an interruption to end users. Subscriptions allow users to receive email or text updates regarding a specific interruption.

Ontology In computer science and information science, an ontology is a set of concepts and the relationships between those concepts for a particular subject. For example, RadLex is an ontology focused on the subject of radiology.

Opacity A measure for how transparent a voxel is, ranging from 0 (completely transparent) to 1 (completely opaque).

Out-of-Band Task A task that is not part of the routine workflow and must instead be performed while normal workflow is suspended. Workers often forget to perform out-of-band tasks.

Outside Study An imaging study that was performed at another institution but needs to be viewed, compared, or dictated locally.

PACS Picture Archiving and Communications Systems store, distribute, and display digital medical images.

Pain Points The problems that are most troubling to your users. Seemingly small issues can become pain points when they are encountered frequently, for example, needing two extra clicks to open an examination. If you read 200 cases in a day, that's a lot of clicks.

Patient-Facing Healthcare providers who directly interact face-to-face with patients are called "patient-facing." In medical imaging, the technologists who create the images are usually patient-facing, but the radiologists who interpret the images may or may not be.

Penetration Testing Simulate an attack on a network to determine vulnerabilities.

PET Positron Emission Tomography uses cyclotron-produced positron-emitting isotopes including oxygen, carbon, nitrogen, and fluorine, enabling accurate studies of blood flow and metabolism (as with fluorine-19 fluoro-deoxyglucose (FDG)). Positron isotopes are short-lived positively charged antimatter electrons. The main clinical applications are in the brain, heart, and tumors.

Phantom A test object intended to represent the patient in an imaging examination performed for quality assurance.

PHI Protected health information is any health-related data that is specific to an individual and thus could be used to identify the individual. There are 18 specific identifiers listed in HIPAA.

Phishing A form of social engineering in which an email is sent that mimics a legitimate business communication. The goal is to trick the recipient into revealing passwords or accidentally accepting malicious code into the network.

Phoneme A phoneme is a basic block of sound that makes up words. English has about 42 phonemes (different opinions exist on the exact number). For example, the word, "speech," has four phonemes: /s/p/E/ch/.

Physical Security The physical environment around a computer system that prevents unauthorized access to equipment. Examples include locks, security guards, video cameras, and biometric devices. Hospitals are notoriously weak at physical security because they want to appear welcoming to patients and families.

Pipeline A sequence of stages that performs a task in several steps, like an assembly line in a factory. Each stage takes inputs and produces outputs which are stored in its output buffer. One stage's output is the next stage's input.

POCUS Ultrasound machines have become small, inexpensive, and safe for non-radiology personnel to use. These machines may be scattered around the hospital and used by other healthcare providers to augment their physical examinations. This is referred to as point-of-care ultrasound.

Preliminary Report Usually, when an examination is interpreted, a formal report is immediately generated. However, there are situations where a temporary interpretation is rendered and is reviewed and finalized later (e.g., radiology residents on call, nighthawk systems). Curating discrepancies between preliminary and final reports is potentially challenging.

Principle of Least Privilege The concept that any user, process, or application should be granted the bare minimum authorization privileges needed to fulfill its responsibilities.

Problem The underlying cause of one or more service incidents. Problems are tracked separately from incidents.

Procurement The act of researching market solutions and engaging with industry vendors to evaluate and purchase products that keep your organization running optimally.

Project Management The discipline of planning, organizing, and managing resources to provide optimal project outcome.

Project Milestones Key events and deliverables in the project timeline. Milestones are attached to specific tasks' start and end dates.

Project Sponsor The fiscal or administrative entity that has overarching responsibility for the project.

Promiscuous Mode A DICOM receiver can be set to accept data from any network device (promiscuous) or can be set to only accept data from pre-defined, known senders (non-promiscuous). These settings can be useful when troubleshooting errors.

Proof of Concept A small-scale test environment that runs proposed software solutions inside your hospital system. Enables the buyer to see how the system integrates with existing solutions and test functionality before a purchase is finalized.

Pseudoanonymization Anonymization is replacing patient-specific information with blanks. Pseudoanonymization is replacing patient-specific information with fake data of a similar format (e.g., replace the patient's name with "Mickey Mouse").

Qualified Medical Physicist (QMP) An individual who is competent to independently provide clinical professional services in one or more of the subfields of medical physics.

Quality Assurance (QA) A process for monitoring and ensuring quality at an *organizational level*. For example, a department mandates standardized templates to minimize errors in reports.

Quality Control (QC) A process for measuring and testing elements of performance at an *individual level*. For example, a radiologist corrects errors in a radiology report before signing it.

Quality Improvement (QI) A process for improving performance quality at an *organizational level in a systematic and sustainable way*. For example, a department implements a standardized report system with ongoing monitoring, feedback, and accountability.

Quality in Medical Imaging The extent to which the right procedure is done in the right way, at the right time, and the correct interpretation is accurately and quickly communicated to the patient and referring physician.

Radiomics A deep learning algorithm extracts numerous features from a radiologic examination, many of which are not evident to a human observer. The resulting imaging biomarkers may provide novel diagnostic or prognostic information. The term "radiomics" is derived from the term "genomics," which is a battery of genetic biomarkers.

Ransomware A form of cybercrime with indirect financial rewards. Critical data is encrypted, and payment is demanded in exchange for the de-encryption key. The healthcare industry has become a major target of ransomware attacks. Ransomware is the greatest threat most health systems face. When activated, it usually renders all computer systems inoperable. Recovery can take days to weeks.

RECIST The Response Evaluation Criteria in Solid Tumors is an imaging-based system for determining whether a cancer treatment has been successful. Based on changes in size of tumor, the patient is classified as having stable disease, complete response, partial response, or progression.There are automated post-processing systems that can assist with this analysis.

Registration A single anatomic structure may appear in a different place on the image when a study is repeated, or from patient to patient. Registration is a means of identifying specific anatomic points so that two images can be "lined up" with each other and more easily compared.

Reject An image that is not useful for care of the patient. Includes test images and nondiagnostic images.

Repeat Duplicate image obtained because original image was substandard or lost.

Request for Information A document delivered to vendors early in the product selection process. It provides general information about the problem and invites descriptions of potential solutions.

Request for Proposal A document distributed to vendors late in the product selection process, after the type of product is known, to solicit specific information about the vendor's solution. Responses are compared between vendors to select the optimal solution.

REST REST (*RE*presentational *S*tate *T*ransfer) is an architectural programming style that ensures interoperability between computer systems on the Internet, and is used for defining APIs. Made popular in many web-based applications outside of healthcare, it is becoming more and more prevalent in healthcare APIs like FHIR and DICOMweb.

Retention Period Time, mandated by federal, state, or local statute, that medical information must be retained in its original and legal form.

Return on Investment Most purchases require an initial capital investment but (hopefully) reduce operational costs in the long term. ROI is a measure of how long it will take for the operational savings to make up for the initial investment.

RHIO Regional Health Information Organizations are not-for-profit organizations that encourage providers to participate in health information exchanges between competing healthcare enterprises.

Root Cause Analysis A formal review of a medical error or near miss that looks at all the factors contributing to the error. The RCA uses just culture techniques to avoid blaming individuals and seeks to address systemic issues that can result in global changes to avoid future errors.

RPV Resting point of vergence is the distance that the eyes naturally converge when relaxed in total darkness. This is the ideal ergonomic distance between the viewer and the display, typically 35–45 inches.

Safe Haven Data Safe Havens, a.k.a. Trusted Research Environments, are highly secure data storage environments meant for researchers who need to maintain PHI for their work. There are legal standards to ensure adequate security for these databases.

Scope Creep Incremental changes to the project, or the addition of features that were not identified in the original project charter. Scope creep delays the timetable and can prevent a project from ever being completed.

Screening Using medical imaging to detect hidden (occult) disease in patients who do not feel sick. The goal of screening is to detect diseases in an early stage when they can be treated more successfully.

Scrum A type of agile project management that is executed in discrete iterations called sprints. A sprint typically lasts for a few weeks. Requirements for each iteration are defined at the start of the sprint, and the incremental outcome is assessed at the conclusion of each sprint. The process repeats until the final project is delivered.

Second Read When a patient is transferred, radiologists at the new hospital may provide an interpretation of the scans from the other institution. This second read is sometimes billable at a lower rate than the primary interpretation.

Secondary Capture The Secondary Capture (SC) Image Information Object Definition (IOD) specifies images that are converted from a non-DICOM format to a modality-independent DICOM format.

Segmentation The ability to outline and identify specific anatomic structures or pathology on a radiologic image.

Self-Edit Mode Users dictate, edit, and sign reports without the aid of a human back-end transcription. The reports can be completed one at a time or batched.

Server-Based Computing (SBC) A general term for technologies that manage, distribute, and run applications from a server, rather than on individual client desktops.

Service Level Agreement (SLA) A commitment between vendor and client that outlines aspects of the product or service related to quality, availability, and responsibilities of both parties. Service availability is a major component of the SLA.

Service Line Service lines are a method for decentralizing administration into smaller, more manageable components. Healthcare was traditionally broken down by department, but "imaging" is now considered a service line in most hospitals. Related departments, such as neurology and neurosurgery, may combine into a single service line, ideally including neuroradiology and neuropathology.

Similarity Metrics Quantitative measures of how well two images are matched. They are an essential element of image registration.

Single Point of Failure A single point of failure (SPOF) is an IT system element that can cause your entire system to stop functioning if it goes bad. An SPOF can be hardware (e.g., a network switch), software (e.g., an HL7 sniffer), a facility, or even a person. Identifying and classifying SPOFs at the onset of planning will expose vulnerabilities.

SPECT Single-Photon Emission Computed Tomography; a tomographic slice is reconstructed from photons emitted by the radioisotope in a nuclear medicine study.

Speech Recognition Software designed to convert spoken language into written text. The resulting text is often tagged and marked up.

St. Elsewhere Any hospital that is not part of your own enterprise. (It's a reference to a 1980's soap opera.)

Statement of Work Defines fulfillment of contractual requirements for scope of work, location, period of contract, schedule for project deliverables, and acceptance criteria for work performed.

Strategic Plan General plan of action to achieve an overarching goal or outcome in a specific time period (usually 3–5 years).

Structured Data Elements In the context of structured reporting, SDE are tags or labels applied to the words in a report that cannot be seen when you read the report but are helpful for data mining or other computer applications.

Structured Reporting While there is no set definition for this term, there are three attributes structured reporting can have: uniform *format*, consistent *organization*, and standard *terminology*.

Superusers Volunteers who become intimately familiar with the system and can train their peers, both during formal training and during routine use. First adopters are often become superusers.

Sync for Science (S4S) Sync for Science (S4S) is a public-private collaboration to develop a simplified, scalable, and secure way for individuals to access and share their electronic health record (EHR) data with researchers. S4S uses and builds upon open-source standards that allow researchers to securely receive EHR data from a third-party application programming interface (API) used by a patient.

System Availability A metric used to measure the percentage of time a service is operational and available to users.

System Redundancy The opposite of a single point of failure is system redundancy, in which every potential failure point has an equivalent fallback that can be quickly (or automatically) invoked. You should seek ways to replace SPOFs with redundancy.

Tactical Plan Specific projects and process improvements designed to meet the goals of a strategic plan.

Task Allocation Matrix A chart listing QC tasks indicating who is responsible for doing them and the frequency that they are performed.

Template A formatted dictation outline in which blanks can be filled in with pertinent information. Templates are helpful to maintain strict organization in reports. Templates may be pre-populated with negative results or may have blanks where the content is added.

The Joint Commission The TJC accredits and certifies hospitals and other healthcare organizations. The TJC conducts periodic on-site surveys, applying strict criteria across numerous metrics. These site visits typically require substantial preparation from hospital personnel.

Thin Client A software application that does not depend upon any local software components and does not perform any processing on the local host.

Total Cost of Ownership TCO includes the initial cost of a system, plus the costs of installation and maintenance, as well as upgrade costs.

Transcription Mode Users dictate using speech recognition. After each report is completed, both the text and voice files are sent to a human transcriptionist, who then performs edits. The edited report with corrections is sent back to the radiologist, who then finalizes it.

Transform A mapping from the space of one image to the space of another image.

Trojan Horse Malicious code that accompanies useful code onto the system during a download or routine maintenance.

Turnaround Time In radiology, TAT refers to the time between completing a study and when the final report is signed. However, the start time and end time can vary depending on the person and situation. Hence, it is essential to clarify both the start time and end time when TAT is used.

Unsolicited Procedure Record An exam or procedure which has been performed without the request coming from the source system managing a patient's electronic health record.

Utilization Management System A third-party service employed by an insurance company that uses independent physicians to determine whether a procedure or test is medically indicated. The insurance company will refuse to pay for tests that are not "pre-approved" by these systems.

Value Chain The steps and processes that transforms the vision and mission of an organization into products and services.

Veiling Glare Reflection of light sources on a monitor's surface. Items in a room that contrast with room color and tonal values (lightness or darkness) and particularly light sources and other monitors are the major causes of veiling glare.

Ventilation According to the World Health Organization, ventilation is the intentional introduction of fresh air into a space while the stale air is removed. It is done to maintain the quality of air in that space.

Virtual Desktop Infrastructure (VDI) Technology that provides virtual desktops from virtual host servers. Examples of VDI include VMware Horizon and Citrix XenDesktop.

VNA A vendor-neutral archive is a large storage system that maintains image data and can interface with any PACS. This enables multiple PACS interfaces to all access the same data. It permits "best of breed" systems.

Volume Rendering A visualization technique to display a 2D image of a 3D data set that retains access to the original voxel data. Commonly referred to as a "3D reconstruction."

Voxel A portmanteau of the words volumetric and pixel, used to represent the individual elements of a 3D volume data set.

Work Area Zone including PACS monitors and computer system; one or several people seated or standing reviewing the same set of images and data (note: architects often refer to a workstation as being the same as a work area; radiologists often refer to a workstation specifically as the PACS equipment)

Workflow The steps that employees perform as they are getting their work done, and the relationships between those steps.

Workflow Bottleneck The most inefficient step in a process; the step that defines the maximum rate at which the entire process can proceed.

Workflow Token Reminder or indicator that a workflow task requires attention. Usually a physical object is passed from one person to another. Examples include paper exam requisitions and typed dictations to be signed.

XDS One of the integration profiles for IHE. The Cross-Document Sharing profile defines how institutions exchange medical information, including images.

XDS Affinity Domain A group of healthcare enterprises that have agreed to work together using a common set of policies and share a common infrastructure.

Index

© The Author(s), under exclusive license to Springer Science+Business Media,
LLC, part of Springer Nature 2021
B. F. Branstetter IV (ed.), *Practical Imaging Informatics*,
https://doi.org/10.1007/978-1-0716-1756-4